WAYS OF HEALTH

EDITED BY
DAVID S. SOBEL

WAYS OF HEALTH

HOLISTIC APPROACHES TO ANCIENT AND CONTEMPORARY MEDICINE

HARCOURT BRACE JOVANOVICH

NEW YORK AND LONDON

To my parents

Library of Congress Cataloging in Publication Data

Main entry under title:

Ways of health.

Bibliography: p.
1. Medicine—Philosophy. 2. Medicine, Ancient.
3. Therapeutic systems. 4. Health. 5. Mind and body.
I. Sobel, David Stuart.
R723.W34   610'.9   78-14081
ISBN 0-15-195308-2
0-15-694992-x (pbk.)

B C D E F G H I J

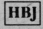

CONTENTS

꩜ ꩜

PART THREE

Unorthodox Medicine

PART FOUR

Techniques of Self-Regulation

Contents

PART FIVE

An Ecological View of Health

By René Dubos

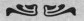

Preface

The history of all civilizations, even of the most ancient, records the names of physicians who achieved great fame by their skill in the treatment of disease. While these medical reputations of the past may have been greatly exaggerated with the passage of time, they certainly have a basis in truth. But it is obvious, of course, that they could not have been built on the kind of medical knowledge available to modern physicians. In fact, scientific medicine—namely, that which was developed during the past one hundred years in association with laboratory research—had little to offer in the way of specific methods of treatment or prevention until a few decades ago. Its first spectacular and unquestionably therapeutic triumph was the introduction of insulin in the mid-1920s. How then did the physicians of the past achieve the cures that made them famous? And similarly, how can one explain the cures brought about by contemporary healers in so-called primitive societies where the treatment of disease has not yet been significantly affected by scientific medicine? This book throws light on these questions by describing and discussing the healing practices of several non-Western cultures. To introduce the topic, I shall define here some conceptual differences between traditional and scientific medicine, and shall also point to similarities in these seemingly different ways of healing.

Regardless of the level of cultural and economic development, all people throughout history and in the different parts of the world have practiced simultaneously two kinds of medicine. On the one hand, they have made use of drugs, surgical interventions and nutritional regimens, to deal with traumatic accidents and with certain organic disorders that they could readily apprehend. On the other hand, they have developed practices of a semimystical or completely religious nature designed to cure physical and mental diseases by influencing the patient's mind. These nonorganic healing practices—such as chants, prayers, pilgrimages, and the like—are usually regarded as irrational by outsiders, but nevertheless they often contribute to the recovery of the patient by helping him to mobilize unconsciously the innate mechanisms for spontaneous self-healing that exist in all living creatures. Faith healing in any form always depends on self-healing.

In any particular culture, the organic and mental elements of the healing process are closely integrated and constitute a coherent medical system characteristic of that culture. The methods used by shamans or physicians are determined, of course, by local conditions and resources—climate, occupations, nutritional habits, drugs with familiar effects, and so on—but the way they are used is profoundly influenced by the locally accepted cultural premises concerning the relation of human beings to the physical and social environment, the cosmos and the deities. The persistence of these basic integrating assumptions assures the continuity of the medical system even when changes occur in the healing practices—for example, following the introduction of a new drug or a foreign influence. Whether traditional or scientific, a particular system of medicine retains its fundamental character as long as the people who use it retain their cultural identity.

Modern scientific medicine has one cultural characteristic that differentiates it from all other systems of healing. Like the other aspects of Western scientific culture, it emphasizes an analytic approach to knowledge and practice instead of depending chiefly on the holistic approach, as is the case for most traditional cultures. This fundamental difference appears with clarity in the comparative descriptions of Western and Chinese medicine presented by Manfred Porkert in this collection of essays.

Ever since the seventeenth century, Western science, including medical science, has been based on the Cartesian analytical philosophy. Its dominant method is to subdivide each anatomic structure, physiological function, and biochemical process into smaller and smaller subunits so as to study each of them separately in greater and greater detail. The most perfect expression of this Cartesian ideal in scientific medicine is the reduction of medical problems to the phenomena of molecular biology, but even the problems of behavior are now being studied by reductionist analysis.

Traditional Chinese medicine, in contrast, seems more concerned with the interplay among the components of biological systems than with the description of these individual components. For example, it studies the way in which the liver relates to the other functions of the body rather than the anatomic or physiologic characteristics of the liver considered as an isolated organ. It also pays much attention to the relationships between the living organism and its environment—the place, the seasons, the weather, the time of day, the social milieu. To a large extent, all systems of medicine except those based on modern Western science are almost exclusively based on a holistic concept integrating the body, the mind, and the total environment.

Western scientific medicine is not more rational than traditional Chinese medicine, which has a rationality all its own, but it is certainly more analytical. There is no doubt in any case that the analytical approach has yielded phenomenal achievements in preventive and therapeutic medicine during the past half-century. On the other hand, it is also true that scientific medicine is not as purely Cartesian as commonly claimed. In fact, some of the greatest medical triumphs of Western medicine emerged not from the reductionist analysis of etiological factors or of pathological mechanisms, but from a holistic view of disease and of man's relation to his total environment.

Jenner had no concept of the specific viral causation of smallpox or of immunological processes when he introduced his technique of vaccination. Rather, the discovery derived from his keen observation of man-environment interactions—namely, that dairymaids exposed to cowpox were not susceptible to the more virulent smallpox. Essentially the same can be said of Pasteur when he generalized Jenner's approach and developed other vaccines for the prevention of microbial diseases. Similarly, Max von Pettenkofer did not believe in the germ theory of disease; yet he made Munich the healthiest city of nineteenth-century Europe and practically eliminated typhoid fever from it simply by bringing clean water from the mountains, disposing of garbage and sewage, planting trees and flowers to create a healthier and more pleasing urban environment.

It would be easy, but wrong, to assume that the successful medical and public health practices of the past were empirical, nothing but lucky accidents. Nor were they simply the outcome of idle, passive observations. In most cases, they involved an implicit, if not explicit, awareness that living organisms respond to environmental challenges by active processes that had adaptive value. The practice of vaccination as applied by Jenner and developed by Pasteur was based on the belief that exposure to a small amount of virus (using the word with its original broad meaning of poison), or to an attenuated form of it, could increase the resistance of the human organism to this agent. Pettenkofer believed that a "good" environment, one that is clean and pleasant, would render the human organism more resistant to a variety of stresses.

If space permitted, example after example could be cited to illustrate that the successful practices of the past were based on processes of organismic and social adaptation. They were empirical only to the extent that they were not based on the kind of reductionist laboratory experimentation that is identified with medical science today, but they were nevertheless rational, because they were derived from attempts to conceptualize logically the interplay between the whole organism and the total environment.

A holistic approach to medicine based on concepts of organismic and social adaptation, is certainly compatible with theoretical and practical scientific developments. The essays presented here are not meant to imply a rejection of the use of science in medicine. Rather, they point to the fact that there is more to medical science than the reductionist analysis of cellular structures and chemical mechanisms, more to medical care than procedures derived from the study of isolated body systems. In fact, the holistic attitude leads to the conclusion that the scientific medicine of our times is not yet scientific enough because it neglects, when it does not completely ignore, the multifarious environmental and emotional factors that affect the human organism in health and in disease. Reducing the normal and pathological processes of life to the phenomena of molecular biology is simply not sufficient if we are to understand the human condition in health or in disease.

WAYS OF HEALTH

Introduction

Contemporary Western medicine is a valuable but incomplete approach to health. It has concentrated on disease and neglected health. It has emphasized individual medical care and slighted the influence of environment and behavior. It has been preoccupied with physiochemical processes and remained insensitive to psychosocial factors in health and disease. And it has tended to regard itself as the only effective form of medicine, thus dismissing alternative systems of healing, both ancient and modern. In short, Western scientific medicine has a severely narrowed view of the health field.

This view is based on several faulty assumptions: (1) Health equals Medical Care, (2) Medical Care equals Western Scientific Medicine, and (3) Western Scientific Medicine equals The Biomedical Model. Although these assumptions are often disguised by the rhetoric of contemporary health care, they show up clearly in the practice of medicine, training of health care providers, behavior of health professionals, expectations and behavior of the public, research priorities, as well as the evaluation of health care. In short, although we may disagree in theory with these assumptions, we act as though they were true.

This book is an attempt to redefine our concepts of health, disease, and medicine—not by abandoning the advantages of modern medicine but by drawing attention to areas that have been neglected and undervalued. It is intended to restore certain perspectives that have been overshadowed by the technical focus of contemporary biomedicine. The topics discussed here suggest that an open, yet critical, examination of ancient healing systems may reveal approaches that can complement and extend contemporary Western medicine. In some instances, this may involve a broadening of the boundaries of medicine; in others, a recognition of the limits of medicine as a determinant of health.

HEALTH EQUALS MEDICAL CARE

Our view of health is paradoxical. Although we put our faith (and money) into medical care, our health is largely determined by factors operating outside the domain of medicine. The dramatic decline in the death rate during the nineteenth and twentieth centuries was due mostly to a decline in deaths from infectious diseases. Although it is tempting to credit medical science with this improvement, most of the reduction in mortality occurred well before the introduction of specific preventive or therapeutic interventions. For example, well over 90 percent of the decline in death from the major killer tuberculosis occurred before the first effective antibiotics were introduced in 1948.

The most significant determinants of our better health are behavioral and environmental: namely, improved nutrition; more effective sanitation; less hazardous living and working conditions; and limited population growth, which preserves the benefits of improved nutrition. People are healthier not so much because they receive better treatment when ill but because they tend not to become ill in the first place, thanks to healthier environments and ways of living.

Disease, however, has not disappeared. With the reduction in mortality from acute infectious disease in most, but not all, parts of the developed world, illness has shifted toward the chronic and degenerative diseases, like cardiovascular disease, stroke, cancer, arthritis, cirrhosis, emphysema, chronic bronchitis, and mental illness. In the United States today, 50 percent of all people suffer from one or more chronic diseases, which now account for over 80 percent of all illnesses. These diseases are sometimes referred to as "diseases of civilization" to highlight their association with the environmental and behavioral aspects of modern industrial societies. Against this new pattern of chronic disease, modern medicine has not been very effective. Nevertheless, the equation of health with medicine suggests that the way to improve health is to provide more medical care. Exponential increases in medical care expenditures (from $12 billion in 1950 to $160 billion in 1978) have not, however, yielded correspondingly impressive improvements in health, at least not in terms of the various health status indicators such as life expectancy of adults.

Mortality and morbidity statistics, of course, do not tell the whole story. We are all aware of numerous instances where medical interventions have saved or aided sick individuals. These *individual* interventions, however, do not necessarily translate into a decline in mortality statistics for the whole population. Furthermore, medicine performs functions other than curing disease that do not show up in the figures, such as comforting the sick and reassuring the well. Ironically, many of these important humanistic and psychosocial functions have been neglected in modern medical care.

This, then, is an age of diminishing returns whereby more medical care will probably contribute only marginally to health. In fact, some such as Ivan Illich claim that further increases in medical care may be detrimental, producing more adverse drug reactions, unnecessary surgery, hospital-acquired infections, and dependency on health care professionals.

This is not to deny the valuable contributions of modern medicine—the antibiotics, the surgical advances, or the future benefits that may accrue from biomedical research. Nevertheless, biomedicine must be placed in perspective, balanced by more attention to the nonmedical determinants of health—our environment, physical and social, and our lifestyles. The equation of health with medical care fosters an inappropriate dependence on medical care and creates unrealistic expectations of health professionals. The evidence is overwhelming that our health depends more on what we choose to do and not to do, and the socioeconomic restraints on those choices, than on the ministrations of health professionals. A broader view of health suggests new roles for patients in actively caring for their health, and new roles for professionals in enhancing the public's competence in self-care. The future role of physicians may again focus more on education and thereby reflect the origin of the word doctor, which comes from *docere,* "to teach."

Health then is more than medical care and more than the absence of disease. What is now called *health care* is, in fact, *sickness or disease care.* Even the fields of preventive medicine and public health share a disease-orientation with modern medicine and neglect the promotion of health. The fact is we know very little about health. We even lack a suitable vocabulary to describe the phenomenon of health. When it comes to discussing health, we can do little better than the ancient Chinese notion of a balance of vital energies or the Greek concept of internal harmony. Our lack of understanding, however, should not be surprising given that the phenomenon of health has not been explored with nearly the same intensity, resourcefulness, or commitment applied to the study of disease. What is health? Why are some people healthier? Why are some people better able to withstand similar challenges? What aspects of physical and social environments enhance health? These are a few of the questions deserving attention. To begin, we might consider how some of the ancient and alternative systems of medicine view and promote health. A study of these systems, which do not share the same preoccupations of modern medicine, may reveal complementary strategies to the disease-oriented approaches of Western scientific medicine.

MEDICAL CARE EQUALS WESTERN SCIENTIFIC MEDICINE

There is a marked tendency to equate all of medical care with Western scientific medicine. However, this ignores the fact that even in the developed countries 70 to 80 percent of all illnesses are managed outside the formal medical care system. Furthermore, many individuals and groups rely heavily on folk medicine and make extensive use of marginal and unorthodox practitioners, despite lack of recognition within the orthodox mainstream.

Until recently, ancient and traditional systems of healing have been viewed by health professionals as archaic, superstitious, interesting perhaps to a few medical historians or anthropologists, but irrelevant to contemporary health care. The prevalent assumption within the medical community has been that Western medicine long ago surpassed the ancient systems, having incorporated everything from them of value.

An alternative interpretation is that Western scientific medicine is not *the* medicine. Ancient medical systems, as well as the modern unorthodox systems, have evolved in independent and different directions from the mainstream of contemporary Western medicine. In many cases, these systems have specialized in areas and approaches neglected by Western medicine. It may be possible to identify valuable perspectives and techniques that can *complement* the specializations of our current medical effort.

A new willingness is emerging within the mainstream of Western medicine to reconsider some of the older systems of medicine in light of contemporary science and present-day health needs. The task, however, is not an easy one. It demands a fine discrimination to separate the essential contents from the admittedly strange packaging of some of the alternative systems. It necessitates interdisciplinary investigation and teamwork both in research and in practice. It also requires an openness to new and often discordant world views and ways of thinking about human health and disease.

However, what is being suggested here is not a rejection of contemporary medicine and a return to ancient practices. The wholesale importation or adoption of medical practices designed for other times and other peoples is not likely to yield much of value. Many ancient practices *are* ineffective, others have been superseded, while still others require specific cultural contexts that are absent in contemporary Western societies.

We don't necessarily want to bring Navaho medicine men into the hospitals, but we should try to understand the basic principles at work in Navaho and other forms of symbolic healing. By extracting relevant perspectives and practices from these older disciplines, a new synthesis, one that combines the special insights of ancient and unconventional medicine with the technical excellence of contemporary scientific medicine, can be promoted.

This book contains some early examples of such a synthesis. For example, many of the ancient systems of medicine were based on strengthening and supporting the organism's inherent powers of recovery, what the Greeks called *vis medicatrix naturae,* "the healing force of nature." Recent scientific studies of ancient yogic meditation techniques as well as new developments in biofeedback technology suggest that we may have seriously underestimated human capacities for self-healing and conscious control of physiological and psychological states. A new science of psychosomatic self-regulation is developing, in which ancient practices combine with modern scientific technology to thereby create new opportunities for individuals to participate actively in their own healing and health maintenance.

Similarly, the ancient Hippocratic concern for the quality of human-environment interactions has re-emerged in the contemporary concern for ecology. New interest is being directed toward the impact on health by the radically different environmental conditions and behavioral patterns to which modern man must try to adapt. Although the evidence is incomplete, it does suggest that changes in eating habits, physical activity, biological rhythms, air ionization, and light may have unrecognized health consequences. The importance of such factors is hinted at in many of the ancient systems of medicine.

Other examples of the merging of ancient and modern medicine are the recent scientific investigation into the biological effects of healing by the laying on of hands and the search for the basic psychotherapeutic features underlying the diverse healing rituals of Western and non-Western societies. There is also growing interest in the theoretical foundations of traditional Chinese medicine, which may form a complement to the analytic methods of Western medical science. These examples discussed in this book, although preliminary in nature, point toward the emergence of a more balanced and complete approach to health and healing.

WESTERN SCIENTIFIC MEDICINE EQUALS THE BIOMEDICAL MODEL

Modern medicine has increasingly become impersonal and technical as scientific medicine has been identified with the biomedical model of health and disease. This model assumes that all aspects of human health can be understood in physical and chemical terms. The aim of medical science, therefore, is to analyze the structure and function of the human body in finer and finer detail. Anatomy, physiology, biochemistry, and molecular biology are considered the "basic sciences." Consideration of the mind is separated from or reduced to a study of the body. Organic diseases become the "real" diseases. Therapy is defined as physical and chemical interventions into the body machine. And, medical science is equated with the analysis and quantification of somatic processes.

The success of this biomedical model is undeniable. But so, too, are its limits. The human experience of health and disease, the personal and psychosocial dimensions of illness, are either neglected completely or reduced to technical concerns. As Abraham Maslow once observed, "If the only tool you have is a hammer, you tend to treat everything as if it were a nail."

This general disregard for the psychosocial environment has been likened by George Engel to the attitude in the days when surgeons ridiculed the concept of antisepsis and persisted in performing surgery in unclean surroundings, sometimes defiantly sharpening their scalpels on the soles of their shoes to show contempt for the power of the invisible germs. Similarly, the current ignorance and insensitivity to the "invisible" symbolic messages of the social and cultural environment limits the effectiveness of contemporary medicine.

With contemporary medicine focusing primarily on technical rather than humanistic concerns, some have criticized medicine as being *too* scientific. The problem, however, is that modern medicine has not been scientific enough. The biomedical model has been unduly restrictive, and we need a broader view of scientific medicine—one that includes a scientific investigation of the psychological, social, and cultural, as well as the physiochemical, factors relevant to health.

This book is, then, an attempt to challenge the assumptions that have markedly restricted our view of the health field. It is an invitation to rethink some of our basic concepts of health and disease by examining other systems of medicine. The discussions of traditional healing practices, Navaho medicine men, Chinese and Greek concepts of medicine, and yogic therapy may seem at first far afield from the present concern over the "health care crisis." However, the crisis itself arises, in part, from limited concepts and strategies. Our current problems can provide a valuable opportunity to reassess our basic assumptions, which, after all, determine in large measure how we structure our health care system and how we behave with regard to our own health and illness.

The subjects covered in the book are diverse, spanning centuries as well as disciplines. At one point the reader is invited to consider the linguistic derivation of a technical Chinese medical term; at another, the physiology of relaxation; and at still another, the physical properties of air ions. The purpose, however, is not to present isolated bits of exotica or an array of alternative health practices. Rather, the first part of the book attempts to develop a framework that allows for the integration of the varied specializations of different systems. The sections that follow are drawn from areas that have been slighted and undervalued in the mainstream. The juxtaposition of these varied systems produces a cumulative effect perhaps greater than any single system and suggests the possibility of a more comprehensive approach to health.

We are now at a frontier of health. The way forward lies not in an extrapolation of the present, nor in a resurrection of the past, but in a new synthesis—an integration of medical and nonmedical approaches to health, Western scientific medicine with alternative systems of healing, and physiochemical investigations with a scientific understanding of human behavior and psychosocial factors in health and disease.

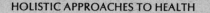

HOLISTIC APPROACHES TO HEALTH

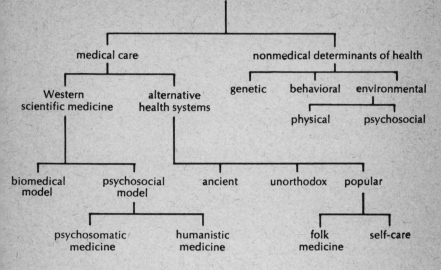

PART ONE

HOLISTIC APPROACHES TO HEALTH

Introduction

Nasrudin was not feeling very well. He called in a doctor.
"You need a purgative," said the physician.
"I want a second opinion," said Nasrudin.
"An operation," said the second doctor.
"Send for another doctor," said Nasrudin.
"Massage is the only answer in cases like this," said the third doctor.
"Now we have the prescription," said Nasrudin. "A third of a cut, a third of a purge, and add one-third of a massage. That should clear things up nicely!"

Idries Shah, *The Subtleties of the Inimitable Mulla Nasrudin*

The term "holistic," or "wholistic" as it sometimes appears, is becoming increasingly fashionable. Unfortunately, it is all too often equated with anything exotic, unorthodox, foreign, alternative, counterculture, mystical, or oriental. It has become the catchword for a varied and uneven collection of fringe practitioners whose major shared characteristic is often no more than an antiscientific bias or a vague endorsement of mind, body, and spirit. Some refer to a discipline of *holistic medicine* as though it were an established body of medical knowledge which one could study like surgery, neurology, or acupuncture. Such misuses of "holistic" represent an unfortunate degeneration of a useful term and concept.

"Holistic" more properly and most simply describes an *attitude* or *mode of perception* that attempts to view *the whole person in the context of the total environment.* The term is perhaps uniquely suited to convey this attitude by virtue of its rich etymology. Lewis Thomas has noted that "holism" suggests something biologically transcendent because it is associated with "holy," even though the word was originally intended to mean simply a complete assemblage of living units. It derives from the Indo-European root word *kailo,* meaning "whole," "intact," and "uninjured." *Kailo* in turn fathered a family of terms, including hail, hale, health, hallow, holy, whole, and heal, all of which remain related in our minds. Thus the word "holistic," by virtue of its lineage, expresses something of the essence of health and healing, namely, a quality of wholeness that we associate with healthy functioning and well-being.

Although the basic concept of wholeness underlying the term "holistic" extends far back into the early history of human thought, the word itself was coined in 1926 by Jan Christiaan Smuts in his book *Holism and Evolution.* He conceived of holism teleologically as "the motive force behind Evolution" and maintained that biological organisms have a tendency toward wholeness, toward righting imbalances, and that these self-healing properties give evidence of the holistic tendency in nature. He further maintained, as others did before him, that a study of parts of any system cannot explain the whole because "the whole is more than the sum of the parts."

The holistic attitude is not new to the life sciences. The holistic or "organismic" approach can be traced throughout the development of modern biology and psychology and is often associated with such names as J. B. S. Haldane, A. N. Whitehead, J. H. Woodger, F. S. C. Northrop, A. Meyer, Kurt Goldstein, Andras Angyal, Abraham Maslow, Paul Weiss, and René Dubos. The holistic approach perhaps finds its most comprehensive development in modern science as part of General Systems Theory, introduced in the 1930s by Ludwig von Bertallanfy. Despite the recent misuses and popularizations, the holistic attitude maintains a respected and valuable place in contemporary scientific thought.

In the health field a holistic approach offers a conceptual alternative to the physiochemical reductionism, materialism, and mind/body dualism that dominates much of contemporary medical thought. However, a holistic approach is not to be confused with various alternative systems of medicine per se. In fact, many unorthodox practitioners who reject completely the technical advances and methods of Western scientific medicine are, by definition, anything but holistic. One cannot afford to discount the methods of modern biomedicine any more than one can afford to overlook the complementary modes of ancient systems of medicine.

A holistic approach to health also differs substantially from piecemeal eclecticism as portrayed by Nasrudin in the story that opens this introduction. The mere addition of a few techniques or practices to the tool kit of modern medicine is more likely to be confusing than effective. Instead, we need to rethink our current ideas of health, disease, and medicine. We need to develop a conceptual framework that bridges disciplinary, professional, and cultural boundaries and integrates into a meaningful whole the specializations of various approaches to health, East and West, ancient and modern.

It is for these reasons that the book begins at a conceptual level rather than with specific techniques. Each essay of this first part attempts to establish the need for a more holistic approach to health as well as offers a perspective on some elements of such an approach.

René Dubos manages to combine the most relevant aspects of medical history and the philosophy of medicine with a unique perspective shaped by many years of research as an experimental biologist. The result is no dry recounting of historical facts, but a dynamic interpretation of the development of the major ideas underlying contemporary scientific medicine. In the chapter reprinted here from his book *Man Adapting,* Dubos traces the evolution of ideas about health and disease beginning with primitive theories of disease and continuing through the influential Hippocratic doctrines to the rise of the doctrine of specific etiology and physiochemical reductionism. While crediting the successes of the specific and analytic approach, Dubos also notes its limitations: "In the most common and probably the most impor-

tant ~~phenomena of life, the constituent parts are so interdepend-~~
ent ~~that they lose their character, their meaning, and indeed~~
~~their very existence, when dissected from the functioning whole.~~"
He calls for the development of an organismic and environmental
biology that takes as its subject the responses of *whole living
organisms* to environmental challenges. Perhaps more than any
other contemporary writer, Dubos is able to express the necessity
of a holistic approach.

Our current strategy for improving health is primarily to
provide more personal medical services despite evidence suggesting that medical care after a point produces only marginal gains
in health. In "The Boundaries of Health Care," Robert Haggerty argues that ~~social and environmental factors are the major~~
~~determinants of health,~~ referring to the way ~~we live, our diet,~~
~~life stresses, housing, environmental pollution and hazards, polit-~~
~~ical and social structures.~~ Addressing the role of the medical
profession, Haggerty contends that working in these "boundary"
areas is likely to contribute more to health than further concentration on curative, personal medical care. Despite the considerable barriers to enlarging the scope of health care, the health
problems of today demand a broader, biosocial approach and a
willingness to work in interdisciplinary areas.

In the essay that follows, John Powles reinforces this position
by evaluating the effectiveness of the current medical effort—an
effort aimed largely at physical and chemical interventions in sick
individuals. As an alternative to this "engineering" strategy,
Powles describes an "ecological" approach that emphasizes the
importance of ways of living in health and disease. He argues that
an ecological approach aimed at populations, not at sick individuals, promises to be more effective in preventing the diseases
of maladaptation that are now predominant in the industrialized
societies. Aspects of this ecological approach, including biological rhythms, air ionization, exercise, and nutrition, will be the
subject of the last part of this book.

Powles also calls attention to traditional healing practices,
highlighting the nontechnical side of medicine, the caring and
"helping to cope" functions. Medicine in all cultures serves not
only to master disease technically but also to help people cope

meaningfully with the emotional and existential significance of disease. All too often this human and nontechnical side of medical care is slighted as the technical side is overvalued.

The major problem with a holistic approach is translating this admittedly vague and abstract ideal of wholeness into a practical strategy for addressing the complex problems of health and disease. While many agree, at least in theory, with the value of a holistic approach, in practice, fragmentation and reduction still hold sway. Part of the problem stems from the lack of a conceptual framework and vocabulary for discussing interdisciplinary approaches. To conclude Part One, Howard Brody and I outline a systems view of health and disease. Our intent is to provide an integrative framework that can inform the actions of a wide variety of health practitioners and help co-ordinate the many elements comprising a more comprehensive approach to health. This framework also helps clarify the complementary techniques and approaches of contemporary Western medicine and other systems of healing.

By René Dubos

Medicine Evolving

All ancient people of whom we have records formulated theories to account for disease and developed practices of prevention and treatment. Many of these practices certainly operated by suggestion and were most effective against disease states of psychic origin. But others had a more physical basis and dealt with the ailments of the body. Baths, massage, blood-letting, dry cupping, cauterization, the setting of fractures, trephining, the use of many drugs derived from plants or from the earth, even vaccination against snake bites and infectious diseases, are among the many therapeutic procedures primitive man discovered empirically and learned to use skillfully. It is possible that some of these procedures originated from an innate health instinct. Just as wild animals instinctively choose the right food, eat certain herbs when they are sick, treat themselves by licking their wounds or by extracting foreign bodies, so did primitive man probably have "medical" instincts which were essential for his survival. Eventually some of these instincts may have evolved into magical practices incorporated into primitive doctrines of health and disease.

Medical theories have changed greatly in the course of time, but not according to a continuous and orderly process of evolution. Rather the changes have occurred as discontinuous steps, the direction of which was determined by the prevailing view of man's nature and of his relation to the cosmos. Emphasis has been placed at times on the whole man and on his relationship to demons or

From *Man Adapting*, pp. 319–43 (New Haven: Yale University Press, 1965). Copyright © 1965 by Yale University Press. Reprinted by permission of René Dubos and the publisher.

to God. In contrast, the focus under other circumstances has been on fragments of man's nature, either on his mind or on the components of the body machine. Throughout the history of medicine, the "ontological" doctrine, which regards diseases as specific entities, has alternated with the "physiological" view, according to which disease is simply an abnormal state experienced by a given individual organism at a given time. In one form or another, the ontological attitude has probably been the most consistently dominant among both laymen and physicians. It assumes that disease is a thing in itself, essentially unrelated to the patient's personality, his bodily constitution, or his mode of life. This concept reasserts itself repeatedly in everyday language when it is said that the patient has *a* disease or that the physician treats *a* disease.

To think of disease as an entity separate from oneself and caused by an agent external to the body but capable of getting into it and thereby causing damage seems to have great appeal for the human mind. This attitude is perhaps a consequence of projection, a process whereby what is felt or experienced as uncomfortable, painful, or dangerous is ascribed to a bad influence from the outside. In prescientific medicine, such explanations took the form of demonological concepts, disease being regarded as resulting from the malevolent influence of taboo violation, sorcery, revengeful ghosts, witchcraft, hostile ancestors, or animal spirits. A man became ill because he had an enemy who cast a spell or because he was being punished for breaking a taboo or for some other transgression.

Similar psychological concepts still influence today the interpretation of phenomena established by scientific medicine. Regardless of their level of education and sophistication, patients are prone to blame their illness on something they "caught" or ate, or which happened to them. They think of disease as something apart from themselves, and many account for it in terms of punishment. "Physicians also find attractive such ways of thinking, particularly if they can see the 'cause' of disease as something which they can attack and destroy" (Engel, 1962a).

Irrespective of medical philosophy, ancient man acquired many practical skills for the treatment of disease. Empirical mastery of a wide range of medical techniques can be observed even today among people who are still in the Stone Age culture, for example, the pygmies of Central Africa or the Australian aborigines; their medicine men perform therapeutic feats that do not depend on suggestion alone. Ineed, so great were the practical skills of ancient people that only during very recent times has medicine come to differ significantly from what it was in the distant past. The differences in medical and surgical procedures as practiced in ancient Egypt, in post-Socratic Athens, in a medieval palace, at the Versailles court, or in a primitive African tribe today correspond not so much to differences in factual knowledge as to differences in medical philosophy of the physician. In one case he believes or pretends to believe that disease comes from demonic forces. In another case he regards health as a gift of God, or as the expression of a harmonious relationship between man and his environment.

Primitive societies developed very early a large stock of practical experience having to do not only with the treatment but also with the prevention of disease. All the great leaders of men, such as Moses, formulated strict sanitary regulations for camp life. In the words of the medical historian Field Garrison, "The ancient Hebrews were in fact the founders of prophylaxis, and their high priests were true medical police." The admonitions in Leviticus, the various kinds of taboo that rule and restrict the activities of primitive people, and so many codes of behavior based on folklore that persist in a concealed form among us are the perennial expressions of empirical practices which served a useful purpose at the time when they were first enacted in the countries of their origin.

In all ancient civilizations, medical wisdom and skills have been symbolized by the attributes of certain gods and goddesses of health. For example, the complex structure of ancient Greek medicine was personified by Asclepius, who was first regarded as the perfect physician, then as a god of health. His cult persisted longer than that of any other Greek god and, instead of being destroyed by Christianity, it progressively was integrated in Christian tradition. The two Christian saints of medicine and pharmacy, Cosmas and Damian, appeared as did Asclepius in the dreams of those who sought help in the temples for the ills of the body and the mind.

While it is customary to emphasize Asclepius' knowledge of the healing arts, his activities in the Greek legend went beyond that of a healer. From the third century on, Asclepius is shown in most of Greek iconography with his two daughters, on the right Hygeia (Hygiene) and on the left Panakeia (Cure-All). The two maidens symbolize the main attitudes modern medicine has retained from this ancient heritage, which it is trying to convert into exact sciences. Panakeia was a true healing goddess, learned in the use of drugs derived either from plants or from the earth; her cult is still alive today in the universal search for a panacea. In contrast, her sister Hygeia, one of the many personifications of Athena, was the goddess who taught the Greeks that they could remain in good health if they lived according to reason, with moderation in all things. Men still honor her memory in the use of the word hygiene. They pay lip service to the wisdom she symbolizes by attempting, even though without much success so far, to formulate ways of life conducive to health yet compatible with their appetites, inertia, and lack of discipline.

Eventually, all the attributes of Asclepius, Hygeia, and Panakeia came to be synthesized in the legends attached to the name of Hippocrates. Although it is likely that the several treatises attributed to Hippocrates were written in reality by different persons at different times, there is no doubt that a distinguished physician by this name did exist and practice medicine on the island of Cos. He was then so well known that Plato mentions him by name in two of his dialogues.

The many stylistic genres and doctrinal contradictions in the Hippocratic Corpus make it certain that its multiple fragments were composed at very different times by physicians of different schools. This multiple origin naturally constitutes a source of great complexities for the historian and detracts somewhat from the fame attached to the man Hippocrates. On the other hand, it accounts for the multifarious and lasting influence the Hippocratic Corpus has exerted on Western medicine. The Corpus, in fact, does not represent merely the doctrine of the school of Cos, with which Hippocrates is identified, but also that of the rival school of Cnidos. More broadly it defines an attitude and states a series of facts and concepts that constitute the summation of Greek medical knowledge, derived in large part from Egyptian sources. The Hippocratic Corpus constitutes even today the essential basis of modern medicine because it encompasses the various complementary aspects of medical science and practice. These can be summarized as follows:

Disease is not caused by demons or capricious deities but rather by natural forces that obey natural laws. Hence, therapeutic procedures can be developed on a rational basis. These procedures include the use of regimens, drugs, and surgical techniques designed to correct the ill effects of natural forces.

The well-being of man is under the influence of the environment, including in particular air, water, places, and the various regimens. The understanding of the effect of the environment on man is the fundamental basis of the physician's art.

Health is the expression of a harmonious balance between the various components of man's nature (the four humors that control all human activities) and the environment and ways of life.

Whatever happens in the mind influences the body and vice versa. In fact, mind and body cannot be considered independently one from the other.

Health means a healthy mind in a healthy body, and can be achieved only by governing daily life in accordance with natural laws, which ensures an equilibrium between the different forces of the organism and those of the environment.

Medicine is an ethical profession and implies an attitude of reverence for the human condition.

Paraphrasing Whitehead's remark on the debt of European philosophy to Plato, one might say that modern medicine is but a series of commentaries and elaborations on the Hippocratic writings. The comprehensiveness of their coverage is such that they have retained a universal appeal for 2,500 years. The scientist recognizes in them the first known systematic attempt to explain disease phenomena in terms of natural laws, on the basis of objectively made and carefully recorded observations. The clinician admires in them a shrewd description of the signs and symptoms characteristic of each disease, a knowledge of prognosis based on clinical experience, and a penetrating concern for the patient considered as a whole, integrated organism. The student of public health points to the clear statement in the Hippocratic doctrine that diseases are determined by the total environment and by the ways of life. The student of man's natural history is impressed by the statement in the Hippocratic Corpus that the general characteristics of populations in the normal state are conditioned by the topographic and climatic factors of the locality.

Thus, the Hippocratic Corpus has a significant message for almost every thinking person concerned with man in health and in disease. But in reality, each person and each age has emphasized some particular aspect of this message at the expense of the others. The practicing physician with the gold-headed cane, the sanitarian concerned with public health, the student of physiological functions and chemical structures, can all trace their scientific ancestry to the Hippocratic teachings, but otherwise their attitude and professional activities have little in common.

SPECIFIC ETIOLOGY AND HOST RESPONSE

The belief in natural causation of disease has led to a multiplicity of scientific attitudes which differ so profoundly that they appear at first sight to be almost incompatible. Some schools of thought have emphasized the unique importance of particular organs or functions, whereas others have claimed that pathogenesis cannot be understood, or disease treated, without considering the patient as a whole. Some believe that the key to medical progress is a knowledge of molecular biology, while others are just as convinced that the most urgent task is to study the response of the body-mind complex to the total environment. Depending upon the time and place, the center of the medical stage has been occupied by anatomy, physiology, cellular pathology, molecular biology, concern with the unique experience of the individual patient, or with the responses of the social group considered as an integrated unit. All medical faiths continue to proclaim allegiance to Hippocrates even though the Hippocratic Corpus, like the Bible, is often invoked but hardly ever read.

Whatever their differences of opinion, all the physicians of Greco-Roman culture have long accepted the concept that diseases are caused by natural forces. But the history of this faith could be written as a debate that has lasted more than two thousand years, between the proponents of the doctrine of specific etiology and those who regard disease as the outcome of a constellation of factors acting simultaneously. . . .

There is no more spectacular phenomenon in the history of medicine than the rapidity with which the germ theory of disease became accepted by the medical profession. This acceptance was due in part to the vigor of the personalities of its two leading proponents, Louis Pasteur and Robert Koch, but in part only. The triumph of the germ theory would not have been as immediate and decisive if the medical public had not been prepared for it by the observations and reflections of several great clinicians throughout the early part of the nineteenth century. . . .

. . . The time was right, because this intellectual departure was consonant with two great themes of early nineteenth-century biology. On the one hand, the Linnean classification of plants and animals was then becoming generally accepted, and it seemed natural to extend it to other natural phenomena, including those of disease. In addition, cause-effect relationships had come to be taken as a matter of course in biological thinking; the principle of causality was replacing vitalism at least among experimenters. On this dual basis, it became possible to construct the theory that each particular disease has its particular cause, and that each noxious agent exerts a characteristic pathological effect.

. . . Acute infectious diseases, . . . then known as "the fevers," were extremely prevalent in Europe; in particular there had been disastrous outbreaks of diphtheria and scarlet fever. . . . The overwhelming importance of acute microbial diseases during the nineteenth century thus constituted the historical accident that gave its first form to the doctrine of specific etiology.

Furthermore, these diseases provided ideal models to demonstrate the validity of the concept of specific causation. Nutritional deficiencies, which were then also widespread, constituted another type of pathological material, which soon proved well suited for studies on specific etiology, and in many cases for the development of specific methods of control. Once proven in these particular situations, the doctrine extended progressively to all fields of medicine. Biochemical lesions, molecular pathology, congenital anomalies, and genetic disorders are direct linear descendants of the doctrine of specificity. Even certain mental diseases are being shown to result from identifiable chemical disturbances or from specific life situations.

The doctrine of specific etiology has thus constituted the most powerful single force in the development of medicine during the past century. But there is now increasing awareness that it fails to provide a complete account of most disease problems as they naturally occur, and especially of those which are most important in our communities today. In general, pathological states are the consequence of several determinant factors acting simultaneously; moreover, the manifestations of any given agent differ profoundly from one person to another. Causality and specificity are therefore much less apparent in clinical situations than they are in the laboratory. A few acute infectious diseases and nutritional deficiencies of course present clinical pictures so characteristic that they can be identified without difficulty; but few are the pathological states that can be classified as true biological entities. What the patient experiences and what the physician observes constitute generally a confusing variety of symptoms and lesions rather than a well-defined entity. In most cases, a syndrome such as anemia, cardiac insufficiency, gastric disturbance, and depression is more in evidence than the unique pathological manifestations of a specific etiological agent.

Furthermore, each noxious agent can express itself by a great variety of different pathological states. The phthisis studied by Laënnec had little in common with the primary infection that is now the most common form of tuberculosis in our communities; yet both are caused by tubercle bacilli of the same virulence. Syphilitic aortitis, paresis, and tabes, syphilitic roseola, a gumma or a chancre, can all be caused by identical forms of *Treponema pallidum*. A traumatic accident that would be fatal for an aged person might have but trivial consequences for a young adult. Thus, the characters of a disease are determined more by the response of the organism as a whole than by the characteristics of the causative agent.

To complicate matters still further, different agents can elicit similar reactions. Bacterial endocarditis in man and mastitis in cows used to be caused almost exclusively by streptococci. Now that streptococcal infections can be successfully treated with penicillin, other microbial species commonly become established in the lesions and thus give a new microbial etiology to these ancient diseases. Similarly, congestion and hypersecretion of the nasal mucous membranes can be caused by viral and bacterial infections; by inhalation of smoke, dust, allergens, or cold air; by migraine of vascular origin; by the administration of parasympatomimetic drugs; by sorrow and tears. Or again, urticaria can be caused by sunlight and cold, by contact with wool, by many types of foods and drugs.

Since the body has only a limited range of reactions, its response to assaults of very different origin and nature is rather stereotyped. For example, an intestinal pathology which mimics that of typhoid fever and shows the typical lesions of the Peyer patches can be produced by injecting into the mesenteric nodes almost any irritating substance, even a rose thorn! More generally, a stimulation of the neurovegetative system can produce important lesions not only in the viscera directly affected but also in others with indirect and distant anatomical connections. The General Adaptation Syndrome seems to constitute an irrefutable denial of the doctrine of specificity.

As is well known, furthermore, the response of the human organism to many noxious agencies is profoundly conditioned by adrenal and other hormones. The secretion of these in turn is affected by psychological factors and by the symbolic interpretation the mind attaches to environmental agents and stimuli. This interpretation is so profoundly influenced by the experiences of the past and the anticipations of the future that the physicochemical characteristics of noxious agents rarely determine the characters of the pathological processes they set in motion.

These facts might lead to the conclusion that the doctrine of specificity has been discredited, but a more useful interpretation seems to be that its meaning must be enlarged to include not only the operations of external agents but also factors that govern the responses of the organism. In its original form, the doctrine of specificity was focused on external noxious agents—microbes, poisons, nutritional deficiencies, ionizing radiations. In its more sophisticated form, it concerns itself not only with the direct effects of these noxious factors on the target organs but also with the organism's responses.

The ancient belief in the healing power of nature, Hippocrates' Naturae vis Medicatrix, is an expression of the faith that the integrated organism can respond in an adaptive manner to environmental insults. But this large philosophical concept of biology will not become part of scientific medicine until precise knowledge is available of the physiological, immunological, and psychological mechanisms through which the healing power operates. Similarly, while the concepts covered by the words "diathesis" and "epidemic constitutions" denote real characteristics of the organism and real ecological situations, they will not evolve beyond the level of understanding reached by Hippocrates and Sydenham until their determinant factors have been identified. Thus the doctrine of specificity still remains the indispensable key to the understanding of all problems of pathogenesis; it must be applied now to the factors of the internal environment as well as to the various cosmic forces that affect mankind.

The experimenter, the epidemiologist, and the clinician approach the phenomena of disease with different attitudes. The experimenter selects from these phenomena a few aspects closely related to his scientific interests; in fact, he must learn to eliminate all others as completely as possible, even while remaining aware of the complexity of phenomena as they naturally occur. Such an attitude involves choices which are intellectually difficult and often painful, but which are the inescapable price of scientific progress. The epidemiologist in contrast must observe and study the biological phenomena in all their natural complexity; he tries to identify the various components of ecological situations and to recognize their interrelationships in the hope of being able to select among the various control methods that are available to him those which are most practical and effective in a given environment at a given time.

Whereas the experimenter selects a simplified model for detailed analysis and the epidemiologist deals with large human groups, the clinician must appreciate the subtleties that determine the response of each individual person. Physicians have long known, for example, that healing tends to be slow and relapses to be frequent in the anxious and irritable person. Experience with diabetic subjects has taught that bereavement and disappointment in love or business can increase insulin requirements as much as does an infection or a physiological disturbance. A person may blush, perspire, tighten his fist, or even collapse following a trivial incident that goes unnoticed by his companion. The underlying mechanisms of those differences in response are poorly understood, but this does not decrease their importance for the physician. They illustrate that each person exists as it were in a private world, and furthermore responds to environmental forces according to a highly individual pattern. These complexities pose to human medicine problems that can usually be ignored by the student of general biology or veterinary medicine.

Finally, the clinician has the responsibility to decide the relative importance of the many different factors that impinge simultaneously on his particular patient, and what aspects of the external and internal environment he can modify usefully. As most clinical decisions must be made on the basis of insufficient information, the practice of medicine retains necessarily some of the characteristics of an art.

The complexity of the problems encountered by the clinician may help to forecast the future trends of the doctrine of specificity. Simple cause-effect relationships involving only one variable are rarely sufficient to account for the natural phenomena of disease. The total environment and the *milieu intérieur* constitute a multifactorial system, each component of which must be studied with regard not only to its own characteristics but also to its effects on the other components of the system. There is reason to hope that a better understanding of multifactorial systems would eventually give concrete meaning and practical usefulness to concepts such as Naturae vis Medicatrix, defense mechanisms, constitution, telluric factors, etc., which medicine has honored since the time of Hippocrates, but which have remained too vague to be practically useful. The concept of multifactorial causation is in reality but an extension of the doctrine of specificity that brings scientific understanding a little nearer to the complexities of the real world.

Theories are like living organisms that can survive only by evolving in order to adapt themselves to new demands. If the doctrine of specificity were restricted to its initial narrow formulation, it would experience the fate of other theories and wither away or at best become mummified. It would constitute another illustration of Thomas Huxley's statement that new truths commonly begin as heresies and end as superstitions. Fortunately, the doctrine is acquiring new life and becoming even more fruitful of understanding, because its scope is being widened. At first focused on a few noxious factors of the external world, it is now taking cognizance of the multiplicity of internal mechanisms through which the body and the mind attempt to respond adaptively to environmental stimuli and stresses. Seen from this broader point of view, the doctrine of specificity will stimulate the development of methods for the study of the response of the organism as a whole, in other words for a truer apprehension of disease. "Science," Pasteur wrote, "advances through tentative answers to a series of more and more subtle questions, which reach deeper and deeper into the essence of natural phenomena."

ORGANISMIC AND ENVIRONMENTAL BIOLOGY

The very process of living is a complex interplay between the organism and the environment, at times resulting in injury and disease. To study this interplay and its effects, medical scientists have naturally adopted the general method that has been used by experimental biologists since the seventeenth century, namely, to devise models as simplified as possible, preferably involving only one variable.

The beginning of the modern era in scientific biology is commonly traced to René Descartes. This is not because his name is associated with discoveries or scientific generalizations of biological importance. In fact, some of his biological ideas were rather primitive or even outright erroneous, as when he challenged Harvey's theory of the blood circulation and proposed instead that the heart worked as a heat engine. Descartes opened a new era in medical science simply by asserting with logical force and literary skill that all the structures and operations of the human body are reducible to mechanical models, while the soul is a direct gift of God and is therefore out of the range of scientific understanding. These assertions encouraged scientists to focus their efforts on the body machine and to study it by the methods used for studying the inanimate world. Removing the mind from scientific concern greatly simplified the study of life and particularly of man.

One of the essential principles of Descartes' famous method was to divide each of the difficulties presented by the system under consideration into as many parts as possible, and then analyze these parts separately, in the faith that knowledge of the more complex aspects would eventually emerge from the reductionist analysis. The obvious objection to this method is that one-variable systems can never represent the complexity of living processes. Human life particularly, in health or disease, is the resultant of countless independent forces impinging simultaneously on the total organism and setting in motion a multitude of interrelated responses. In this light, most medical problems appear so complex as to be beyond the range of experimental science.

However, the Cartesian analytical approach is so powerful that innumerable discoveries immediately emerged from its application to medicine. The immensely complex problems posed by living man were converted into much simpler questions focused on the mechanical aspects of structures and functions isolated from the body machine. To a very large extent the history of modern medical science consists in an attempt to pursue the reductionist analysis until it reaches into smaller and smaller fragments, or simpler and simpler functions. The study of life has thus become almost identified with the study of the molecules of which the body is made.

While the operations of the mind have not yet proved amenable to description in terms of molecular events, it seems that Descartes was too timid when he placed this field outside the realm encompassed by his method. On the one hand, nerve action can be described in much the same terms as muscular action. Even more striking is the fact that the most glamorous achievements in the study of behavior bear the stamp of the Cartesian scientific philosophy. Pavlov and the behaviorists after him have reduced complex responses into simple conditioned reflexes. And Freud taught that the mind of each individual person could be explained if one tried with enough skill and patience to identify the particular events that had shaped it early in its development.

Unfortunately, the very success of the reductionist approach has led to the neglect of some of the most important and probably the most characteristic aspects of human life. Starting from a question singled out for study because of its medical importance, the modern medical investigator is likely to progress seriatim to the organ or function involved, then to the single cell, then to the cellular fragments, then to the molecular groupings or reactions, then to individual molecules and atoms; and he would happily proceed, if he knew enough, to the elementary particles where matter and energy become indistinguishable. There is no doubt, of course, that fascinating and important problems continuously emerge at each step in the analytical disintegration of a complex biological phenomenon. But experience shows that all too frequently the original phenomenon itself is lost on the way. Many are the investigators who descend from man to molecules, but few are those who ever try the more difficult task of using molecular knowledge to deal with the problems of real life.

From a more practical, even if narrow, point of view, there is the obvious limitation that life is too short to make it possible to reduce all problems to their elementary constituents. As stated by Latham in his *Aphorisms:*

It is all very fine to insist that the eye cannot be understood without a knowledge of optics, nor the circulation without hydraulics, nor the bones and the muscles without mechanics: that metaphysics may have their use in leading through the intricate functions of the nervous system, and the mysterious connections of mind and matter. It is a truth, and it is also a truth that the whole circle of science is required to comprehend a single particle of matter: but the most solemn truth of all is that the life of man is threescore years and ten.

Many scientists who dedicate themselves to medical research tend to shy away from the problems peculiar to man's nature, and even from those posed by other complex *living* organisms. They fear that the uniqueness of each individual person makes the kind of generalizations on which science thrives all but impossible, and for this reason they deal by preference with questions pertaining to lifeless fragments of the body machine. Yet while it is true that the responses of living man are extremely complex, they exhibit nevertheless patterns that can be described in the form of scientific laws. Such patterns, however, can be recognized only if scientists devote to the study of man's responses to his environment the intellectual effort and technical skill they presently devote to the analysis of fragments isolated in a lifeless form.

Awareness of the limitations of the reductionist approach in medicine expresses itself in the ever-increasing emphasis on the "whole man." But in practice this interest has not yet been converted into an active field of science. One of the reasons for this failure is the ambiguity of the word "whole." It is used on the one hand to denote those aspects of the organism that make it function as an integrated structure; on the other hand, it refers also to the summation of all the constituents and properties of the organism, including their individual relations to the total environment. Shrewd judgment based on experience will be needed to decide the extent to which the "whole" can be investigated by scientific methods. But unfortunately the research activity in this field is so limited that there is little chance for developing the experience needed.

It is certain in any case that, in comparison with the enormous effort devoted to the components of the body machine, living as a process has hardly been studied by scientific methods. The reason commonly given for this failure is that the proper techniques are not yet available and that such study must await the completion of more "fundamental" steps. But the truer reason is that this field of research does not fit in the reductionist philosophy that has prevailed since the seventeenth century. Many phenomena that have long been known empirically have been neglected by biological and medical investigators, not for lack of techniques but because their study was not fashionable. Such is the case with adaptive processes, conditioned reflexes, the subconscious manifestations of the mind, the effect of sensory deprivation, imprinting, and other phenomena of behavior.

Pavlov, Freud, Frisch, and Lorenz opened the scientific analysis of the responses made by man and animals to various situations, not so much by introducing new techniques as by accepting the fact that many aspects of life cannot be studied except when the organism functions as a living entity. Most of the techniques they used could have been developed long ago. The areas of knowledge to which they devoted themselves could have blossomed into full-fledged sciences long before the physicochemical sciences. Similarly, techniques could now be developed to study the living process in the full complexity of its manifestations, without waiting for further advances in the knowledge of the unit structures and reactions through which the body machine operates. . . .

Living man presents of course very special obstacles to those who attempt to investigate him scientifically. By the exercise of free will, he constantly introduces unpredictable complications into the study of his behavior and the effect that environmental factors exert on him. For these reasons, knowledge of human life cannot reach the level of precision and predictability achieved with regard to the inanimate world, or even to other living organisms in which the exercise of freedom can be kept under control. Granted these difficulties, man's responses to his environment pose problems of such urgency that scientists cannot long remain indifferent to them. The social pressures building up all over the world bid fair to force biological and medical sciences into new directions, focused on the manner in which individual persons and human populations respond to their total environment.

Until the nineteenth century, most educated men believed that it was within the power of analytical science to reach a complete understanding of life, and to provide health and happiness for all. Few are those who have retained this euphoric attitude and believe that the accumulation of detailed knowledge can provide in any foreseeable future a reductionist explanation of man's special attributes. Expression of skepticism on this score might be regarded as a form of the antiscience movement, but the worst form of anti-intellectualism may turn out to be the unwillingness to acknowledge the present limitations of science, with its vested ideas and its neglect of certain problems of human life. Indeed, this self-satisfied attitude is likely to retard the development of scientific methods applicable to many of the problems that have direct relevance to the future of mankind, especially in the areas of human biology, psychology, and sociology.

There is no need to belabor the obvious truth that, while modern science has been highly productive of isolated fragments of knowledge, it has been far less successful in dealing with the complexity of human problems. The high degree of specialization required for professional effectiveness accounts in part for this difficulty since no one person can give thorough attention to the multiple facets always found in any human situation, or can control its multiple determinants. But above and beyond these techical complexities, the life sciences present other difficulties of a more philosophical nature, which do not fit readily in the usual conceptual attitude of scientists.

In the most common and probably the most important phenomena of life, the constituent parts are so interdependent that they lose their character, their meaning, and indeed their very existence, when dissected from the functioning whole. In order to deal with problems of organized complexity, it is therefore essential to investigate situations in which several interrelated systems function in an integrated manner. Multifactorial investigations will demand conceptual and experimental methods different from those involving only one variable, which have been the stock in trade of experimental science during the past 300 years. It is widely acknowledged that such methods are needed to bring sociological problems within the scientific fold; but it is less frequently recognized that the need is just as great for other biological problems. The most important aspects of life fall outside the net of reductionist analysis.

Two examples . . . will serve to illustrate types of biological problems that require an organismic and environmental approach. . . . normal human beings placed under conditions where they are sheltered as completely as possible from external stimuli soon develop abnormalities in perception and behavior. The profound pathological effects caused by sensory deprivation, as well as by certain psychotomimetic drugs, demonstrate beyond doubt that the maintenance of personality structure depends upon, and indeed is an expression of, the responses that the organism as a whole makes to the bombardment of stimuli that is a constant feature of normal life. A similar conclusion emerges from an entirely different kind of facts. Animals raised under germ-free conditions, or deprived of their indigenous microbiota by prolonged treatment with antimicrobial drugs, develop gross histological and physiological abnormalities; the structural and functional integrity of many essential organs and structures depends, in other words, upon the constant stimulus exerted on them by the presence of microorganisms.

These two examples, so different in nature yet so concordant in their implications, illustrate the fundamental fact that organisms cannot be understood unless they are studied in their integrated responses to the environment. Oversimplified systems, involving only one variable, may be adequate for the analysis of the structures and chemical reactions found in the isolated components of the body machine, but they are not sufficient to study the complex manifestations of the processes and experiences of living. Yet these manifestations are the very subject matter of life, in health and in disease.

The physician ministers of course to the human body, but he is concerned also, and even more perhaps, with life as experience—physical, social, and mental. In final analysis, the success of his action is measured by the happiness and performance of his patient in a certain environment. One of the responsibilities of medical science is therefore to study the effects on the body and the mind of the new threats created by technological civilization; the constant exposure to environmental stimuli and pollutants; the estrangement of the human organism from the natural cycles under which evolution occurred; the solitude and emotional trauma of life in congested cities; the monotony and the boredom of regimented existence; the compulsory leisure ensuing from automation. These are the influences that are now at the origin of many medical problems characteristic of Western civilization. Most of the disorders of the body and the mind are expressions of inadequate response to environmental influences.

The scientific knowledge of man's environment and of his response to it is much less developed than the precise knowledge of body structure gained by one century of scientific research or than the empirical art of the healer gained from age-long experience. Like other biologists, any physician worth his salt knows that all the features and all the manifestations of an organism are influenced as much by the environment as they are by the genes. ~~Genes determine not characters or traits, but reactions and responses. Health and disease are manifested in the phenotype of the organism. And in practice the phenotype is modifiable, or controllable, much less by the alteration of the genotype than by manipulation of the environment and by adaptive efforts.~~

A few examples . . . will be briefly reviewed . . . in the following pages to illustrate what kind of knowledge is required to foster the ~~growth of organismic and environmental medicine~~.

Laboratory methods exist or can be developed for studying the effects of most substances or stimuli on tissue cultures, biochemical systems, or isolated cells. In other words, certain biological aspects of the influence that technological innovations exert on the constituents of the human body can be brought within the field of cellular and molecular biology. This analytical approach leaves unexplored, however, the effects that have the most direct bearing on the actual life of man, as well as of animals. It does not provide the kind of knowledge that would be relevant to the various forms of response that the intact living organism makes to the actual conditions of exposure over long periods of time.

One of the reasons for this failure is that most effects of environmental forces are extremely indirect and delayed; they are transformed and magnified through a chain of reactions in which almost every organ is involved. Time is an essential component of the system, because exposure to a stimulus or to a substance that appears innocuous today may result after many months or years in crippling secondary effects, whether these be allergic reactions, malignant neoplasms, or psychotic states. Man fortunately has a wide range of adaptive potentialities and thus can achieve some form of adjustment to many different stressful situations. There are limits, of course, to the range of his adaptabilities, but they are unknown.

The problems posed by indirect and delayed effects, as well as the questions raised by adaptability and its limits, involve the responses of the organism as a whole. The effects on man of the conditions created by urban and industrial life in modern societies thus transcend the phenomena that can be recognized by the study of simplified experimental systems using only cells or isolated chemical reactions. They demand the use of more complex biological models observed over long periods of time.

The increasing concern with iatrogenic diseases, especially those caused by drugs, has the quality of a caricature in accentuating the new kinds of threats to health arising from technological innovations. It is a painful but richly documented paradox that each and every drug of proven worth in the treatment of disease can itself become a cause of disease, even when used with understanding, skill, and moderation.

Some of the toxic effects exerted by drugs are direct and can be studied by the orthodox toxicological techniques, using short-term tests in simple laboratory systems. In most cases, however, the toxic effects are extremely indirect and delayed. They result from disturbances in the physiological and ecological equilibrium of the organism. Their mechanism does not reside in chemical or physiological reactions involving direct cause-effect relationships, but rather in complex interrelated responses made by the whole integrated organism, including its indigenous microbiota. Clearly these forms of toxicity can be understood only through an organismic and ecologic approach.

The problems of behavior are of course among those which require complex organisms for investigation. Many different kinds of substances are known to modify behavior not only in human beings but also in animals; the effects of the nutritional state and particularly of amino acid metabolism on mental processes are especially well documented. Furthermore, while behavioral response to any given situation is under genetic control it is also conditioned by various forms of deprivation during early life. Early associations and experiences, training, and crowding are among the many factors that modify behavior in animals and thus provide experimental techniques for behavioral studies.

It goes without saying that such investigations acquire their full scientific significance and practical usefulness only if carried out under a wide range of conditions, for long periods of time, even extending into several generations.

... the size of the world population is conditioned by many biological and social factors that are poorly understood. It is known, on the other hand, that many animal species automatically adjust their populations to levels low enough not to overtax their resources. However, these homeostatic mechanisms of population control do not always operate effectively. The understanding of the factors that control population dynamics is still very meager.

Another aspect of the population problem is that any association of living things creates new properties that transcend the properties of each one of them. The individual members of a population interact with each other, and the consequences of this interplay affect their anatomical, physiological, and behavioral characteristics. For example, the degree of crowding affects reproduction, growth, learning, and resistance to stress. The magnitude and direction of the effects cannot be predicted from even the most detailed knowledge of the individual components of the biological system. Crowds and even small groups respond differently from isolated organisms to almost any kind of stimulus.

Progress in the different aspects of population problems can be made only by studying experimental groups maintained under a wide range of conditions. By necessity such studies must be focused not on the component parts of the organisms, not even on the individual organisms themselves, but rather on their interplay as affected by the environment.

Harvey Cushing is reported to have taught that "a physician is obligated to consider more than a diseased organ, more even than the whole man—he must view the man in his world." So sweeping a statement expresses a lofty medical and scientific ideal, which is difficult if not impossible to fulfill in practice. But it is consistent with the view that medical sciences must concern themselves with complexities that are not encountered in most laboratory disciplines.

It has been observed, for example, that certain people within a given social group are much more vulnerable than others to almost any etiological variety of disease—whether it be infections, neoplasms, gynecological troubles, or mental disorders. Among these vulnerable people, diseases are more frequent and severe during periods when the environment is regarded by them as threatening, depriving, or overdemanding. Such facts obviously transcend the orthodox concept of etiological specificity. They cast doubt furthermore on the view that there exists a consistent relation between certain kinds of bodily disease and personality type. As stated by Hippocrates 2,500 years ago and by Harvey Cushing more recently, the physician "must view the man in his world."

One of the most puzzling but also most important aspects of the healing art is that the physician can exert a healing effect by his very presence, even without using any objectively effective method of treatment. The maintenance of health also requires certain kinds of human experience and contact above and beyond the biochemical and physiological conditions required for cellular metabolism. Despair, grief, and other trials certainly have a part in the genesis of disease, and many physicians have stressed the role played by faith and hope in recovery. To a large extent, however, this kind of dependence of the organism on psychological forces has been dealt with exclusively in religious or spiritual terms.

Attempts have been made during recent years to accumulate evidence that helplessness, hopelessness, unresolved griefs, and "giving up" are attitudes likely to generate or aggravate many illnesses, even neoplasms. (Reviewed by Engel, 1962a and b; Schmale, 1958; Wolff, 1960b; Wolf, 1961, 1963). But despite improved insights into the workings of the mind, the problems of psychology and their bearing on health have remained on the whole outside the main channels of biological thinking and experimentation. Indeed, there is a widespread feeling that these problems cannot be studied by the usual scientific approach because each human being is unique with regard to his life experience, his attitude, and his values.

In reality, however, most members of any given culture share a number of attitudes, values, and modes of thought, which make their behavior largely predictable; furthermore, many fundamental traits are common to all of mankind. It should be possible, therefore, to base the study of man's responses on a large body of working assumptions and thus to assess the effect of certain environmental conditions on his health and performance.

The scientific exploration of these fields is rendered even more promising by the fact that most aspects of human life have their counterparts in some animal species. The response of experimental animals to a variety of insults and stimuli, and the incidence and severity of disease among them, can indeed be profoundly modified by loneliness, separation of the young from their mothers, and other conflict situations that present close analogies to the stresses of human life. Even the uniqueness of the individual is not peculiar to man, as every pet owner knows (reviewed in Engel, 1962b). . . .

Thus, observations in human beings and experiments with animals establish beyond doubt that health and disease are influenced by life situations that transcend the direct impact of physicochemical forces. The mechanisms involved are different from those revealed by the concepts and operations of physicochemical biology; and consequently different experimental methods are required for their investigation.

BIBLIOGRAPHY

Ackerknecht, E. H. 1942 (a). "Primitive Medicine and Culture Pattern." *Bulletin of the History of Medicine* 12:545–74.

———. 1942 (b). "Problems of Primitive Medicine." *Bulletin of the History of Medicine* 11:503–21.

Cannon, W. B. 1957. "Voodoo Death." *Psychosomatic Medicine* 19:182–90.

Edelstein, L. 1956. "The Professional Ethics of the Greek Physician." *Bulletin of the History of Medicine* 30:391–419.

Edelstein, E. J., and Edelstein, L. 1945. *Asclepius.* Baltimore: Johns Hopkins University Press.

Engel, G. L. 1962 (a). "The Nature of Disease and the Care of the Patient: The Challenge of Humanism and Science in Medicine." *Rhode Island Medical Journal* 45:245–51.

————. 1962 (b). *Psychological Development in Health and Disease.* Philadelphia: W. B. Saunders.

Harlow, H. F., and Zimmerman, R. R. 1958. "The Development of Affectional Responses in Infant Monkeys." *Proceedings of the American Philosophical Society* 102:501.

———— and ————. 1959. "Affectional Responses in the Infant Monkey." *Science* 130:421–32.

Hinkle, L. E., and Wolff, H. G. 1958. "Ecologic Investigations of the Relationship Between Illness, Life Experiences and the Social Environment." *Annals of Internal Medicine* 49:1373–88.

Latham, P. M. 1962. In *Aphorisms from Latham.* Collected and edited by W. B. Bean. Iowa City: Prairie Press.

Lorenz, K. 1952. *King Solomon's Ring.* New York: Crowell.

Reilly, J. 1942. *Le Role du systeme nerveux en pathologie renale.* Paris: Masson.

Richter, C. P. 1943. "Total Self-regulatory Functions in Animals and Human Beings." *The Harvey Lectures,* pp. 63–104. Lancaster, Pa.: The Science Press.

————. 1957. "On the Phenomenon of Sudden Death in Animals and Man." *Psychosomatic Medicine* 19:191–98.

Saunders, J. B. 1963. *The Transitions from Ancient Egyptian to Greek Medicine.* Lawrence: University of Kansas Press.

Schmale, A. H., Jr. 1958. "Relationship of Separation and Depression to Disease." *Psychosomatic Medicine* 20:259–77.

Selye, H. 1956. *The Stress of Life.* New York: McGraw-Hill.

Sudhoff, K. 1926. *Essays in the History of Medicine.* New York: Medical Life Press.

Whitehorn, J. C., and Betz, B. 1960. "Studies of the Doctor as a Crucial Factor for the Prognosis of Schizophrenic Patients." *International Journal of Social Psychiatry* 6:71–77.

Wolf, S. 1961. "Disease as a Way of Life: Neural Integration in Systemic Pathology." *Perspectives in Biology and Medicine* 4:288–305.

————. 1963. "A New View of Disease." *Journal of the American Medical Association* 184:143–44.

Wolff, H. G. 1953. *Stress and Disease.* Springfield, Illinois: Charles C. Thomas.

————. 1960 (a). "The Mind-Body Relationship." In *An Outline of Man's Knowledge,* ed. L. Bryson, pp. 41–72. New York: Doubleday.

————. 1960 (b). "Stressors as a Cause of Disease in Man." In *Stress and Psychiatric Disorder,* ed. J. M. Tanner, pp. 17–33. Oxford: Blackwell.

By *Robert J. Haggerty*

❧ ❧

The Boundaries of
Health Care

National priorities have now been set for health services in our country: they are to increase access, to moderate cost, and to maintain or improve quality.[1] Most of the current efforts are directed to the first two of these goals—getting existing types of services to those who do not now receive them and reorganizing and financing care to improve efficiency and contain costs. Solutions to these first two goals are in sight although considerable struggles still lie ahead before they are achieved.

While the public and the professions are most concerned with these two issues today, I suspect that the next crisis will center around the issue of quality—and by quality I mean effectiveness of the whole process of health services and what factors produce health. I will review a few studies that bear on this and then discuss what role medicine can play in the production of health as opposed to merely providing health services. This will lead me on into several areas not now a part of traditional medical care. This future oriented area, I think, is appropriately titled "The Boundaries of Health Care."

From *The Pharos* 35 (July 1972):106–11. Reprinted by permission of Robert J. Haggerty and the editor of *The Pharos* of the Alpha Omega Alpha Medical Society.

HEALTH SERVICES AND THEIR
EFFECT ON HEALTH

First, I would like to review some evidence as to the effectiveness of health services in changing health. Health itself is difficult to measure, but there can be little argument that it is somehow the reciprocal or absence of mortality, morbidity, disability and distress. I will start with two studies in underdeveloped areas where we might expect the evidence to be clear. If 20th century curative medicine is introduced into a primitive society, surely some improvement in health should occur. But the data are not very convincing. The first study was a controlled trial in three villages in Guatemala carried out by N. S. Scrimshaw and his colleagues.[2] In the three villages, modern medical care was delivered to one, nutrition and medical care to a second and neither to a third. After five years the data were discouraging. Among the preschool population episodes of illness were actually higher in the village receiving medical care, while there was little difference between the village receiving nutritional supplements and the control village.

In a second study by Walsh McDermott and colleagues from Cornell Medical College,[3] modern medical care was introduced and delivered for five years to a population of about 2,000 Navaho Indians who had primitive living conditions and little medical care, but adequate nutrition. The data are not quite so discouraging. Tuberculosis and otitis media were reduced, some surgically treated conditions, especially trauma, benefited from medical care, but trachoma, pneumonia and diarrhea were unaffected—neither their morbidity nor mortality—nor were other less common illnesses. To quote from their conclusions:

> Thus, the delivery of this carefully organized and well received primary health care system to Many-Farms Rough Rock Community had relatively little influence on disease here. The two conditions that did not require changes in household practices for their control—otitis media and the transfer of the tubercle bacillus—were significantly influenced, but the two (diarrhea and pneumonia) that did require such changes were not.

In contrast in urban areas of our own country, where absence of medical care is unusual, studies of effectiveness must compare some new form of care (often called comprehensive) with average available care (albeit often fragmented, episodic and uncoordinated as it is). There are few people with no care in America today. We like to think that medical care does something for people and I doubt that anyone could or should do a study comparing no care with care. At best one can only study different types of care with resultant diminished chance of showing changes. But the methodological problems of such studies are difficult. Random assignment of patients to two groups is unusual and it is very hard to keep an experiment going for the three to five years minimum necessary to show changes. Measurement of end results is also not easy. There are a few studies, however.

In one such study, we were able randomly to assign indigent families to a comprehensive care program and to maintain a control group who received care from emergency rooms and scattered other sources. After three years there was no difference in the mortality nor prevalence of disease in the two groups.[4]

In another study, the "welfare medical study" in New York[5] carried out by C. H. Goodrich and G. S. Reader, there was also no difference in mortality or morbidity among the aged after the experimental group had received high quality care at New York Hospital and the control group had received only fragmented services at a variety of sites. Still a third negative bit of data is the fact that for all our curative care, longevity for men who reach 50 years in the United States has not changed for half a century.[6] Average life span has increased during this period only because infant mortality has been reduced thereby increasing the average age of death.

In contrast to these unsuccessful global attempts to improve health through medical care, it should be possible in selected illnesses to show the benefits of medical care. But even that is not easy! A recent report of a well controlled but small study compared home treatment of myocardial infarction with care in a hospital intensive care unit and showed no difference[7]—a bit shaking to us clinicians.

One of the problems of proving the benefits of overall care is the large population needed.[8] For example, to show a 5 per cent change in child mortality (a statistically significant change) one would have to study 6.25 million children. But in spite of all these problems, occasionally studies have shown positive results. Mortality of hospitalized patients with selected illnesses was found to be lower in teaching as compared to nonteaching hospitals in Britain in a study by J. A. H. Lee, et al.[9, 10] Infant mortality has also been shown to be somewhat responsive to new forms of organization and delivery of care in H.I.P. groups compared to non-H.I.P. in New York[11] and in areas of inner cities where maternal and infant care programs have been introduced compared to other similar areas of these cities without such programs. These studies are subject to considerable criticism on methodological grounds, however. On a national scale there is evidence that input of medical care plus all other factors do affect infant mortality. Infant mortality, which had decreased by only 5 per cent in a decade (1956–65), dropped from 24.7 in 1965 to 19.8 in 1970 (20 per cent in five years)—a period when several special programs were introduced to deliver better maternal and child health care. But we are forced to look very long and hard to find evidence that medical care makes much difference to mortality or morbidity (i.e. presence of disease). When we look at the level of human functioning with disease the picture is a little brighter.

Most impressive are a few well designed studies, such as the one by C. E. Lewis and B. A. Resnick,[12] which demonstrated that one can improve function of patients. In this study nurse clinicians were able not only to deliver most of the care to adult patients with chronic illnesses such as hypertension, diabetes and arthritis, but these patients actually had less days of loss of work, less bed days, than a control group managed by a physician.

In the absence of our ability to show much reduction in death, disease and only occasionally in disability as a result of medical care, most of us have turned to measure other factors that we felt might be more responsive to care—costs, utilization of services such as hospitals, office visits and compliance with preventive or curative regimens. Here the evidence that different types of medical care have different effects is much better.

In the Boston study mentioned above[4] we did carry out a carefully controlled trial with random assignment and blind assessment of data. The significant increase in receipt of preventive services, reduction in costs of laboratory and prescription medications, hospitalizations, operations and illness visits were all what we had predicted.

Likewise in Rochester E. Charney and his colleagues have been studying the effectiveness of our neighborhood health center introduced into a black poverty area. Here we have a comparison —although not a control group—another, physically separate black ghetto of approximately the same size and socio-economic status where to date there is no comprehensive care medical program. Again we have not been able to show any differences in mortality or morbidity, but there have been other important changes. Emergency room visits have been reduced for children by 30 per cent,[13] and hospitalizations for children have been reduced by about 30 per cent among the users of the health center. All of the reductions occurred in the respiratory-infectious illnesses group—those conditions for which early medical care and office and home management could be expected to make a difference. Surgical admissions actually increased as correctable conditions such as hernias, squints, and others were discovered.

Another micro-study illustrates the effectiveness of certain aspects of health care. At Yale J. K. Skipper and R. C. Leonard[14] studied several physiological measures in children undergoing tonsillectomy and adenoidectomy. In the experimental group open discussion was carried out by a special nurse and the child before operation. The interesting finding was that compared to a control group of children who went through the usual procedure at Yale, New Haven Hospital, the rate of return of temperature to normal and reduction of nausea, vomiting and blood pressure were significantly greater in the experimental group. Yes, there is some proof that comprehensive, compassionate and skilled care has beneficial results!

In sum, we can say that there is not much evidence that illness care (which is what most medical care consists of) reduces mortality or morbidity very much. When well organized, it can reduce utilization of expensive facilities such as hospitals and emergency rooms and can reduce other costs such as laboratory and pharmacy without any measurable difference in health status. In other words, the effect of illness care after a point produces only marginal gains in health.

I need to make perfectly clear that I am well aware that we do have some data on the effectiveness of specific aspects of curative medicine—penicillin for pneumonia, antimicrobial treatment of meningitis, drug therapy for essential hypertension and a few other conditions that have been shown by controlled clinical trials to be positively affected by modern therapy. And I certainly do not wish to belittle the very important effects of our role as relievers of pain and distress. Individuals and society need someone who provides hope by not giving up when the outcome is death. They need the comfort that there is access to such people as physicians even for conditions that will be self-limiting. Medicine satisfies a deep human need for someone else to provide help. I need also to make clear that I, as a clinician who has spent my entire professional life caring for children and their families, like to practice medicine. I am not disillusioned, bitter or tired of practice. But I also believe that we need to be humble about what we clinicians accomplish and raise our sights a bit to see if there may not be other things that we or someone in society could do to improve health much more than we are doing today.

As René Dubos has described so magnificently in *Mirage of Health*,[15] the great advances in health in the 18th and 19th centuries were largely the result of social reforms that alleviated some of the pollution, dirt, poor housing and crowding, and malnutrition that had come from the industrial revolution. The fact that in the past 50 years center stage in the promotion of health has been held by the laboratory scientist should not blind us to the fact that he was not there throughout the period of most rapid improvement in health. As Dubos, a microbiologist states, ". . . the monstrous specter of infection had become but an enfeebled shadow of its former self by the time serums, vaccines and drugs became available to combat microbes. Indeed many of the most terrifying microbial diseases—leprosy, plague, typhus, and the sweating sickness, for example—had all but disappeared from Europe long before the advent of the germ theory." To go on in Dubos' words, "When the tide is receding from the beach, it is easy to have the illusion that one can empty the ocean by removing water with a pail. The tide of infectious and nutritional diseases was rapidly receding when the laboratory scientist moved into action at the end of the past century."

David Mechanic, who expresses so many things so well, said that "medicine has three principal tasks: (1) to understand how particular symptoms, syndromes or disease entities arise, either in individuals or among groups of individuals; (2) to recognize and cure these or shorten their course or minimize any residual impairment and (3) to promote living conditions in human populations which eliminate hazards to health and thus prevent disease."[16] The first of these tasks has generally been the province of biomedical research, and second of curative medicine and the last of public health and social medicine. The time is now at hand to join these three and to move into what I like to call the boundaries of health care.

The problem is simply stated. Where do health services end and other human services begin? Or, what factors affect health? The answers are far from clear. Let me first discuss the evidence.

SOCIAL AND ENVIRONMENTAL FACTORS EFFECT ON HEALTH

On a superficial level it is easy for everyone to accept that the way we live, our diet, our pace of life, our housing, our political and social structure, all contribute to health—perhaps sharing only with our genes predominance as the factor most responsible for our state of health. In comparison, what we as doctors do for people is rather insignificant. Let me spend just a few moments documenting this bold statement since it is said with a good deal more conviction than the facts often allow.

Lead poisoning is an easy example with which to start. Most lead poisoning in children results from ingestion of paint from housing with high lead content paint. The outcome of therapy, once symptomatic poisoning occurs, is bad—mortality and especially late intellectual morbidity are high.[17] We can now diagnose body lead burdens above normal before symptoms appear and have fairly good chelating agents to accelerate its elimination, although we still do not know the long term consequences of asymptomatic lead burdens. But the poisoned child usually must remain in his same environment where he will continue to ingest lead. To date no cure for his desire to eat paint has been found to be successful. We must remove him from the lead. Even if we move him, however, another family with a small child is likely to move into the same house and become poisoned. Getting landlords and even parents to remove the paint from the housing has been disappointing—it is costly, time consuming and, with absentee landlords and poorly prosecuted housing codes, often impossible to accomplish. What is medicine's role? Should it stop at treatment of the symptomatic child? At surveillance programs to detect and then treat the asymptomatic child? At getting social workers to move the child to a new home? At enforcing housing codes that may require the physician's attendance in court if he pushes hard enough? At promotion of building new, safe housing for his community? At political action? At building the new house himself? Clearly, each of us stops somewhere along this spectrum, usually before building the new housing himself. But until new housing has been built to replace all the old, or complete renovation of the old achieved, there will not be a solution to lead poisoning, any more than there was a solution to the problem of rickets until vitamin D was put in all milk.

Environment. A second example of the effect of physical environment on health is the nice work of H. Sultz and W. Winkelstein in my neighboring city of Buffalo. They showed that on days when there was high air pollution, there were also many more asthmatic children having acute attacks and coming to physicians. What role should we as clinicians play in air pollution control when it directly affects the health of our patients?

One of the most strikingly successful stories of such a role in altering environment by a physician is that of L. Colebrook, a surgeon in Britain, who became incensed that little girls were frequently severely burned by standing close to open hearth fireplaces and catching their clothes on fire. He collected data, presented it and got legislation passed requiring that every fireplace have a grate six inches in front of the fire.[19] Such burns were significantly reduced as a result. As a clinician he contributed more to health by this move than by all his surgical skills.

Way of Life: Let me now take a third example from adult medicine. L. Breslow and his colleagues in California have been engaged for some years in the Human Population Laboratory conducting a longitudinal study of the health status of a random sample of people and correlating this with various aspects of life style. He found that five factors in the way people live—the amount of sleep (less than six hours/night vs. 7–8), diet (erratic or regular), alcohol consumption (less or more than five drinks per day), regular exercise and tobacco use—were significantly associated with health.[20] Good health practices were associated with good health, and the relation was cumulative—the more of these factors that were "good" the better the health. In fact, people of 55–64 who had had these "good" habits had the health, as determined by their functioning, of 25–34 year olds who had these "bad" habits. To the epidemiologists there are, of course, many missing links. Most important to the clinician is the question, can such "bad" habits, if present, be changed and how; and if changed, will that alter a person's health? For the purpose of this discussion the issues I would like to have you think about include, "Is it medicine's job to educate people on how to sleep, eat, drink, exercise and smoke?" Is this within or beyond the boundary? The implications are that if we could change men's function this much by altering life habits, we would accomplish more than through all of our therapeutic medicine.

Schools and Health: The next example I would like to mention is the role of medicine in schools. Traditional school health programs of "laying on of hands," inspections, referrals without follow-up have been shown to be a waste of time.[21, 22] But at the same time one quarter of the referrals of children to our pediatric clinic are now sent for "school learning problems." We find very few traditional medical problems among such children. But the suffering of the child and family with such problems is still just as real, and the management requires that we alter the child's environment—the school and the home. We have been quite unsuccessful, even after doing rather complete work-ups in the clinic, if we only make recommendations or treat with drugs. When we have moved out of our offices into the schools, we have achieved greater success. We need to join with teachers to help them understand how children grow and develop, with psychologists to understand how they learn, and sociologists to learn how the organization of the school affects learning. While the data to support the effectiveness of such new programs are not all in, we as doctors either have to decide that we do not have anything to offer such parents and children or we have to join forces with other professions to seek solutions to the problems by crossing the boundaries of traditional health services.

The schools also offer remarkable settings for health education to achieve more healthy patterns of living that may then affect health. The boundary between medicine and education is not difficult to accept, but few of us have crossed it.

POPULATION VS INDIVIDUAL HEALTH CARE

Most of these examples could be thought of as in the range of traditional public health—that is population medicine—and the clinician would be quite correct to say that the boundary problem is largely one between population medicine, where responsibility for such things as housing, group health in schools and community wide health education is the province of the public health physician, while the provision of curative medicine of individual patients is his domain.

One of our own studies[23] illustrates that the problem of boundaries exists even for the clinician dealing with individuals. For some time we have been interested in the clinical observation that family-life stress seemed to be positively related to illness and also to the timing of seeking health care related to such stress. We have studied two types of family stress—long term or chronic, such as poverty, divorce, poor housing, unemployment, and short term, such as quarrels in the family, deaths in near relatives, loss of jobs, moves and interpersonal problems outside the family. As part of our system for monitoring the state of health of children in our area, we selected a random sample of over 500 families with children from Monroe County, N.Y., and interviewed the mother about illness in the family, their use of health care, and long term stress, and also we asked her to keep a diary for 30 days covering the same topics. Long term or chronic stress is very strongly associated with illness—in fact it accounts for as much as 80 per cent of all illness in families with children. Likewise short term stress has a strong association with illness, but little over-all relation to when people seek health care. There are interesting and important differences in the relation of stress (controlling for the amount of illness) and where care is sought. Telephone, emergency room, and OPD contacts are two to three times more likely if there is family stress, while office visits show no difference.

There is a considerable body of other data in this field of stress and illness. L. E. Hinkle's[24] documentation of the greater occurrence of illness in workers in a telephone company at times of stress, and a study by R. H. Rahe, I. D. McKean, and R. J. Arthur of navy men's greater illness at times of life changes (moves, deaths of close relatives, job changes)[25] give credence to our view that life stress is an important cause of physical illness.

The important point is again the boundary problem. If this type of family-life stress and life change is a major factor in causing illness and in determining when and where people seek care, what should be the physician's role in helping families to avoid or learn to cope in more healthy ways with stress? What is the physiologic pathway by which such stress works its havoc? What could social changes, such as income maintenance, or various educational efforts, such as operant conditioning (to teach families how to manage life crises without the stress that leads to illness), do to improve health? What should be the doctor's role in these boundary problems? Should we become engaged in these areas? I think it is clear that, as a society, we must find ways to manage boundary problems if we are to improve health. As physicians we do have another reason for involvement.

G. Caplan many years ago proposed the crisis intervention theory.[26] In brief, he postulates that at these times of crisis, people are more amenable to changing ways of life that are unhealthy than at more stable times. If this is so, and we obviously need data to prove or disprove it, then crisis-related illness and crisis-related use of health services bring the clinician into the middle of social medicine.

By working in these boundary areas it seems likely that we will contribute more to health than we will by sticking purely to our curative, traditional medical care. Another important facet of the boundary problem is the plight of developing countries. They have generally adopted western curative medicine, a relative luxury. Countries with limited resources might do well to limit their investment in curative medicine and invest more extensively in the boundary areas.

BARRIERS TO WORK IN BOUNDARY PROBLEMS

What are the problems or barriers in moving into these boundary areas? Clearly one of the problems is the lack of data on the causal chain from social factors to physiologic change, to disease, and the lack of studies of the effectiveness of any proposed intervention. It is a special role of academic medicine, in collaboration with practitioners, to develop such data.

A second major barrier is the current constricting atmosphere that results from our mania for efficiency in health services. All new financing plans for illness services, such as the Health Maintenance Organizations, encourage limiting the time and effort of health care personnel to as little as the public will tolerate, rather than encouraging them to take on new tasks—especially if these new tasks may not result in improved health for many years. We are clearly in danger of exchanging the short-term goal of lowered costs for the longer-term effect of better health. Physicians working in prepaid programs with an annual capitation fee will think twice about spending time to deal with school learning problems, housing problems to eliminate lead poisoning, lengthy court proceedings to place battered children or crisis intervention to reduce stress.

In our current enthusiasm for efficiency many critics have lost sight of what is the essence of medicine—an open door for distressed people to enter, and improved health. The role of social-psychological distress is so great in the whole care process that I doubt that much of it will be solved with technological means, such as automated multiphasic screening to reassure the "worried well." Health will more likely be improved by utilizing additional people in the caring process, such as nurse practitioners and family counselors to help families deal with these problems of living, than by such technological devices.

A third barrier is our reluctance and lack of experience in working with other professions. Clearly the boundary areas are not the province of any one group. Our academic institutions and our training set up departmental and attitudinal barriers to effective collaborative efforts.

A fourth barrier is man's lack of future orientation or deep concern about prevention. As Dubos said,[15] "... men as a rule find it easier to depend on healers than to attempt the more difficult task of living wisely." He goes on to point out that in Greek mythology Hygeia, the goddess of health, was always pictured as subservient to Asclepius, the god of healing. It is clear that a great deal of attitudinal change must occur before we can effectively work in these boundary areas.

THE FUTURE

For the present, general medical care programs should not pay for these as yet unproven services. The immediate short term goal of health services is to meet the public demand for equity of access at reasonable cost. But we must be honest with the public that provision of such traditional curative services will not greatly affect the outcome or health of our people. But somewhere in our social system, and I believe that somewhere is in the university, there must be some groups who are more future oriented, who look ten to 20 years ahead, and who seek to explore the boundaries of health services in an effort to improve quality and understand what works in these poorly understood boundary areas and why. We must be careful not to assume arrogantly that we as physicians know what is best for people nor to decide by ourselves what the boundaries are to be. In the long run society will decide this. As E. Freidson has so eloquently said in his book

Profession of Medicine,[27] "... the public should be brought into this process much more than it has. In the past what was once labelled the province of religion is often now in the medical domain." There is no reason why what is now in medicine's province will remain there forever, any more than it did with religion. Certainly medicine must advance in technology, but I believe at this moment we need to provide an opportunity for some people in medicine who, together with other disciplines, can carry out carefully controlled studies of the effects of intervention in these social boundary problems.

But we must also try to avoid the twin perils of too constricted a view and a too global one. At age 45 Metchnikoff changed his interests after a distinguished career in microbiology to focus on the global effort he called "orthobiosis," which did not get very far. There is clearly the danger of adopting too broad a point of view. It is the danger of substituting meaningless generalities and weak philosophy for the concreteness of exact knowledge.

Perhaps the major thing medicine has to contribute is the ability to meld biology and social sciences—drawing people from both disciplines to work on the complex problems of social and family life and how they affect health. We and society may then end up by developing new helping groups or professions that actually deal with or deliver the care at these boundaries. But at the moment my medical chauvinism leads me to believe that physicians have a special role. They are often more acceptable as agents of change. They do have access to methods for studying the physiologic consequences of environmental manipulation, and they are highly acceptable to people in distress.

The boundaries of medical care offer exciting challenges to the future oriented biosocial physician. By successful blending of social and biologic research we may finally, as physicians, contribute to improved health and not merely to the production of health services.

ACKNOWLEDGMENT

Supported by Children's Bureau Research Project Number 104 and Public Health Service Grant No. HS 467.

REFERENCES

1   "Towards a Comprehensive Health Policy for the 1970's." A White Paper. U.S. Dept. H.E.W., Government Printing Office, May, 1971.

2   Scrimshaw, N. S., Gerzman, M. A., Flores, M., *et al.:* "Nutrition and Infection Field Studies, Guatemalan Villages, 1959–64. V. Disease Incidence Among Preschool Children Under Natural Village Conditions, With Improved Diet, and With Medical and Public Health Services." *Arch. Environ. Health* 16:223–34, 1968.

3   McDermott, W., Deuschle, K. W. and Barnett, C. R.: "Health Care Experiment at Many Farms: A Technological Misfit of Health Care and Disease Pattern Existed in This Navaho Community." *Science* 175:23–31, 1972.

4   Robertson, L. S., Kosa, J., Heagarty, M. C., Haggerty, R. J. and Alpert, J. J.: *Changing the Medical Care System.* New York, Praeger Publishers, 1974.

5   Goodrich, C. H., Olendzki, M. C. and Reader, G. S.: *Welfare Medical Care.* Cambridge, Harvard University Press, 1970.

6   *Leading Components of Upturn in Mortality of Men, U.S., 1952–1967.* National Center for Health Statistics, Series 20, No. 11, P.H.S., H.S.M.H.A., Department of Health, Education and Welfare Pub. No. 72-1008, September, 1971.

7   Mather, H. G., *et al.:* "Acute Myocardial Infarction: Home and Hospital Treatment." *Brit. Med. J.* 3:334–38, 1971.

8   Lewis, C.: "Does Comprehensive Care Make a Difference?" *Am. J. Dis. Child.* 122:467, 1971.

9   Lee, J. A. H., Morrison, S. L. and Morris, J. N.: "Fatality From Three Common Surgical Conditions in Teaching and Non-teaching Hospitals." *Lancet* 2:785–90, 1957.

10 Lipworth, L., Lee, J. A. H. and Morris, J. N.: "Case Fatality in Teaching and Non-teaching Hospitals." *Medical Care* 1:71–76, 1963.

11 Shapiro, S., Weiner, L. and Densen, P. M.: "Comparison of Prematurity and Perinatal Mortality in a General Population and in a Population of a Prepaid Group Practice Medical Care Plan." *Am. J. Pub. Health* 48:170–87, 1958.

12 Lewis, C. E. and Resnick, B. A.: "Nurse Clinicians and Progressive Ambulatory Patient Care." *New Eng. J. Med.* 277:1236–41, 1967.

13 Hochheiser, L., Woodward, K. and Charney, C.: "Effect of the Neighborhood Health Center on Use of Emergency Departments." *New Eng. J. Med.* 285:148–52, 1971.

14   Skipper, J. K. and Leonard, R. C.: "Children, Stress and Hospitalization: A Field Experiment." *J. Health Hum. Behav.* 9:275–87, 1968.

15   Dubos, R.: *Mirage of Health; Utopias Progress and Biological Change.* New York, Harper & Row Publishers, 1959.

16   Mechanic, D.: "Response Factors in Illness: The Study of Illness Behavior." *Social Psychiat.* 1:11–20, 1966.

17   "Acute and Chronic Lead Poisoning. Report of Committee on Environmental Hazards and Subcommittee on Accidental Poisoning and Committee on Accident Prevention." *Pediatrics* 47:950–51, 1971.

18   Sultz, H., and Winklestein, W.: *Long-Term Childhood Illness.* Princeton, Princeton University Press, in press.

19   Colebrook, L. and Colebrook, V.: "Prevention of Burns and Scalds: Review of 1,000 Cases." *Lancet* 2:181–88, 1949.

20   Belloc, N. B., and Breslow, L.: "Relationship of Physical Health Status and Health Practices." *Preventive Medicine* 1:409–21, 1972.

21   Yankauer, A. and Lawrence, R. A.: "A Study of Periodic School Medical Examinations. II. The Annual Increment of New 'Defects.' " *Am. J. Pub. Health* 46:1553, 1956.

22   Yankauer, A., Lawrence, R. A. and Ballou, L.: "A Study of Periodic School Medical Examinations. III. The Remediability of Certain Categories of 'Defects.' " *Am. J. Pub. Health* 47:1421, 1957.

23   Haggerty, R. J., Roghmann, K. J. and Pless, I. B.: *Family Stress and the Need for Child Health Services.* Presented at the International Epidemiology Association Meeting, Primosten, Yugoslavia, 1971.

24   Hinkle, L. E., Jr., *et al.*: "An Investigation of the Relation Between Life Experience, Personality Characteristics, and General Susceptibility to Illness." *Psychosomat. Med.* 20:278, 1958.

25   Rahe, R. H., McKean, I. D., Jr. and Arthur, R. J.: "A Longitudinal Study of Life-Change and Illness Patterns." *J. Psychosom. Res.* 10:355–66, 1967.

26   Caplan, G. (ed.): *Prevention of Mental Disorders in Children.* New York, Basic Books, 1961.

27   Freidson, E.: *Profession of Medicine.* New York, Dodd, Mead and Company, 1970.

By John Powles

On the Limitations of Modern Medicine

One of the more striking paradoxes facing the student of modern medical culture lies in the contrast between the enthusiasm associated with current developments and the reality of decreasing returns to health for rapidly increasing efforts. As this paradox involves both the technical and nontechnical aspects of medicine, any attempt to unravel it must involve an exploration of each of these two sides of medicine—the "science" and the "art." It must also take as its field of enquiry the wider medical culture of modern societies, encompassing as it does a complex web of explanations and activities accepted by both doctors and their patients.

DIMINISHING RETURNS

The resource requirements for medical care have been increasing rapidly since World War II. In England and Wales for the two decades to 1969 the number of hospital workers per thousand population increased by 54 percent [1]. In the U.S.A. the increase over the two decades to 1970 was 60 percent [2]. Price in-

Revision of his article in *Science, Medicine and Man* 1, no. 1 (1973):1–30. Reprinted by permission of John Powles and Pergamon Press Ltd.

flation makes the monetary increase even more alarming. But even in 1970, before the acceleration in general inflation rates, hospital expenditure in the U.S.A. was increasing by more than 15 percent per year [3].

What effect has this rapidly-increasing effort had on health? The only reliable measures of community health levels that are comparable over time are death rates. Long-term mortality trends show that it is precisely during the last two decades — when scientific medicine has blossomed and when the quantity of resources devoted to medical care has increased rapidly — that the decline in mortality that has been associated with industrialisation has tapered off to virtually zero. It is males who have fared the worst, especially in middle-age. Continuing slight gains for females only serve to extend an already lengthy average period of widowhood.

The very real problem of diminishing returns in health is, of course, partly due to the approach to natural limits. But to a significant extent it also reflects an evolving balance between the two contrary effects of economic development on health. On the positive side an improvement in material conditions (especially nutrition) and increased medical effectiveness reduces vulnerability to infection in early life. But as economic development takes man further and further away from the conditions under which he evolved and to which he is therefore genetically adapted, so it produces increasing derangement of the human organism. These maladaptations, or diseases of civilisation, have their most serious impact in middle life and are probably responsible for at least two-thirds of all deaths in middle age. Leading examples are degenerative cardiovascular disease (heart attacks and strokes), chronic bronchitis, diabetes and much cancer (including cancer of the lung and probably also of the large bowel and breast).*

We may now ask: What has been the strategy for tackling this new disease burden? Why has it not been more successful?

* A fuller discussion of the determinants of human health, including the reasons for the modern decline in mortality, is given in the original version of this paper.

THE CURRENT MEDICAL REPORT

Much of the recent increase in resource consumption for medical care has been for short-term hospital care and drugs. Ischaemic heart disease is the paradigmatic disease of maladaptation and the response to it typifies wider trends within medicine. As a preliminary it may be noted that the underlying disease process (atherosclerosis) progresses with age and tends to be generalized throughout the body. The terminal "heart attack" results from an occlusion of a coronary artery. The major thrust of the medical response to this problem has been towards the hospital treatment of heart attack. This has been elaborated in complex and expensive intensive cardiac care units. For the U.S.A. it has been estimated that 3000 such units were established by the end of 1971 and that they were using 10 percent of all trained nurses [4]. And yet this major effort has been mounted in the absence of convincing evidence of benefit. The only randomised controlled trial which has compared treatment at home with hospital treatment, with which this author is familiar, failed to show any benefit from hospital treatment [5].

A consideration of the natural history both of the acute episode and of the underlying process points to the implausibility of significant gain from the hospital treatment of heart attack. Results from Belfast and Edinburgh indicated that:

About half of the deaths occurred within 2 hours, and more than half before the doctor arrived. Most of the delay took place before the doctor was even called, so one may say that at present about 50 per cent of fatal heart attacks are outside the possible reach of medical treatment. In such cases hope must lie with prevention [6].

Moreover, the individual who has survived one acute episode is still a "coronary-prone" individual and therefore much more likely than average to succumb to another.

Why then this apparent technological "over-reach" in the response to heart disease? Was it just a simple mistake encouraged by genuine gains in other fields? Or has the perception of the problem been seriously constrained by limits inherent in contemporary medical thinking? If so what is the nature of these limitations?

Thomas McKeown has noted the extent to which the contemporary medical effort is based on an "engineering" approach to the improvement of health:

The approach to biology and medicine established during the seventeenth century was an engineering one based on a physical model. Nature was conceived in mechanistic terms, which lead in biology to the idea that a living organism could be regarded as a machine which might be taken apart and reassembled if its structure and function were fully understood. In medicine, the same concept lead further to the belief that an understanding of disease processes and of the body's response to them would make it possible to intervene therapeutically, mainly by physical (surgical) chemical, or electrical methods [7].

In view of the limited effectiveness of this approach, it is worth examining its origins. At least four things have been important. They are: (1) the nature of the doctor-patient relationship, (2) the limitation of medical theory to the "biology of the individual," (3) the germ theory of disease and (4) institutional and political factors.

Given the traditional form of doctor-patient interaction, it was inevitable that doctors would strive to get better and better at intervening in their patients' illnesses. This is the historical foundation of the engineering approach. When doctors drew from the emerging biological science of the nineteenth century, they chose that strand which had the most obvious relevance to their ability to treat their patients: They chose what Crombie refers to as the "science of the organised individual" and were singularly uninfluenced by the other strand—"the science of populations." This theoretical bias is the second important factor [8]. In medicine this theoretical foundation lent support to the view that it was the doctor's role to intervene chemically (by drugs) or physically (by surgery) in order to restore the patient's disordered system or systems to normal.

The extent to which human population biology—for example evolutionary theory, historical demography and medical ecology —has failed to influence medical theory is quite remarkable. The resulting inability to deal theoretically (as distinct from statistically) with biological phenomena at levels of organisation above a single organism has left medical theory seriously deficient. Medicine has deprived itself of the only possible theoretical basis on which criteria for biological normality in man could rest. It hesitates to call progressive health-compromising processes—such as arterial degeneration, rising blood pressure and tendency towards diabetes—"diseases" because they are associated with a way of life it feels bound to accept as "normal." The limits of "normality" in blood pressure are endlessly debated. The serious issue of whether a bodily change that is induced by our way of life and predisposes to overt disease should be regarded as pathological has been reduced to the trivial one of whether the distribution of blood pressures in the population is unimodal or bimodal. . . . It hardly needs to be added that the debate gains its significance not from a felt need to prevent the development of the abnormal but from the felt imperative to knock it into line with drugs.

With little understanding of the way of life to which man is biologically adapted, modern medicine is unable to predict the possible harmful consequences of departures from it. It was "surprised" to find that the repeated inhalation of tobacco smoke actually harmed the lungs and caused cancer. It was led to this conclusion by the investigation of the observed rise in deaths from lung cancer and the exclusion of other possible causes [9]. Until quite recently it was not widely suspected that large bowel cancer, a major cause of cancer death, might be associated with dietary habits that have become far removed from those of our forebears.* The fourteenth edition of Bailey and Love's famous *A Short Practice of Surgery,* published in 1968, contains 7 pages of discussion on cancer of the colon and 8 on cancer of rectum. Much of it is naturally concerned with operative techniques for the removal of the tumours. In the case of rectal cancer it includes

---

* The removal of dietary fiber and a high intake of refined carbohydrates that is typical of diets in industrialized countries is associated with a much slower transit of food through the gut and this may be significant in the increased incidence of large bowel cancer associated with economic development [10].

a paragraph and a diagram on the complete removal of all pelvic organs (under the appropriate heading "More Extensive Operations"). In contrast to this readiness to consider drastic attempts at cure there is no discussion of aetiology and there is no acknowledgement of the possibility that these cancers might be caused by our way of life and therefore be preventable. . . .

The limitation to individual biology also handicaps consideration of the role of genetic factors in disease. Frequently, naive interpretations are placed on the relative contributions of nature and nurture to disease processes. Epidemiological studies, say on ischaemic heart disease, are carried out on populations with an industrial way of life which is implicitly assumed to be "normal"; on the basis of findings a certain weight is accorded to the influence of heredity on the disease. The fact that these inherited characteristics may only become relevant to the aetiology of the condition under stresses that are in evolutionary terms novel—and that it is therefore the interaction between the stresses and the inherited variation in body build that is important—is often not acknowledged [11]. This fallacy has been nicely exposed by Gleave and Campbell. In populations that wear shoes the inherited variability of the build of the foot may well make some individuals more likely than others to develop bunions—but bunions only occur in populations who wear shoes [12]. Exactly the same point could be made with respect to heart disease, diabetes and some cancers.

The third factor contributing to the dominance of the "engineering" approach within modern medicine was the rise of the germ theory of disease. It identified discrete, specific and external causal agents for disease processes which were usually thought of as acute and short-lived. The theory gave support to the idea of specific therapies, and failed to emphasise the importance of general resistance to infection. By contrast one could now describe the preindustrial situation with respect to infection, as one of chronic predisposition to infection due to poor nutrition and environmental conditions. Thus the appropriate model for infectious disease need not, as is often suggested, be fundamentally different from that for the degenerative diseases. A fatal infection, like the occlusion of a coronary artery is often a terminal event to which the individual involved is strongly predisposed by his social experience.

The germ theory also coincided with a high point in the view that progress was to be secured by the mechanical domination of nature. The response to the problem of infection was not thought of principally in terms of a strengthening of natural forces of defence—for example improved nutrition and population control. Even the preventive implications were taken up in what were literally engineering terms. Primitive man, it was imagined, lived amongst his own filth. Modern man, by means of sewers, piped water and antiseptics would cleanse himself of germs.

The fourth group of historical influences on the rise of the engineering approach are professional and institutional ones. Rosenberg has recorded how the American medical profession in the middle of the last century, hitched its fortune to the rising star of science [13]. The germ theory of disease came just in time to save the faltering public prestige of doctors. Class interest was also important in suppressing an alternative approach. While the well-to-do physicians proffered their clinical skills to the rich, it was social and preventive medicine that was needed most urgently for the poor. Unfortunately, the prestigious physicians dominated the teaching hospitals and medical education, and therefore, the theoretical and practical development of public health and preventive medicine received little encouragement.

... The engineering approach to the improvement of health has been dominant over an alternative approach which would emphasise the importance of way of life factors in disease—an approach which could be described as "ecological." While it is to changes with which this latter approach is concerned that industrial man largely owes his current standard of health, it is in the engineering approach that he has placed his faith. Curative medicine has not been very successful in reducing the impact of diseases of maladaptation. Against heart disease there has been almost no real progress. Surgery has secured some modest gains against cancer but the overall burden has not been significantly reduced. While it may be argued that the current strategy still offers the most hope—especially as significant changes in the pattern of life seem unlikely—the nature of the underlying disease processes involved makes it improbable that curative interventions will be very successful. Nor can there be any guarantee that industrial populations have already exhausted the possibilities in respect of diseases of maladaptation. If technological advances continue to be pursued and implemented with little regard for their impact on man's biology there may well be an additional twenty-first-century equivalent of the current epidemic of ischaemic heart disease. Medical technology may have to run fast just to compensate for increased insults to the human organism.

It is therefore concluded that the problem of diminishing returns is a real one. It results from the nature of the contemporary disease burden and the limited front on which medical effort has been concentrated. These technical considerations cannot, however, explain modern medicine's considerable cultural momentum. To do so it will be necessary to explore the relationship between medicine's technical and nontechnical sides.

THE NONTECHNICAL SIDE
OF MEDICINE

. . . Medical institutions can be identified by their purpose— they mediate between man and his vulnerability to disease. It is clear that medical cultures differ from one another as radically as do the wider cultures of which they are a part. Further, differing medical cultures have a certain internal consistency—that is, the way in which any individual copes with disease is largely socially determined.

Magical medicine would be widely regarded as the most primitive element of medical culture. But how is magic to be interpreted? Western rationalism has placed great emphasis on the importance within man's mental life, of gaining as accurate as possible a picture of the objective world. Within this approach it is the logical and empirical content of a belief rather than its function within the mental lives of individuals which is considered important. Thus magic involves a set of very stupid beliefs ("superstitions") from which there is nothing to learn. An alternative and more fruitful approach is to focus on the function of magical beliefs and practices. Lévi-Strauss has shown that this is, in fact, what the practitioners of magic do [14]. If the members of such a community are presented with empirical evidence which is inconsistent with their magical beliefs, they do not deny the evidence—but nor does the evidence weaken their faith in magic. Belief in magic then, is not critically dependent upon the empirical status of magical propositions. For primitive man, magic helps to impose order on the Universe, to reduce ambiguities and to neutralise and reduce perceived threats and actual misfortunes [15]. Communities that are constantly exposed to natural forces that may appear to be random and beyond man's control need means of coping with their incomprehension and vulnerability. Magic is an active response to that need.

Religion and medicine were closely associated in Europe until relatively recent times. In the medieval period, it was the religious orders that maintained the hospitals and infirmaries and this association has continued in some institutions to the present day. Religious interpretations were placed upon illness and relief from suffering was sought in the healing rites of the church. The central theme in the theistic response to man's vulnerability to disease and suffering is resignation to the will of God. Belief in an afterlife helps the sufferer to make little of the cruelties of this earthly realm. It is worth noting that there was also a fatalistic character to nonreligious interpretations of illness during the medieval period. The movement of the heavenly bodies was widely believed to be responsible for epidemics and for individual episodes of illness. If the social reinforcement of resignation to misfortune is the functional core of religious medicine, then this core can be seen to be common also to nontheistic mysticism such as Buddhism and even to some atheist philosophies such as Stoicism.

The emotive mainspring for much of the social response to disease lies in man's capacity for compassion. There must be few who are not frequently distressed by the suffering of a fellow creature and it seems unnecessary, if not offensive, to look for any functional significance in the behaviour that this sentiment inspires. Tolstoy, however (in *The Death of Ivan Ilyich*), shows how sympathy can be far from peripheral to the task of helping the patient.

Something dreadful was happening to Ivan Ilyich, something novel, something of such great moment that nothing of greater moment had ever happened to him. And he alone was aware of this: the people about him either did not understand or did not care to understand, and went on thinking that everything in the world was just as it had always been. It was this that tortured him more than anything else [16].

Unfortunately, there is another side to the emotive response to the sick: They may be perceived as an unwanted reminder of the vulnerability of the well to diseases that they dread, and so evoke apprehension and disquiet. This applies particularly to those whose behaviour is bizarre and unpredictable (the insane) and to those who are physically deformed or mentally handicapped. In these instances, social mediation may well work against the interests of the sick individual—as for example, when they are incarcerated in longstay hospitals to relieve others of the disquiet that their presence creates. As such incarceration often has an adverse effect on the patient's health [17, 18, 19], the usual justification—that it was necessary for the effective treatment of the patient's condition—deserves to be treated sceptically.

So far, four modes of mediation between man and his vulnerability to disease have been identified—magic, religion, compassion and rejection. Together they may be regarded as constituting the nontechnical or "helping to cope" side of medicine. By none of these means is the natural history of disease processes within individuals predictably and specifically changed for the better. That has been the achievement of the fifth mode—the technical mastery of disease. All medical cultures can be regarded as being made up of these five elements [20]. For some centuries, in the West, the technical mode of response has become increasingly manifest. There has been a progressive increase in the understanding of the structure and function of the human body and, to some extent, of the nature of disease processes within it.

Disease has been described in increasingly scientific terms. But it needs emphasising that until very recently indeed, doctors could do little to alter the natural course of events [7]. Thus the response to disease came to be described in technical terms well before the technical capacity to master disease became significant. The vocabulary and activities changed but the functional content of doctor-patient interaction remained that of the "helping to cope" side of medicine.

In recent decades, and especially since World War II, scientific medical technology of an "engineering" kind has gained overwhelming dominance in the mediation between industrial man and disease. The situation of the sick is increasingly defined in scientific terms, and by this means ambiguities and uncertainties are reduced. Major crises are responded to in a confident and surehanded manner. The victim of a heart attack is taken to an intensive cardiac care unit; the victim of a car accident to an accident and emergency unit; the cancer patient "has to go to hospital for an operation." And the minor illnesses too. For upper respiratory infections there are antibiotics; for depression and anxiety, psycho-active drugs.

This particular ("engineering") kind of technical response to disease pervades the whole of contemporary medical culture—the organisation of medical care, the education of doctors and the character of doctor-patient interaction. The social costs of this style of medicine are not limited to its considerable and rapidly rising resource demands. It concentrates the medical effort on the large acute hospitals while the ordinary citizen finds access to primary care ever more difficult. It concentrates resources on patients with technically interesting conditions while the insane, the handicapped and the elderly are frequently left to live out their lives in overcrowded and unpleasant conditions. Medical education detours doctors from the areas of greatest need by emphasising technical challenges rather than moral ones. Concentration on the technical (biological) problem deflects attention from the emotional and existential significance of disease.

The doctor said: this-and-that indicates that this-and-that is wrong with you, but if an analysis of this-and-that does not confirm our diagnosis, we must suspect you of having this-and-that. If we assume that you have this-and-that, then . . . and so on. There was only one question Ivan Ilyich wanted answered: was his condition dangerous or not? But the doctor ignored that question as irrelevant. From the doctor's point of view, such a question was unworthy of consideration. One had only to weigh possibilities: floating kidneys, chronic catarrh, or an ailment of the caecum. There was no question of the life of Ivan Ilyich—nothing but a contest between floating kidneys and the caecum. In the presence of Ivan Ilyich the doctor gave a brilliant solution of the problem in favour of the caecum, with the reservation that the analysis of his water might supply new information necessitating a reconsideration of the case [16].

And yet, in spite of deficiencies of this kind, discontent with health services does not usually lead into criticism of the basic characteristics of contemporary medicine. The system is strongly legitimised. This legitimacy is strengthened by medicine's consonance with the wider culture of which it is a part. Its technical aspects are themselves consonant with the general pattern of interaction between industrial man and his environment. So too is the idea of progress. Progress is seen to be the simple sum of what are taken as its component parts. Thus, if the hospital treatment of heart attack really did show a significant, if marginal, improvement over treatment at home, this would be regarded as progress. An increase from, say, 50 to 70 percent in patients surviving 5 years following treatment for cancer would be regarded as further evidence of medical progress. So also in economic life; $a+b$ cars per thousand population is better than a cars; $x + y$ television sets better than x, and so on. But in terms of real human welfare, neither whole is the simple sum of parts such as these. There is as little reason for believing that the health of the population is being significantly improved as there is for believing that the material conditions for human life are becoming more favourable (see for example [21]).

The original paradox remains. Enthusiasm for the system has outpaced its concrete achievements and its indirect costs tend to be underplayed. Despite the evidence to the contrary, it is widely believed by both patients and their doctors that industrial populations owe their higher health standards to "scientific medicine," that such medical technology as currently exists is largely effective in coping with the tasks it faces and that it offers great promise for the future. To unravel this paradox it is helpful to explore further the complex and subtle relationship between the truly technical, the apparently technical and the nontechnical elements of modern medicine. This will be done by focusing on the nature of the interaction between the sick and the purveyors of high technology medicine in two typical cases—firstly the hospital treatment of heart attack and secondly the treatment of upper respiratory infections with antibiotics.

A heart attack is one of the gravest threats that faces middle-aged men of the industrial world. The surehandedness of the technical response to this problem and its elaboration in coronary care units has already been noted. Thanks to television, the drama of the battle with death within these units is part of public experience—the faltering heart rhythm traced on the oscilloscope screen, the mysterious fluid funnelled into the veins, the white-coated doctors fussing around the passive victim. This technical response seems both impressive and credible. And yet, as noted earlier, there is no convincing evidence that this energetic intervention secures any more favourable an outcome than simple treatment at home. What then is going on?

Death may follow a heart attack either because the heart is left too weak to pump the blood or because the rhythm of its contractions becomes disrupted. It is the latter possibility that intensive cardiac care is designed to prevent. By monitoring the heart rhythm electronically, it is thought possible to get an early warning of imminent disruptions. Chemical, electrical or physical interventions may then be rapidly instituted in order to stabilise the heart rhythm again. It is on these engineering type interventions that scientific attention has been focused. It is claimed that dangerous disturbances in rhythm may sometimes be reversed. But everyone is aware that the heart is easily excited by emotion. Is it not likely, therefore, that by rushing the victim into an environment that is so strange; by placing him with others who are dying from the same condition, and by fussing around him and connecting him up to machines and intravenous drips; that, by doing all these things, the "treatment" might be introducing as many disturbances into the heart rhythm as the drug and electrical shocks are able to get out? This may be why it has been difficult to show any overall objective gain.

What is notable is the preoccupation with an engineering style of response and the reluctance to compare outcome with that from a low technology (home treatment) response. The scientific testing of this high technology response was widely regarded as unethical until the publication in August 1971 of the study (already referred to) by Mather and others [5] which failed to show any benefit from it. Despite this, specialists have been willing to encourage massive expenditure on intensive cardiac care.... Some of this expenditure would almost certainly have secured much greater reductions in mortality if it had been used to persuade people to change those elements of their way of life (such as smoking and overeating) which increase their risk of heart disease. (Sceptics see [22].)

The development of coronary care units has far outpaced what would have been justified in terms of a rational programme to reduce the toll from ischaemic heart disease. It has a momentum which is almost detached from considerations as rational as this. How different, *functionally,* are the activities involved from the rituals of the magicians of old? Both are active responses to forces threatening well-being. In neither case is there much enthusiasm amongst the operators for the empirical testing of the effectiveness of their treatment and, in any case, such considerations do not seem central to the worthwhileness of the activity. The operators work in ways that are credible within their wider cultures. Their activities provide means of coping with some threat which, if not coped with, would leave its victims exposed and, equally important, would remind the other members of that society that they, too, were defenceless before the same threat.

One of the recurrent annoyances of urban life are upper respiratory infections which frequently leave one feeling miserable. Patients, therefore, expect their doctor to "do something." Now most of these infections are viral and nearly all doctors, if questioned at a scientific meeting, would admit both that antibiotics are ineffective in altering the course of viral infections and that they should not be used indiscriminately. Yet the prescription of antibiotics is now widely expected by patients when they present themselves to their doctor with an upper respiratory infection—and most doctors oblige. This author was once called to task by a general practitioner for whom he was deputising for failing to prescribe antibiotics to a woman with the classical signs and symptoms of a viral upper respiratory infection. The woman was feeling very miserable and her general practitioner felt that she "deserved" antibiotics. Whilst few general practitioners would offer such a blatantly nonscientific justification for prescribing antibiotics, most are more convinced, as it were, of the human value of this type of exchange between doctor and patient than they are of its effectiveness in altering the natural course of events. But they would prefer not to be pressed on this latter issue. ... Such an attitude may annoy rationalists who believe that it is wrong to be guided by beliefs which are not logically consistent. This behaviour is, however, quite consistent with the view that men seek first of all to cope with the immediate world of experience.

The argument therefore is that the almost exclusive concentration, within modern medical culture, on the technical mastery of disease is more apparent than real. For in addition to countering the challenges to human well-being on the biological level, this technology is serving also to meet the emotional and existential challenges that disease involves. The problem of disease cannot be reduced to the purely technical one of the prevention and correction of biological malfunctioning. Nor is it sufficient just to add on the dimension of emotion—of symptomatology. For in addition to the distress that disease causes directly and to such emotional distress as is itself regarded as a disease, there is the threat that disease poses to the individual's sense of his own integrity and well-being. This existential challenge, in the ultimate, is the threat of oblivion.

At this point it is desirable to clarify, in the terms of this analysis, the nature of symptomatic treatment. Such treatment may serve to counter disease on all three levels. Firstly, there are medical interventions which relieve symptoms by means of specific and predictable physiological effects. The use of aspirin in a muscular sprain is a good example. Secondly, there are nonspecific but nonetheless physiological responses that could not be predicted from the known properties of the drug. This is frequently referred to as a psychosomatic or placebo effect and may be observed, for example, in the effect of dummy tablets in lowering blood pressure or relieving tension and anxiety. Thirdly, there are those doctor-patient interactions which do not alter the observable course of events but which both parties nevertheless feel to be worthwhile. By means of "explanation," ritual and symbol, such interventions are serving principally to counter the existential threat. The patient's situation is defined, ambiguity is reduced and "reassurance"—as doctors frequently call it—results. Psychotherapy and much prescribing behaviour would appear to be serving this objective.

In this attempt to explore the interrelation of the technical and nontechnical aspects of modern medicine, two sets of distinctions have been drawn. Firstly, five different modes of mediation between man and disease have been identified—magic, religion, compassion for the suffering, rejection of the abnormal and the technical mastery of disease. The first four of these may be taken as constituting the nontechnical or "helping to cope" side of medicine. Secondly, it has been argued that disease challenges well-being on three main levels—biological, emotional and existential. Clearly, these two sets of factors are interrelated. Thus, the technical mastery of disease is serving to reduce biological malfunctioning. Further, the "helping to cope" side of medicine is principally serving to reduce the emotional and existential challenge. But the essence of this argument is to point out that these interrelationships are not simple or self-evident. For example, magical ritual may strengthen the organism's capacity to recover (or conversely, "black magic" may cause the victim to pine away and die). And most importantly of all, not all that is manifestly about the technical mastery of disease is serving merely to counter biological challenges to well-being. To an increasing extent medical technology is serving as a mask for nontechnical functions. It carries a large symbolic load. The more attention within medicine is focused on the technical mastery of disease, the larger become the symbolic and nontechnical functions of that technology. This process has been intensified by the decline of theistic religion.

THE FUTURE OF MEDICINE

It has been suggested that the character of medical culture is largely determined by that of the wider culture of which it is a part and that the medical beliefs and behaviour of individuals are largely socially determined. It would be wrong however to ignore the scope for voluntary activity. For one thing, current developments do not always fulfill past expectations. Thus strains are created, both in the sphere of practice and the sphere of theory. The old ways of seeing the world are fractured and through the cracks the real world becomes more visible. The scope of human freedom expands. Within the wider sphere of productive life, as indeed within medicine, the most serious emerging strains derive from industrial man's relation to the natural world.

It is clear that the increase in human numbers and the increase in material consumption per capita must reach limits in a finite world. Currently each is increasing at around 2 percent per year, with global levels of material production thus rising around 4 percent and doubling in less than 20 years. Because of the momentum inherent in demographic growth and of the effect of rising global expectations in sustaining economic growth, some studies have suggested that the global "population-capital system" seems bound for "overshoot and collapse" before re-stabilising within the limits nature imposes on man [23]. This is not a problem that will go away if it is ignored and an increasing awareness of it is likely to lead to a fundamental reassessment of the wider constraints on human action. As ecology is central to health, it would be surprising if such a reassessment did not also involve re-examination of the assumptions underlying modern medicine. In any case medicine contains its own particular expression of the wider crisis—diminishing returns and a self-defeating dependence on economic growth to solve the health problems associated with such growth.

How then might medicine respond to these emerging strains? In which direction will thinking need to develop if it is to reorient itself within these newly recognised constraints? The technical side of medicine involves fewer conceptual problems and for this reason it will be considered first. The problem facing the "experts" is to identify those means of increasing biological wellbeing that are not dependent on measures (such as continued economic growth) which are likely to aggravate the wider ecological problem. This will almost certainly involve a switch away from emphasising the potency and potentiality of high technology clinical interventions towards an emphasis on the importance of way of life factors in disease. For medical theory to meet this challenge it will need to broaden its scientific base. Lessons relevant to the improvement of health will need to be learned from human evolution; from the study of the health consequences of the transition from hunter-gathering to agriculture and from agriculture to industry; from historical demography and the debate about the regulation of numbers in animal populations. The health aspects of the relationship between human communities and their environments need much more detailed study. There is a need for good comprehensive epidemiological studies on groups with widely differing ways of life. The critical importance of an understanding of health and disease in hunter-gatherers to a fuller appreciation of the human experience of disease, and therefore of our own health problems, deserves urgent recognition—especially because many of these groups are being subject to rapid acculturation [24].

It would however be unrealistic to expect all doctors to be expert not just in comprehending biological phenomena at an individual level but also at a population level. The principal concern of the clinician will continue to be the treatment of the sick. It is understandable that clinicians, in their day to day practice, should take the general way of life of the community for granted and judge the significance of behavioural factors in individual illness against that background. But if the burden of the diseases of maladaptation is to be reduced by changing those elements of our way of life that are most to blame (and this is the most effective strategy currently available for these diseases) then clinicians need to have a much more sophisticated understanding of the relationship between behaviour and disease. Human population biology is essential to that understanding.

The greatest theoretical challenge within contemporary medicine lies with those responsible for the health of communities—specialists in public health or . . . community medicine. Such specialists cannot afford to take any way of life for granted. They will need a comprehensive understanding of the experience of disease in different communities with differing ways of life—that is they should be experts in the biology of human populations. Unfortunately, there is, as yet, little recognition of the need to develop the theoretical basis of community medicine in this way. The dominance of an empiricism devoid of theoretical pretensions is arguably doing more to hold back than to develop the practice of community medicine. For this reason the concentration of intellectual effort onto the development of the theoretical basis of community medicine is an urgent precondition for the articulation of an alternative—"ecological" strategy for the improvement of health.

It is often argued that such a strategy is not feasible because it lacks public acceptability . . . But it seems as mistaken to interpret our current medical strategy as the product of a conspiracy by patients as it is to see it as a conspiracy by doctors. When health problems are perceived differently they may be responded to differently. For example, despite health propaganda efforts that have been very modest in comparison to the promotional activities of the tobacco interests, tobacco consumption per adult British male had fallen by 1971/2 to its lowest level since 1916 [22]. Anti-smoking propaganda does seem to be having an effect—given its low intensity it would have been unreasonable to expect more. The current rates of decline in tobacco consumption are likely to prevent several thousand premature deaths each year [22]. Their impact on health is therefore of an order of magnitude that bears comparison to major hospital-based activities.

Much of the impact of diseases of maladaptation may be reducible by changes in our way of life that are not too onerous. Habits can be changed. It is relatively easy to increase the amount of high residue food in the diet and although we've become accustomed to helping ourselves, for example, to more and more sugar and salt, it is possible to wean oneself back down to more modest intakes without loss in the palatability of food. If a reduction in the intake of saturated fats is shown to reduce the risk of heart disease, then the substitution of polyunsaturated margarine for butter and the avoiding of fatty meat need be no great hardship. Avoiding obesity and keeping fit both have their own immediate rewards as well as the long-term health ones. The fundamental task is to change thinking about disease and about what can be done about it. Given that, significant further gains in health may well be possible. In Victorian times there was a happy synergism between the germ theory of disease and the wider puritan culture which lead to the successful war against the germs. That battle has been largely won. Is it too much to expect a similar future interaction between specific advice on changing health damaging habits and a wider culture which is increasingly sensitive to the need for man to treat the natural world with respect?

None of this is meant to imply that the improvement of biological well-being should take automatic precedence over other human goals. Individuals and the wider community may well be prepared to pay a biological price for the achievement of competing objectives. But such choices should be both deliberate and well-informed. At the moment they are usually neither.

A switch in technical strategies away from high technology hospital medicine may have a major impact on the nontechnical, "helping to cope" side of medical culture. The placing of deliberate constraints on the further development and deployment of such technology would seem to deny its potential for the alleviation of human suffering. It would be compromised as a source of hope and thus divested of much of its current symbolic load. One of the lines of defence especially against the existential challenge of illness would be weakened. Such a change would however make possible other major gains on the nontechnical side. With a more realistic assessment of the capabilities of medical technology there might be less of the tendency to interpret the problem of illness in purely technical terms. The emotional and existential aspects of its challenge to well-being could be given more open recognition. It has often been argued that a more balanced response to illness is, in any case, more effective. By being more sensitive to the patient's situation doctors are likely to obtain better information about the problem, provide more relevant advice and treatment and secure more co-operation.

Little has been said so far in this chapter about the very large categories of people whose illnesses and disabilities have not (and often could not have been) prevented and who cannot be easily restored to health—those with congenital and acquired handicaps, the mentally ill, the chronic sick and the disabled elderly. This is because the argument has been principally concerned with the major forces at work in the evolution of contemporary medical culture. Meeting the needs of these handicapped groups for humane care and rehabilitation has not in practice been a major objective [25, 26]. Resources and energy have been directed elsewhere—to the high technology short-stay hospitals; to the patients with "interesting" conditions for whom "something" (i.e. a technical "something") can be done. The needs of the handicapped comprise a large and growing proportion of the work load of the health services. Within a more balanced medical culture, there would be less need to translate their frequently nontechnical needs into technical ones. The challenge that they pose to the compassion of the healthy could be confronted and responded to more directly. And the resources to improve their lot can only be made available—especially if economic growth is to be phased out—by carefully constraining the further development of expensive high-technology medicine. There is, in fact, a growing recognition that the "care" function of the health services is in direct competition for resources with the "cure" function and that hitherto "cure" has had more than its fair share [27, 28].

One of the most important preconditions for improving the care of the mentally ill is an increased tolerance on the part of the "normals" for bizarre and unpredictable behaviour. Given such tolerance the need for institutionalisation and its attendant harm to the "patient" is reduced. Currently it is often felt necessary to represent this essentially ethical problem as a technical one—to try and make mental illness respectable by insisting that it is "just like other illness" and "needs treatment just the same." The problem would benefit from a more direct and honest confrontation.

CONCLUSION

In much discussion of the current state of medicine the wider medical culture is often accepted as given. This confers an unnecessary aura of inevitability to current ideas about how to improve health and about the relation between the technical and nontechnical aspects of medicine. Medicine is the product of man and can be as he chooses to make it. It is, in any case, possible to argue that there have always been two conflicting approaches within medicine—one emphasising the potency of clinical intervention (the "engineering approach"), the other the importance of way of life factors (the "ecological approach"). The Hippocratic tract *Airs, Waters and Places* gives a good summary of the latter:

[The physician who is an honour to his profession is one] who has a due regard to the seasons of the year, and the diseases which they produce; to the states of the wind peculiar to each country and the qualities of its waters; who marks carefully the localities of towns, and of the surrounding country, whether they are low or high, hot or cold, wet or dry, who moreover takes notes of the diet and regimen of the inhabitants, and, in a word, of all the causes that may produce disorder in the animal economy [29].

This approach is currently finding expression in the works of René Dubos [29, 30], Thomas McKeown [7, 27], A. L. Cochrane [28], Stephen Boyden [31, 32] and Macfarlane Burnet [33]. It is, however, grossly underdeveloped in relation to other kinds of medical knowledge.

Medicine may be expected to come under increasing pressure from the wider culture, which is in turn likely to change as a result of increasing confrontation with material and biological constraints on human action. With a rising proportion of illness evidently man-made and increasing restrictions on the further increase of resource consumption for medical care, medicine seems bound to move in an "ecological" direction.

If it does, biological well-being may be expected to benefit. Emotional problems in relation to illness may be increasingly respected. But the sense of exposure of the existential threat that disease represents may, by contrast, be heightened. It will be more difficult to say such things as "don't worry, doctor, by the time I get lung cancer they'll have a cure for it." Faith in the effectiveness of society's defences against death might be weakened. With less confidence in his ability to master nature man will have to learn to live more openly with his vulnerability to forces he cannot control and with the frailty of the individual human existence. Man's domination of nature has been the central impetus of modern industrial culture. Further pursuit of this within the already industrialised countries is likely to be self-defeating and could well be disastrous. Could it be that man will return instead to the development of his inner life?

Mary Douglas has characterised the primitive world view as one which interprets the universe in terms of human needs [15]. The belief that expansionary economics and technical advance will solve the most pressing human problems, often contains the un-supported assumption that the material and biological worlds will help sustain the drama of human expansion—by supplying virtually unlimited raw materials and energy sources, by absorbing pollutants and by allowing the constraints implicit in man's biological constitution to be easily transcended. Such thinking might be considered to involve interpreting the universe on the basis of human needs—that is, as being "primitive." The thinking of modern man should rather be directed towards identifying his best available options in a universe indifferent to his welfare, but sensitive to his insults.

REFERENCES

1. Department of Health and Social Security, *Digest of Health Statistics for England and Wales, 1971,* H.M.S.O. (1971): Tables 1.2 and 3.2.
2. *Statistical Abstract of the United States, 1973,* pp. 5, 75.
3. Rice, D. P., and Cooper, B. S., "National Health Expenditures, 1929–70," *Social Security Bulletin* (U.S.) (January 1971):3–18.

4. Holland, W. W., "Clinicians and the Use of Medical Resources," *The Hospital* (London) 67 (July 1971):236–39.

5. Mather, H. G., et al., "Acute Myocardial Infarction: Home and Hospital Treatment," *British Medical Journal 3* (1971): 334–38.

6. Rose, G., "Epidemiology of Ischaemic Heart Disease," *British Journal of Hospital Medicine* (March 1972):285–88.

7. McKeown, T., "A Historical Appraisal of the Medical Task," in *Medical History and Medical Care*, ed. G. McLachlan and T. McKeown (London: Oxford University Press for the Nuffield Provincial Hospitals Trust, 1971), p. 36.

8. Crombie, A. C., "The Future of Biology: The History of a Program," *Federation Proceedings 25* (1966):1448–53.

9. Doll, R., and Kinlen, L., "Epidemiology as an Aid to Determining the Causes of Cancer," Cancer Research Campaign, *49th Annual Report* (London: 2 Carlton House Terrace, 1971):42–46.

10. Burkitt, D. P., "Epidemiology of Cancer of the Colon and Rectum," *Cancer 28* (1971):3–13.

11. Sonksen, P. H., "Aetiology and Epidemiology of Diabetes," *British Journal of Hospital Medicine* (February 1972):151–56; and Kannel, W. B., Castelli, W. P., McNamara, P. M., and Sorlie, P., "Some Factors Affecting Morbidity and Mortality in Hypertension, the Frammington Study," *Milbank Memorial Fund Quarterly* XLVII, *3*, Part 2 (1969):116–42.

12. Cleave, T. L., and Campbell, G. D., *Diabetes, Coronary Thrombosis and the Saccharine Disease* (Bristol: Wright, 1966), Chapter 1.

13. Rosenberg, C. E., "The Medical Profession, Medical Practice, and the History of Medicine," in *Modern Methods in the History of Medicine*, ed. E. Clarke (London: The Athlone Press of the University of London, 1971), pp. 22–35.

14. Lévi-Strauss, C., "The Sorcerer and His Magic," in *Magic, Witchcraft and Curing*, ed. J. Middleton (New York: Natural History Press, 1967).

15. Douglas, M., *Purity and Danger* (Harmondsworth: Penguin, 1970).

16. Tolstoy, L., "The Death of Ivan Ilyich" (trans. Margaret Wettlin), in *Lev Tolstoi, Short Stories* (Moscow: Progress Publishers), pp. 108–67.

17. Barton, R., *Institutional Neurosis* (Bristol: John Wright, 1966).

18. Lieberman, M. A., "Relationship of Mortality Rates to Entrance to a Home for the Aged," *Geriatrics* (October 1961):515–19.

19. Aldrich, C. K., and Mendkoff, E., "Relocation of the Aged and Disabled: A Mortality Study," *Journal of the American Geriatric Society* (March 1963):185–94.

20. I have derived this analytic model from that used by Mark Field. To his four types of "societal response" I have added "rejection." See: Field, M., "The Health Care System of Industrial Society: The Disappearance of the General Practitioner and Some Implications," in *Human Aspects of Biomedical Engineering*, ed. E. Mendelson, J. Swazey, and I. Taviss (Cambridge: Harvard University Press, 1971), pp. 156–80.

21. Mishan, E. J., *The Costs of Economic Growth* (New York: Praeger, 1967).

22. It is often suggested that health education has little effect. However tobacco consumption has recently been falling at around 5 percent per year (*The* [London] *Times*, 1/12/1972). The Chief Medical Officer of the Department of Health and Social Security has estimated that there are approximately 100,000 premature deaths due to smoking in the United Kingdom each year (Department of Health and Social Security, *On the State of the Public Health; The Annual Report of the Chief Medical Officer . . . for the Year 1969* [London: H.M.S.O., 1970], p. 9). As the health damage from smoking is roughly proportional to the quantity of tobacco consumed (Royal College of Physicians of London, *Smoking and Health Now* [London: Pitman Medical, 1971]), the current decline may be saving around 5,000 premature deaths each year. And this is the result of a small-scale campaign. The Health Education Council spent £120,000 on its smoking and health campaign in 1970–71 (The Health Education Council, United Kingdom, *Accounts,* 31st March, 1971, Appendix IV, Wembley: Middlesex House). By contrast the tobacco industry spent £52 million on sales promotion in 1968 (Royal College of Physicians of London, *Smoking and Health Now* [London: Pitman Medical, 1971]).

23. Meadows, D. H., Meadows, D. L., Randers, J. and Behrens, W. W., *The Limits to Growth* (New York: NAL, 1972). Also see Mesarovic, M., and Pestel, E., *Mankind at the Turning Point* (New York: E. P. Dutton & Co., 1974).

24. Dunn, F. L., "Epidemiological Factors: Health and Disease in Hunter-Gatherers," *Man the Hunter,* ed. I. DeVore and R. B. Lee (Chicago: Aldine, 1968), pp. 221–28.

25. Mead, T. W., "Medicine and Population," *Public Health* (London) 82 (1968):100–110.

26. Department of Health and Social Security, Information Division, Intelligence Section, *National Health Service Notes,* 13 (figures for 1949–50) and Department of Health and Social Security, *Digest of Health Statistics for England and Wales* (1971):Table 2.3 (figures for 1969–70).

27. McKeown, T., *Medicine in Modern Society* (London: Allen & Unwin, 1965), pp. 21–58.

28. Cochrane, A. L., *Effectiveness and Efficiency, Random Reflections on Health Services* (London: Oxford University Press for the Nuffield Provincial Hospitals Trust, 1972), pp. 39–40.

29. Quoted in: Dubos, R., *Man Adapting* (New Haven: Yale University Press, 1965), pp. 36–37.

30. Dubos, R., *Mirage of Health* (New York: Harper, 1959).

31. Boyden, S. V., "The Human Organism in a Changing Environment," in *Man in His Environment,* ed. R. T. Appleyard (Perth: University of Western Australia Press, 1970), pp. 1–20.

32. Boyden, S. V., "Cultural Adaptation to Biological Maladjustment," in *The Impact of Civilization on the Biology of Man,* ed. S. V. Boyden (Canberra: Australian National University Press, 1970).

33. Burnet, M., *Genes, Dreams and Realities* (New York: Basic Books, 1971).

By Howard Brody and David S. Sobel

A Systems View of Health and Disease

Western scientific medicine, long used to an information explosion within its own territory, is now confronted with a barrage of information from other disciplines and medical systems. Within the Western scientific tradition, disciplines such as psychology, sociology, and ecology are turning up new factors that influence human health and disease but that fall outside medical boundaries as traditionally defined. Also from outside the Western tradition there is increased interest in ancient, non-Western and alternative approaches to healing.

Western medicine has to decide whether and how to incorporate this new information. The analytic and reductionistic tendencies that have served scientific medicine so well up to now suggest two possible strategies—either to reject this new information as perhaps interesting but not relevant; or to accept it in a condescending way, meanwhile being confident that it will soon be replaced by "hard" knowledge once the "real" physical-chemical underlying processes are understood. Both strategies amount to turning one's back on important, different ways of knowing more about human health.

Information becomes knowledge only when it is fitted within a

Supported in part by a Fellowship from the Institute on Human Values in Medicine, Philadelphia, funded through the National Endowment for the Humanities, grant EH-10973-74-365.

wider framework, so that the relationship between the new information and existing knowledge becomes more useful and clearer. The framework that we have found most helpful for this purpose we call a systems view of health and disease. The systems view shows how the scientific-medical, the scientific-nonmedical, and the non-Western ways of knowing the world all complement one another, each providing pieces of a puzzle that would otherwise remain incomplete. Our version of the systems view is adapted largely from Ervin Laszlo [1], who works within the school of general systems theory pioneered by Ludwig von Bertallanfy [2]. But the use we make of the systems view is more similar to what Churchman calls the "systems approach" [3]. That is, we are not postulating new scientific laws that hold true for all phenomena in nature that display systems organization, be they atoms or galaxies. Our most modest goal is to provide a structured way of shifting one's viewpoint, so that the same phenomenon can be looked at from a number of different perspectives, and the resulting data can be assembled in an orderly manner instead of remaining fragmented. Although the systems approach has been used widely in many areas, including health care management, there have been few attempts to apply it as a framework for understanding health and disease [4–9].

To begin, the terms "system," "hierarchy," "information," and "environment" need to be clarified, for we will be using them in a somewhat technical way. A system is an organized set of components that is conveniently regarded as a whole consisting of interdependent parts. It is characteristic of a system that if one part or subcomponent is replaced by a different but similar part, the system functions as before; if the organization among the parts is changed, however, the system's function is altered even though the parts remain the same. Any system (for example, the liver) can be viewed as a whole composed of parts (for example, cells) or as a component part of a higher-level system (for example, the body), depending upon what is most convenient for the purpose of inquiry.

When systems are ranked in order of increasing complexity we have a hierarchy—that is, atoms are subcomponents of molecules, which are subcomponents of cells, which are subcomponents of

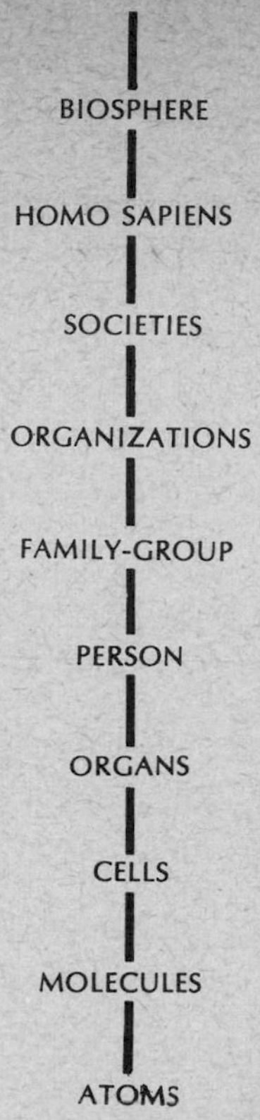

BIOSPHERE

HOMO SAPIENS

SOCIETIES

ORGANIZATIONS

FAMILY-GROUP

PERSON

ORGANS

CELLS

MOLECULES

ATOMS

Figure 1. A Hierarchy of Living Systems

tissues, which are subcomponents of organs, and so on. Biologists are accustomed to thinking in terms of such a systems hierarchy that begins with atoms and molecules and moves up in complexity through organelles, cells, tissues, organs, organ systems, and finally to the individual organism. It is useful, however, to continue the hierarchy beyond the individual level, with persons viewed as subcomponents of still-higher-level systems such as families, communities, and nations [10].

This hierarchical pattern can be illustrated by a variety of graphic conventions, including concentric circles, nesting boxes, or a linear array. Figure 1 demonstrates one simplified way of depicting the levels of a hierarchy of living systems. As Paul Weiss has noted with regard to this concept of hierarchical level:

The "level" we are speaking of signifies really the level of attention of an observer whose interest has been attracted by certain regularities of pattern prevailing at that level, as he scans across the range of orders of magnitude. He scans as he would turn a microscope from lower to higher levels of magnification, gaining detail at the expense of restricting the visual field, and he finds noteworthy constancies on every level. As long as we remain conscious of the fact that any geometric image (or verbiage) that we might choose as a visual (or verbal) model of hierarchical structure is a simplified artifact reflecting the inadequacy of our faculty for visualizing abstract concepts, it becomes rather immaterial which one we use [11].

While the order of levels in a hierarchy is not arbitrary—for example, organs are always made up of cells and not vice versa—the labeling of the levels is arbitrary. For instance, each level depicted in Figure 1 could be further subdivided and different labels could be affixed to the various levels. In using the conceptual device of a hierarchy of systems, it is important to remember that such terms as "hierarchy" or "higher-level system" refer to the level of complexity; they are not judgments about the intrinsic value or worth of the various levels of organization. To designate one level as the primary system for analyzing a certain problem is not to say that level is more important, only that it may be more appropriate for understanding the phenomenon in question. For example, to understand certain features of heart disease, we may wish to focus on cell membranes and electrical potentials; but to investigate whether certain personality patterns are correlated with increased incidence of heart disease, we would do better to shift our attention to higher-level systems.

The concept of hierarchy tells us that organs are made up of cells, but it does not by itself tell us how cells organized into an organ differ from cells merely collected together. For this we need to describe the patterns of information flow within the system. Here, we define "information" in a very broad sense as that which has the potential to change the activities of a component of the system. The patterns of information flow determine the orderly organization among the subcomponents permitting the system to function as more than a random collection of parts [10].

The flow of information commonly takes the form of feedback loops, in which component A influences component B and the new state of B then "feeds back" to influence A. There are two basic types of feedback regulation [12, 13]. The first, known as negative feedback, acts to reduce any deviations and return the

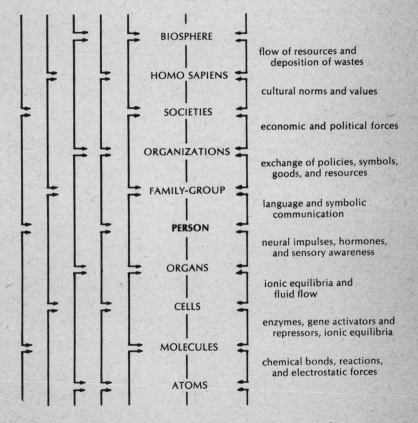

Figure 2: Information Flow in the Hierarchy

system to equilibrium. For example, in the human organism each organ depends upon a certain level of blood flow to carry out its particular activities. When the heart begins to pump too slowly or too quickly, a complex series of neural and hormonal feedback mechanisms is activated to return the heart to homeostatic normal limits. Thus, each subsystem has the freedom to function within certain limits, but once it crosses these limits the negative feedback mechanisms act to return it to its proper role in the functioning of the larger whole. The second type of feedback mechanism is called positive feedback because it tends to amplify, rather than dampen, deviation within the system. Most growth and maturation processes are regulated in this manner [13].

The general patterns of information flow appear to exist at all hierarchical levels, but the actual nature of the information will be different at each level. Atoms maintain equilibrium configuration within a molecule by means of electrostatic attractions and repulsions; family members relate to each other largely through language and symbols; and organizations regulate individual behavior by enforcing rules and social norms (see Figure 2). Information flows not only within a given level or between adjacent levels but also between widely spaced levels, as, for example, when a nation communicates directly with an individual via income tax laws or requirements for immunization.

Living systems are continuously exchanging matter, energy, and information with their environments and must periodically adapt their internal processes to accommodate changes in the environment [1]. Here, environment is simply and relatively defined as everything outside the boundaries of the system we are studying. Factors we label as environmental may, therefore, occur at any level of the hierarchy, so that we can speak of our physical environment, our chemical environment, our social environment.

HEALTH AND DISEASE DEFINED

The description of a hierarchy of living systems suggests characteristic features of a concept of "health," which can be summarized as the *ability of a system (for example, cell, organism,* family, society) to respond adaptively to a wide variety of environmental challenges (for example, physical, chemical, infectious, psychological, social).*

This view of health suggests several advantages over more traditional definitions. Health is seen as a positive process, not as the mere absence of the signs and symptoms of disease. Furthermore, this definition is not restricted to biological fitness or somatic well-being; rather, it demands a consideration of the broader environmental, sociocultural, and behavioral determinants of health. Also the level of health is dynamically changing; encounters with environmental challenges result in either a lower level of health, a restoration of customary equilibrium, or a growth-enhancing response. This latter response involves more than a passive reaction or homeostatic adjustment. It refers to a creative adaptation that leaves the organism or system at a higher level of functioning than before the challenge [16]. Immunizations, major life-style changes following illness, and the development of an international peace-keeping force are examples of such adaptations.

Our definition of health clearly does not exclude the central role played by value judgments in evaluating health. In particular, health must be viewed as only one among many possible human values. For example, health is not necessarily equivalent to happiness, and individuals will often sacrifice their health to pursue other goals. Furthermore, what is judged as healthy or unhealthy varies from person to person and, even more dramatically, from culture to culture because of highly individual requirements and relative social norms.

Given this systems view of health, "disease" can be seen as *a failure to respond adaptively to environmental challenges resulting in a disruption of the overall equilibrium of the system.* The disruption may be due to feedback constraints that have become

* Adapted from Dubos, "the states of health or disease are the expressions of the success or failure experienced by the organism in its effort to respond adaptively to environmental challenges" [14] and Audy, "health is a continuing property, potentially measurable by the individual's ability to rally from a wide range and considerable amplitude of insults, the insults being chemical, physical, infectious, psychological, and social" [15].

too rigid to permit compensatory responses of the component parts. More commonly, however, the disruption results from perturbing forces in the environment to which the usual feedback mechanisms cannot accommodate. Perturbations may take the form of an excessive stress (for example, germs or toxins) or a lack of necessary stimuli (for example, food or love). These perturbations may impinge upon one hierarchical level—radiation, for example, primarily affects the molecular level—or they may impact across many levels, as in the trauma of an automobile collision.

As a rule, however, a disease does not stop at one level since all the levels are interconnected by the information circuits. Therefore, unless the homeostatic mechanisms at contiguous levels can restore a level of normal function and "buffer" the disruption, it will tend to spread up and down the hierarchy. For example, in diabetes, genetic and environmental factors interact to produce an initial disruption at a biochemical level that can lead to pathological changes in cellular function and a disruption of organ systems (for example, kidney and eye). Such changes are likely to disrupt the individual's behavior and may strain the family as well as produce a potential resource drain on the community. A disruption can also travel downward through the hierarchy, as when economic or natural disasters produce societal disruptions creating upheavals in community and family function and, in turn, precipitating a variety of psychosomatic or sociosomatic symptoms among individuals.

Therefore, from a systems view diseases are not regarded as discrete entities localized in one organ or tissue but as patterns of disruptions manifested at various levels of the system at various times. Patterns may differ in regard to where the disruption arises, which hierarchical levels are most affected, the type of environmental force that initiated the disturbance, and so on, allowing us to classify diseases by the traditional diagnostic categories [17, 18].

The systems view, however, predicts certain features of disease that traditional classifications do not make explicit. For instance, the systems approach accommodates very well a multiple-causation understanding of disease. The development, expression, and course of disease is seen to depend as much on the stability and adaptive capacity of the host system as on the nature of specific perturbing forces impinging on the hierarchy. In fact, the actual signs and symptoms of disease not infrequently represent the failing efforts of the system to restore order (for example, autoimmune diseases). The systems view also eliminates the sharp distinction between mind and body which has plagued medical thought. If disruptions are seen to move up and down the hierarchical levels, then we might expect that psychosocial disruptions can cause tissue or biochemical manifestations and vice versa.

IMPLICATIONS FOR HEALTH CARE

When a system is disrupted, it may attempt to restore equilibrium by activating special reserve information circuits and subsystems. For example, during an infection white blood cells may be mobilized to remedy the disruption or, at least, to keep it from spreading. If some components die, they can often be replaced by the activation of growth processes. Sometimes, however, the inherent self-regulatory mechanisms alone are not sufficient and some form of therapy is required. In traditional Chinese medicine two distinct and complementary therapeutic strategies have been described: the *liao* approach, involving active therapeutic intervention, and the *yang sheng* approach, aimed at strengthening the natural powers of resistance of the organism [19].

In modern systems terminology the former consists essentially of a disruption from the environment designed to oppose a specific disease-disruption, as when antibiotics are used to treat bacterial infections. The difference between a therapeutic disruption and a disease-producing disruption lies in the value judgments placed on the predicted outcomes of each. However, in practice, the distinction is often blurred because of the so-called side effects, or iatrogenic diseases, produced by therapeutic interventions. Until recently, medical thought has regarded the ill effects of therapy as freak occurrences, or the losing end of a calculated risk, rather than as expected outcomes due to the intrinsic nature of therapeutic measures and the interconnectedness of living systems. On the whole, however, the active therapeutic interventions that characterize modern medicine, whether surgical or chemical, have appeared so dramatic and successful that complementary health strategies have tended to be overlooked.

Ancient systems of healing are replete with examples of another therapeutic approach that attempts to support the inherent healing powers of the body. In systems terms this can be viewed as attempts to improve the information flow in the system in order to accommodate disruptions and facilitate the restoration of equilibrium. For example, such techniques as yogic therapy, meditation, and biofeedback training operate at psychophysiological levels to improve (or, in the case of biofeedback, to add) feedback circuits in order to enhance the self-regulatory capabilities of the organism. Similarly, immunization and the more recent developments in immunotherapy for the treatment of cancer represent methods of stimulating the body's inherent capacities to manage and prevent disease. In the absence of specific disease, this approach can be extended to general health promotion [20]. Improving the feedback and communication among family members, for example, can stabilize the hierarchy at that level, rendering the system more capable of handling challenges and resisting disruption. The same rationale may be applied to other health-promotive measures such as improved nutrition, exercise, and relaxation techniques.

In general, Western scientific medicine has focused on the lower levels of the hierarchy—the biological causes of disease and physical and chemical interventions. This approach has been remarkably successful for diseases in which the primary disruptions are largely confined to the biological levels. But, even here the strict biomedical approach is limited. By failing to attend to the person and sociocultural levels, where disease is shaped into the human experience of illness, contemporary medicine undermines its own effectiveness [21, 22]. The attempt to treat disease as a purely physicochemical dysfunction also ignores that many ailments presented as somatic complaints are due primarily to disruptions at the person, family, or societal levels. But, as Abraham Maslow has observed, "If the only tool you have is a hammer, you tend to treat everything as if it were a nail" [23].

The treatment of human sickness can never be reduced to a completely technical and impersonal matter. Disease most often involves multiple levels, disrupting the person and social group, and therefore requires multiple interventions directed at different levels. Many of the traditional healing systems of other cultures recognize the importance of the sociocultural dimensions of disease. Although these systems often ignore the biology of sickness, we can still learn a great deal from their management of the illness experience as a personal and social phenomenon [21]. Also, a recent approach to the treatment of cancer patients illustrates how standard biological therapies (radiotherapy, chemotherapy, and surgery) can be combined with adjunctive support at the person level (various meditation and relaxation exercises) as well as the family level (group work and counseling) [24].

Intervention at multiple levels, however, must be systematically integrated as part of total patient care, not added on as an afterthought or left to chance. This will require a team effort, for no single individual can be expert in the various modes of interventions at each hierarchical level. At the same time, if the members of the team all share a common language, a common framework, and an understanding of one another's specializations, then a real co-ordination of effort becomes possible. The systems model can potentially provide an integrating framework to inform the actions of the individual members of such a team [5].

The systems approach also emphasizes that prevention and cure are not the only objectives of health-related interventions. When a disease-disruption cannot be prevented or removed, it can often be confined to allow a maximum degree of normal functioning. An individual with organ-level dysfunction can often be supported so as to lessen person-level and family-level disruption. One can therefore speak of "a healthy way to live a disease" [20] and the importance of helping patients develop confidence that they can to some degree control their illness [25].

The systems view also avoids the problem of confusing the level of intervention with the level of disease. While diseases may represent patterns of disruption affecting many hierarchical levels, a therapy aimed at just one level may be highly efficacious because it can affect other levels via the interconnected patterns of information flow. Thus, chemotherapy for depression is often strikingly effective even though depressive disorders are characterized by complex mixtures of genetic, biochemical, behavioral, and social factors [26]. Therefore, to conclude from a clinical trial of a drug that depression is only a biochemical disease would be to ignore the true complexity of the illness. This confusion might also lead to the systematic neglect of other possible preventive or health-promotive strategies that could be directed at higher system levels.

In trying to prevent many of the complex health problems that confront us today, the biomedical approach needs to be broadened and complemented by interventions aimed at higher levels of the hierarchy. The physician has been likened to a man rescuing drowning people from a river, too busy to investigate why all these people were falling in upstream [27]. The systems view encourages us to look upstream, to consider the behavioral, social, political, and environmental, as well as the biological, determinants of health and ill health.

Clearly there is no way that the doctor, or even an interdisciplinary health care team as presently constituted, can address the problems of preserving health across all these levels. For instance, we look to politicians to handle disruptions that occur at the society-nation level; are politicians then to become members of the health care team? On the other hand, we cannot deny that the various hierarchical levels are interconnected and that events at the social level have major implications for the health or sickness of individuals.

These arguments lead to the conclusion that it cannot be the task exclusively of the medical profession to preserve health, but that the efforts and domain of the medical profession need to be placed in perspective and integrated as a part of a more holistic approach to health.

IMPLICATIONS FOR
HEALTH PLANNING AND POLICY

The systems view suggests a more rational approach to planning health interventions and evaluating their outcomes [5, 28]. Ideally, in considering a particular health problem, planners would examine the problem as it relates to each hierarchical level. For example, nutrition presents many different, yet inter-related, concerns at each level. At the molecular and cellular levels we might be concerned with the intricate metabolic roles of nu-trients. At the person level, the question of individual food selec-tion and eating habits arises. At the institutional level, issues concerning agribusiness, food production, processing, and distri-bution emerge. At the level of societies, we must consider cultural beliefs about food and nutrition. And at the biospheric level, ecological considerations about climate, soil, and the limits of the earth in terms of food production become critical concerns. Of course, all the hierarchical levels interact in a systems model: nutrient requirements change with various stressors or drugs, eating habits are influenced by commercial food advertising, climatic and political changes modify food production, and so on.

The systems model provides an orderly and systematic way of inquiring into these interactions between levels and avoids the risk of viewing each level in isolation. For example, if the in-dividual is not viewed in terms of the social, political, and eco-nomic context that constrains and conditions individual behav-ior, we run the risk of developing a policy that "blames the victim" for poor health [29, 30].

With this broader picture in mind, the planner can then look for possible interventions at each level and assess the likely con-sequences, good and bad, of alternative strategies. The interven-tions promising the greatest efficacy at lowest cost and with the lowest level of unwanted side effects would be adopted. Thus, in dealing with lung cancer, appropriate studies might determine, for instance, that a societal policy of buying out tobacco growers and converting the land to other crops might be more effective in the long run than increased efforts in chemotherapy, surgery, radiotherapy, or public health education. The evaluation of alter-native strategies is particularly important since increasing health care costs and the allocation of scarce resources have become critical issues.

The systems approach can also be used to evaluate interven-tions in terms of their short-run and long-run consequences at different hierarchical levels. For example, in testing new drugs, food additives, and pollutants, physiological side effects such as cancer production are often considered, while potential toxicities at a behavioral level are ignored [31]. Similarly, in massive technological interventions like the building of a dam, the promised economic benefits may blind us to the disastrous public health problems that may result [32]. Public policy interventions, therefore, often produce unintentional side effects at a different level than the original intervention and after a considerable time lag. Of course, these unintentional consequences may be positive as well as negative, as when automobile fatalities were reduced following the lowering of the speed limits to save energy.

Thus, the systems perspective, which reminds us of the interconnectedness of the hierarchical levels, not only clearly warns of the probability of short-range and long-range side effects but also provides a checklist of where they might occur. It also reminds us that modest attempts to aid the natural restorative actions of the system generally cause less trouble than heroic interventions. Therefore, longer-range, higher-level changes in the system that make it more adaptable and better able to cope with stresses are preferable to one-shot interventions after disease has occurred. For instance, while antibiotics have been regarded as one of the greatest medical advances of this century, their effect on infant mortality in Western countries has been only a fraction of the effects of general improvement in nutrition, chlorination of water, and pasteurization of milk [33].

IMPLICATIONS FOR THE HEALTH SCIENCES

At each hierarchical level, new functions and properties emerge due to the interaction among the component parts. These properties are "lost" when the system is analyzed at a lower level of organization and the components examined in isolation. This is what is meant by the phrase "the whole is more than the sum of the parts." The "more" arises from the relationship of the components. For example, the human capacities for symbolic communication, decision-making, and goal-setting cannot be fully explained in terms of molecules, cells, or organs. Therefore, from a systems view, it makes no sense to say that the processes of the mind are nothing but biochemical and biophysical occurrences in the brain. It makes very good sense, however, to attempt to investigate which biochemical and biophysical processes are *correlated with* higher-level mental functions. The systems approach is, therefore, not opposed to analysis—breaking complex systems down into component parts—as long as the limits of analysis for understanding whole-system behavior are appreciated [34].

Unfortunately, much of contemporary scientific research is characterized by marked disciplinary rigidity and isolation. This situation is particularly tragic in the study of human health and disease since these subjects clearly demand an understanding that transcends disciplinary boundaries. The current scientific disciplines of biophysics, biochemistry, cellular biology, physiology, psychology, sociology, anthropology, and political science roughly correspond to each of the levels of the hierarchy. The systems approach attempts to bridge and unify, not replace, these levels of study. However, since each discipline requires specialized methods of inquiry and a scientific notation appropriate for its level, it makes no sense to say that the social sciences are less scientific than the biological sciences. The difference between the so-called hard natural sciences and soft social sciences can be attributed largely to the different levels of the hierarchy that each deals with.

Many complex problems, particularly in the health field, involve multiple levels and, therefore, demand multidisciplinary investigation. For example, in examining the efficacy of traditional healing practices, a complete research strategy would include not only pharmacological analyses of the herbs used by native healers but also an assessment of the sociocultural context within which the healers live and practice [21].

Research aimed at the hierarchical levels of the person, family, community, or ecosystem are not meant to replace basic biomedical research. Rather, studies in these areas are likely to stimulate biomedical research as attempts are made to correlate behavior at higher hierarchical levels with changes at the physiological and biochemical levels [35].

The systems approach can provide a framework and language

to facilitate communication across disciplines. It illustrates how the various disciplines can complement one another in addressing complex, multilevel problems such as ecological, sociopolitical, psychosomatic, and ethical questions. Issues concerning human health, because they span the entire hierarchy, can also stimulate information flow between the disciplines and promote a unification of the human and physical sciences. Again, the systems view, while not necessarily providing the answers to the complex problems of human health and disease, can at least provide a useful way of asking the appropriate questions.

REFERENCES

1. E. Laszlo, *The Systems View of the World* (New York: Braziller, 1972).
2. L. von Bertallanfy, *General Systems Theory* (New York: Braziller, 1968).
3. C. W. Churchman, *The Systems Approach* (New York: Delta, 1968).
4. H. Brody, "The Systems View of Man: Implications for Medicine, Science, and Ethics," *Perspectives in Biology and Medicine* 17 (1973):71–92.
5. H. L. Blum, *Expanding Health Care Horizons* (Oakland, Cal.: Third Party Associates, 1976).
6. A. Sheldon, "Toward a General Theory of Disease and Medical Care," In *Systems and Medical Care,* eds. A. Sheldon, F. Baker, and C. P. McLaughlin (Cambridge, Mass.: MIT Press, 1970), pp. 84–125.
7. W. Gray, F. J. Duhl, and N. D. Rizzo, eds., *General Systems Theory and Psychiatry* (Boston: Little, Brown, 1969).
8. W. Buckley, ed., *Modern Systems Research for the Behavioral Scientist* (Chicago, Aldine, 1968).
9. George Engel, "The Need for a New Medical Model: A Challenge for Biomedicine," *Science* 196 (1977):129–36.
10. James Miller, *Living Systems* (New York: McGraw Hill, 1977).
11. Paul A. Weiss, "The Living System: Determinism Stratified," in *Beyond Reductionism: New Perspectives in the Life Sciences,* ed. A. Koestler and J. R. Smythies (Boston: Beacon Press, 1969).

12. N. Wiener, *The Human Use of Human Beings: Cybernetics and Society* (Garden City, N.Y.: Doubleday Anchor, 1954).
13. William Schlenger, "A New Framework for Health," *Inquiry* 13 (1976):207–14.
14. René Dubos, *Man Adapting* (New Haven: Yale University Press, 1965).
15. J. R. Audy, "Measurement and Diagnosis of Health," in *Environmental: Essays on the Planet as Home,* ed. Paul Shepherd and Daniel McKinley (New York: Houghton Mifflin, 1971).
16. René Dubos, "Health and Creative Adaptation," *Human Nature* 1 (January 1978):74–82.
17. George Engel, "A Unified Concept of Health and Disease," *Perspectives in Biology and Medicine* 3 (1960):459–85.
18. Alvan Feinstein, *Clinical Judgment* (Huntington, New York: Krieger, 1967).
19. Joseph Needham and Lu Gwei-Djen, "Chinese Medicine," in *Medicine and Culture,* ed. F. N. L. Poynter (London: Wellcome Institute of the History of Medicine, 1969), p. 286.
20. R. Hoke, "Promotive Medicine and the Phenomenon of Health," *Archives of Environmental Health* 16 (February 1968):269–78.
21. Arthur Kleinman, Leon Eisenberg, and Byron Good, "Culture, Illness and Care: Clinical Lessons from Anthropological and Cross-Cultural Research," *Annals of Internal Medicine* 88 (1978):251–58.
22. H. Fabrega, *Disease and Social Behavior* (Cambridge, Mass.: MIT Press, 1974).
23. Abraham Maslow, *The Psychology of Science* (Chicago: Henry Regnery, 1969).
24. O. Carl Simonton and Stephanie Simonton, "Belief Systems and Management of the Emotional Aspects of Malignancy," *Journal of Transpersonal Psychology,* 7 (1975):29–47.
25. E. J. Cassell, *The Healer's Art* (Philadelphia: Lippincott, 1976).
26. A. S. Akiskal, and W. T. McKinney, "Depressive Disorders: Toward a Unified Hypothesis," *Science* 182 (1973):20–29.
27. John B. McKinlay, "A Case for Refocussing Upstream: The Political Economy of Illness," in *Applying Behavioral Science to Cardiovascular Disease,* Proceedings of an American Heart Association conference, Seattle, Washington, June 17–19, 1974.
28. Tapani Purola, "A Systems Approach to Health and Health Policy," *Medical Care* 10 (1972):373–79.
29. William Ryan, *Blaming the Victim* (New York: Vintage, 1971).

30. Robert Crawford, "You Are Dangerous to Your Health," *International Journal of Health Services,* 7 (1977):663–80.

31. H. L. Evans, and B. Weiss, "Behavioral Toxicology," in *Contemporary Research in Behavioral Pharmacology,* ed. D. J. Sanger and D. E. Blackman (New York: Plenum, 1978).

32. Donald Heyneman, "Mis-aid to the Third World: Disease Repercussions Caused by Ecological Ignorance," *Canadian Journal of Public Health* 62 (1971):303–13.

33. Thomas McKeown, *The Role of Medicine* (London: Nuffield Provincial Hospitals Trust, 1976).

34. A. Koestler and J. R. Smythies, eds., *Beyond Reductionism: New Perspectives in the Life Sciences* (Boston: Beacon Press, 1969).

35. S. Kiritz, and R. H. Moos, "Physiological Effects of Social Environments," *Psychosomatic Medicine* 36 (1974):96–114.

PART TWO

ANCIENT SYSTEMS OF MEDICINE

Introduction

> I declare, however, that we ought not to reject the ancient
> art as non-existent, or on the ground that its method of
> inquiry is faulty, just because it has not attained exactness
> in every detail, but much rather, because it has been able
> by reasoning to rise from deep ignorance to approximately
> perfect accuracy, I think we ought to admire the discoveries
> as the work, not of chance, but of inquiry rightly and cor-
> rectly conducted.
>
> Hippocrates, *Ancient Medicine*

The ancient and traditional systems of medicine are not embryonic forms of Western medicine. Instead, they have followed their
own evolution along separate lines. The result is different em-
phases and specializations. The history of medicine is far from a
linear, cumulative process that culminated in the development
of Western scientific medicine. Rather, the evolution of medical
theory and practice has followed a tortuous course with many
branch points and many avenues bypassed often because of personal, political, economic, and cultural influences. Indeed, the
history of medicine is as much the history of the loss of ideas as it
is the development of ideas.

Unfortunately the predominant understanding of ancient systems of healing has been marked by extreme ethnocentrism and
misinformation. Some believe that any writings with a publication date prior to 1970 are automatically outdated. Most assume
that contemporary medicine now incorporates all that was of

value in ancient medicine, the rest being a collection of superstition, primitive thinking, and ineffective ritualistic behavior. Not a few medical historians have been concerned primarily with identifying in the ancient systems the precursors of modern practice. Much of medical anthropology has been preoccupied with aiding "primitive" societies to adopt Western medicine. Our concerns here, however, are quite different. The selected essays in this section on Navaho, Chinese, and Hippocratic medicine draw attention to techniques and perspectives neglected in Western scientific medicine. The focus is on what we can learn from ancient medicine that can complement and extend our contemporary understanding of health and disease.

As we have seen, Western scientific medicine is largely concerned with objective, nonpersonal, physicochemical explanations of *disease* as well as its technical control. In contrast, many traditional systems of healing are centered on the phenomenon of *illness,* namely, the personal and social experience of disease. Therefore, traditional healing techniques are aimed principally at providing meaningful and understandable explanations of the illness experience. Furthermore, since the symptoms of an individual are often viewed as signs of social disharmony, the treatment is generally applied to the entire social unit in the form of a healing ceremony. The sick individual is not isolated from family and friends; instead social support is mobilized to reintegrate the individual and reinforce the cultural beliefs and values. The medium of this healing process is symbolic, mediating between the individual and social group and bridging physiological processes and cultural events. Where Western scientific medicine focuses on *curing the disease,* traditional medicine aims primarily at *healing the illness*—that is, managing the individual and social response to disease.

In any discussion of traditional healing, one question always arises: Do traditional healing practices actually work? Unfortunately there are few objective studies of the therapeutic success of traditional healers (or of Western physicians, for that matter). With regard to traditional healing, it is clear that any evaluation of efficacy must include not only objective criteria of symptom relief and curing, but also the degree to which the illness experience is shaped, managed, and made personally and socially meaningful. Criteria of efficacy, therefore, are determined, in part, by the particular values of the culture. Perhaps this is best illustrated by the story of a Navaho patient who was treated surgically for gall bladder disease, pronounced cured, and sent home. The patient, however, then insisted on having a healing ceremony to treat the "real" causes of the disease that were not touched by the surgeon's blade. In the extreme, healing may be viewed as successful in a given society even if the patient is not cured, even if the patient dies, as long as the illness is made meaningful. Death is not necessarily a failure if one dies with dignity and meaning. Indeed, much of the criticism of modern medicine comes not from its failure to cure, but from its failure to heal— that is, its neglect of the human reality of medicine. A complete approach to human health includes both the effective control of disease and an attempt to manage the individual and social response to disease.

It will not be possible in this book to represent all the varieties of traditional healing systems. In Part Three Jerome Frank will discuss the common psychosocial features underlying shamanistic practices and religious healing. In this part Donald Sandner, a Jungian psychiatrist, examines the symbolic healing system of the Navaho, the largest surviving Indian tribe in North America. In complex healing ceremonies, called chants or sings, the Navaho medicine men involve patients and tribal members in intensive symbolic dramas portrayed in chants, myths, and sandpaintings. To catch even a glimpse of the significance, meaning, and power of these ceremonies, one must have some understanding of the rich symbolic system that structures the Navaho's experience of the world. For example, the Leightons have noted that to an outsider the dawn landscape after a Navaho healing ceremony is made up of mountains, yellow pines, and a cloudless sky. But, to the Navaho, the sage-covered earth is Changing Woman, one of the most benevolent gods who grows old and young again with the cycle of the seasons. The rising sun is himself a god who with Changing Woman produced a warrior that rid the earth of most of its evil forces. So to the North, South, East, and West the Navaho can see the homes of other deities.

These symbols depend upon a complex interlocking system of meanings specific to Navaho culture and, therefore, cannot be transferred across cultures like universally active pharmacologic agents. We cannot usefully adopt the sandpaintings, chants, or rituals of the Navaho medicine man, but, as Sandner suggests, we may be able to understand the basic principles and mechanisms at work in symbolic healing. Sandner identifies and illustrates four basic patterns of symbolic healing in the Navaho chantways and sandpaintings: (1) return to origins, (2) management of evil, (3) death and rebirth, and (4) restoration of a stable universe. Such thematic patterns may be common to other forms of traditional healing and may permit a theoretical linking with modern forms of psychotherapy. The result may be an enriched appreciation of symbolic healing as a complement to more technical medical interventions.

In the West there has recently been a great surge of interest in traditional Chinese medicine, an interest largely sparked by renewed political contacts with the People's Republic of China. Much of this curiosity centers on the exciting innovations in public health and health care developed in China, some of which combine traditional and modern medicine. Attention has also turned to acupuncture with many theories (psychogenic, neurogenic, immunological, etc.) being advanced to rationalize the ancient technique in terms of Western scientific medicine.

But what of the ancient Chinese medical theories themselves? These have been largely ignored or dismissed as historical curiosities, archaic nonsense, metaphysical or nonscientific speculations. Even from a reading of the writers in the West who are sympathetic to traditional Chinese doctrines, one gains little more than the impression that the ancient Chinese had some rather unusual ideas about the human body. In modern China itself there has been little real effort to integrate traditional Chinese and Western scientific medicine beyond a pragmatic mixing of techniques and practitioners.

There is, however, another approach. Manfred Porkert, a professor of Chinese studies in Munich, has made an extensive study of traditional Chinese medicine, science, philosophy, and language. His conclusions can be summarized as follows: the techniques and practices of traditional Chinese medicine are best viewed within the context and terminology of ancient Chinese medical theory; this theory, in its purist form, represents a logical, consistent, and rational framework for an effective healing science *complementary* to Western medical science. Admittedly a minority position, this viewpoint nevertheless deserves serious consideration both because of the strength of Porkert's arguments and the enormous importance of the view if it is correct.

The examination of traditional Chinese medicine poses many problems. First, the current practice of Chinese medicine is, almost without exception, based upon a poorly understood conceptual framework that has degenerated over the centuries to empiricism. To gain any insight into traditional Chinese medical theory, one must refer to ancient texts written when Chinese medicine was at its height. Attempting to evaluate Chinese medicine on the basis of current interpretations or practices is like trying to judge Western scientific medicine solely by referring to the popularized medical accounts in *Reader's Digest*. The second major difficulty is that the concepts of traditional Chinese medicine cannot be translated into Western medical terms without the loss of meaning. Chinese medicine is based upon a different, yet complementary mode of thinking that demands its own system of notation. Whereas Western scientific medicine employs a linear, sequential, and causal mode of cognition to analyze the material and somatic aspects of the human body, traditional Chinese medicine relies upon an "inductive and synthetic" mode of cognition for examining the simultaneous, dynamic, and functional relationships of the individual organism and the larger macrocosmic environment.* An appreciation of the fundamental difference and mutual exclusiveness of these two modes of perception is essential to any real consideration of the value and potential contribution of traditional Chinese medicine.

* It is interesting to note that recent research on the two cerebral hemispheres of the brain suggests that the human brain is specialized in two complementary and mutually exclusive modes of cognitive functioning. The left hemisphere operates in a more linear, sequential and analytic manner concentrating on component parts. The right hemisphere functions in a more nonlinear, simultaneous, and holistic mode concentrating on whole patterns.

Because Western scientific medicine is largely interested in analysis of material phenomena, it has developed a system of conventional standards for measuring and comparing *quantities* (centimeters-grams-seconds). In contrast, Chinese medicine is primarily concerned with functional relationships, and it has developed another system of conventional standards to allow comparison of various *energetic qualities* (hence, the Chinese system of correspondences of yin and yang and the Five Evolutive Phases of Earth, Air, Water, Fire, and Metal).

These fundamental differences make it undesirable, if not impossible, to translate the ancient Chinese medical terms into the analytic terms of Western science. Therefore, Porkert has undertaken the task of creating a new terminology in English that approximates more closely the technical Chinese medical terms. For example, *tsang* is often translated as "organ" or "viscera." However, this is inappropriate, for it connotes an anatomical structure while the Chinese are referring more to a sphere of activity or cyclical functional pattern. To clarify this meaning, Porkert uses the term "orb." Similarly, the Chinese term *kan* does not mean "liver," as it is usually translated, but is associated with a specific orb of functions that in the Chinese system corresponds to certain colors, seasons, directions, emotions, foods, times of day, and only loosely to any of the organs described in Western medicine. The imagery of these functional orbs (orbisiconography) is, therefore, according to Porkert not a crude or naïve Chinese portrayal of anatomy but a sophisticated and logically consistent way of ordering certain empirical observations about the function (though not necessarily the structure) of the human system. Similarly, the Chinese have developed sinarteriology to describe their observation that certain sensitive points on the skin are able to influence the functioning of the orbs. The sinarteries, or energetic conducts, however, were never intended to be viewed as anatomical structures, like arteries or veins; they are conceptual devices for remembering certain functional relationships.

Porkert maintains that this complex theoretical system is of more than academic interest. It provides a rational, although not analytic, basis for diagnosis and effective therapy. He claims that, because of its methods and cognitive mode, Western scientific medicine is specialized to deal better with acute diseases, organic changes, and diseases caused by physical agents. On the other hand, the strength of traditional Chinese medicine lies in the diagnosis and treatment of preorganic, functional disruptions and diseases due to cosmological and climatic changes.

Such therapeutic claims must be tested, but, to be fair, they should be evaluated with reference to the most sophisticated use of traditional Chinese medical theory, not its current popularizations. In focusing solely on a few techniques or remedies of Chinese medicine, we may lose the opportunity to explore another approach to health and healing that complements Western scientific medicine. The article by Porkert will require more than a single reading. It will take many of the readers into the unfamiliar waters of medical philosophy and epistemology as well as the complexities of traditional Chinese medical theory. The article is an invitation to consider another way of viewing the world and another system of describing observations of the world. It also gives a brief glimpse of the problems and promise of integrating Western scientific and traditional Chinese medicine.

The problems of translating ancient medical texts alluded to above can be illustrated by reference to the Chinese classic *Huang Ti Nei Ching,* which was written and revised sometime between 450 and 100 B.C. but refers to medical practices dating from the third century B.C. Even translating the title of the work is problematic. It is variously rendered as "The Yellow Emperor's Classic of Internal Medicine," "The Yellow Emperor's Manual of Corporeal Medicine," and "The Inner Classic of the Yellow Sovereign." Interestingly, the term "yellow" has nothing to do with skin color; in traditional Chinese thought, yellow corresponds to the idea of centrality or majesty. Comparing passages from the *Nei Ching,* one translated into French and one into English, can be very disconcerting. For example, what in the French appears as "How should one look after the patient?" is translated in English as "How can one prepare soup?" and the French version of "examination of the patient" corresponds with the English "rules of death."*

Unfortunately there is not yet available an English translation

---

* See Guido Majno, *The Healing Hand* (Cambridge, Mass.: Harvard University Press, 1976).

of the *Nei Ching* that meets the stringent criteria oulined by
Porkert. However, we can taste something of the flavor of ancient Chinese medicine from a translation prepared in 1949 by
Ilza Veith, a medical historian. She describes her work as "a rough
translation . . . [by means of which] it would be possible to find
passages which warrant more detailed and careful translation."
The portion of the *Nei Ching* that she has translated consists of
a dialogue between the Emperor Huang Ti and his Prime Minister Ch'i Po, who is quite well versed in the Chinese medical
theory of his day.

I have selected passages from this translation to illustrate the
microcosm-macrocosm theory of Chinese medicine in which the
human body reflects the same patterns of organization as the societal, natural, and cosmic levels. Here we also learn of the ancient
art of pulse diagnosis and different methods of treatment including acupuncture, moxabustion, herbs, breathing exercises, calisthenics, and massage. The preventive focus of traditional Chinese
medicine is clearly in evidence, as is the importance of living in
harmony with the natural order. From these brief extracts we can
gain some sense of the attitude of Chinese medicine, an attitude
finding increasing currency among those interested in re-examin-
ing ancient ways of health and healing.

Next we turn to Hippocratic medicine, which is generally considered the historical precursor of Western scientific medicine.
Perhaps even more striking than the similarities between contemporary Western medicine and its Greek ancestor, are the
marked differences in orientation and the loss of certain valuable
Hippocratic perspectives through the intervening centuries.

Hippocratic medicine was concerned fundamentally with man
in nature (*physis*). Health was to be achieved by living with nature, not fighting it. Disease was viewed in the context of a disturbed relationship between man and the environment. The
physician's task was to support the healing efforts of nature, to
study the effects of environmental forces (airs, waters, places) on
human health, and to teach regimens of personal hygiene that
would strengthen the constitution of the individual. The predominant attitude of humility—"to help or at least do no harm"
—also contrasts sharply with the therapeutic exuberance of our
day.

To illustrate the perspectives outlined above, I have selected some passages from the *Works of Hippocrates,* a collection of writings by various authors and, some say, schools of Greek medicine during the fifth to second centuries B.C. The extracts are not intended to be representative of the whole spectrum of Hippocratic thought and practice; they have been chosen instead to highlight certain perspectives that may have relevance for our contemporary health effort.

This relevance is discussed by René Dubos in the essay that follows entitled "Hippocrates in Modern Dress." Dubos contrasts the environmental approach of Hippocratic medicine with the current medical focus on analyzing the elementary structures and mechanisms of the organism's internal environment. He suggests not a return to Hippocratic practices but a resurgence of the Hippocratic perspective within contemporary medical science. Some examples of this modern ecological view of health will be presented in the last section of the book.

By Donald F. Sandner

Navaho Indian Medicine and Medicine Men

The Navaho Indians are a tribe of well over a hundred thousand members living in or around their reservation in northeastern Arizona and northwestern New Mexico. Their land, though spectacularly beautiful, is part of a high plateau which is arid and highly eroded. They migrated here from the north during the fifteenth and sixteenth centuries, and in spite of the hardships of the environment and the opposition of Indian and non-Indian peoples around them, they have prospered and increased, especially during the last decades. They are now by far the largest, cohesive, actively functioning Indian tribe in North America; part of their success is due to the vitality of their religion, which is still flourishing and still gives unity to their tribe.

Gladys Reichard, a lifelong student of Navaho religion, summed it up: "The Navaho religion must be considered a design in harmony, a striving for rapport between man and every phase of nature, the earth and the waters under the earth, and the sky and the land beyond the sky, and of course the earth and everything on and in it."[1] She also said: "Navaho dogma connects all things, natural and experienced, from man's skeleton to universal destiny, which encompasses even inconceivable space, in a closely interlocked unity which omits nothing, no matter how small or stupendous, and in which each individual has a significant function until at his final dissolution, he not only becomes one with the ultimate harmony, but he *is* that harmony."[2]

The harmony of which she speaks is the core and essence of the

Navaho system of healing. In the past it has been pursued with unremitting vigor, not only by the medicine men but also by the ordinary Navaho man and woman. There is also "evil" or disharmony that threatens the normal balance of nature, causing disease and misfortune. This "evil" must be controlled or banished and goodness restored. To implement this desired state of affairs, the Navahos have created a great body of symbolic rituals called chants or sings. These ceremonies attempt to placate or expel the destructive powers and attract the good, helpful ones. By doing this they reestablish the basic harmony, cure individual illness, and bring general blessing to the tribe. All religious energy, except for minor hunting, blessing and warfare rites, is directed to this purpose. The Navahos do not have an annual round of festivals and communal ceremonies to promote the growth of crops, bring sufficient rainfall, and provide general community benefits as, for instance, their neighbors the Pueblos do. These desirable things are mentioned in the songs and prayers, but essentially all ceremonies are performed for the *individual* who feels the need, consults his family, summons the medicine man, sets the date, and pays the fee. Though hundreds of people may attend chant ceremonials given by well-known medicine men and receive side benefits, it is the individual patient, not the community, who is at the center of this unique religion.

The Navahos were originally organized as nomadic bands without strong, central leadership, so the medicine men were the main carriers of culture and highly influential spokesmen for the group. In recent times their exclusive functions have been eroded by modern medicine, the Christian religions, and the Native American Church, but in spite of such formidable opposition there is still a large body of medicine men practicing in a way that has changed little since it was first described in the late nineteenth century by the father of Navaho religious studies, Washington Matthews.[3]

The material used in this paper is based on such ethnographic works and on personal interviews with individual Navaho medicine men (from 1968 on) to determine their professional attitudes and concerns about what they do. Besides giving a brief description of the Navaho system of healing, I will explore from the viewpoint of its practitioners how it functions dynamically to produce results that are in *some* ways more satisfactory than ours. Further on in this paper I will try to demonstrate the structure and thematic patterns of such a system using the Navaho religion as a basic model. The purpose of my studies and field work has never been to uncover more ethnographic information but to understand and experience a symbolic healing system in theory and active, clinical practice.

MEDICINE MEN

The Navaho medicine man is remarkable in that in him the functions of priest and doctor exactly coincide. In the old days he was the only personage of the tribe to perform religious ceremonies. These were the chants and sings that are still performed today. Each requires so much in the way of knowledge, special equipment, and the exact memorization of songs, prayers, and sandpaintings that a single medicine man usually learns only a few thoroughly in his lifetime. The amount of knowledge required has been compared to that expected of a modern graduate student for his master's degree. Blessingway, a short two-day ceremony, is the cornerstone of the whole ceremonial system.[4] It lends its prayers and myths to all the other chants and controls the meaning and purpose of the whole. Stemming from Blessingway there are three major divisions of the chantway system: Holyway, Evilway (or Ghostway), and Lifeway. Holyway chants attract the good powers to cure illness and repair malfunctions; Evilway banishes the effects of evil things such as witches, ghosts, and foreigners; and Lifeway is specific for physical injuries and accidents. In these three categories there are about twenty-six distinct ceremonial complexes, but only about ten of these are given at the present time.[5]

Most of the medicine men I met were quite old, several in their seventies and eighties, but still in active practice. When I interviewed Denet Tsosi, who was over eighty, he was just returning from an all-night sing, but without any great fatigue he spent the whole morning answering questions. He had begun learning chant practice in his early teens from his brother, Red Mustache. He followed his brother around watching him perform the Male Shooting Chant, and after about eight years he felt he could do it himself. He also had the ceremony sung over himself as the patient four times and paid for it each time.

Alan George on the other hand did not start learning to be a chanter until he was close to fifty. He said he started to learn then because the chant had helped him twice, once as a child when he had been gored by a goat, and once as an adult when he strained his back lifting heavy logs. He said: "I was treated by the medicine man with chants and herbs, and I got better.... I got interested in learning about the chants. I got a feeling about the chants that if nobody knows and learns it, it will die out. I came back then and joined the people to become a medicine man. Later the doctors, hospitals, and clinics came. I respect that, I hold nothing against that, but I still feel that my medicine should be kept up." It took him three years to learn the Night Chant from his instructor, whom he supported during that time with gifts and livestock. His instructor was a clan father to him.

Another important chanter, Natani Tso, said that his instructor was not a relative but "ever since we knew that same chant and performed it, we have been close friends." It took two years of study to learn the Big Star Chant, and he turned the first proceeds over to his instructor. He said it was not hard to learn. "If you're interested in the songs and chants, it comes to you naturally."

This then was the general pattern: the instructor was usually a relative or fellow clan member, but sometimes only a friend. There usually was a close bond between the two men, master and pupil, unless something went wrong (as in one case I observed) and the teaching was broken off. Then the teacher might feel that the student had not completed his training and would not give public approval of his right to practice. There might be considerable enmity between the two. To learn any of the major chants required several years of effort, and payment for the teaching was made in livestock, food, and lodging or the proceeds from the first performances.

There was general agreement that the main qualifications for a prospective medicine man were interest and patience. Natani

Tso said: "He has to have interest. He must not be too lazy. He's got to have patience. If he gets easily discouraged there's no use starting. Young men when they are drunk often ask me what a particular song or prayer means, but there is no use telling them. Their minds are not clear. You really have to be interested to learn the chants." Asked whether medicine men need a special dream or vision, he answered: "It is not necessary to have a vision or a dream. He just has to want to learn." With this the other medicine men were in unanimous agreement; it is knowledge that makes a good chanter, not special visionary or mystical gifts.

Diagnosis, as the Navaho medicine man conceives it, is usually directed toward special causes, not symptoms. It is often done by a hand trembler or stargazer. These persons, often called diagnosticians, do not have special knowledge or training, but they *do* go into a trance to determine what is wrong with the patient and what should be done about it. They never perform the therapy; they are in a different category than the medicine men and do not enjoy the same status and professional dignity. Their ability comes spontaneously, and no learning is involved. Their rite is very short, lasting less than an hour. They sit beside the patient and go into a trance. Then their hand of its own accord starts to shake and tremble. It may seem to point at certain parts of the patient's body. One hand trembler said: "The corn pollen in the hand trembling ceremony is an offering to Gila Monster (the medicine man's special animal). I put the pollen down my arm with two branches to the thumb and forefinger like Gila Monster. I start praying, then singing. Then I work my mind very hard. Then I notice shocks running through my fingers. My hand starts shaking and away I go." When asked how he made the diagnosis, he said: "That depends on what sign your hand is making. I work my mind. I wonder what my hand is referring to. It shakes, sometimes at the patient, sometimes at the ground, until I guess the right answer with my mind. When that is done, it stops shaking."

Some of the chants have definite, rational indications. For instance, in past times the Flint Way (a Lifeway Chant) was performed for persons who had suffered injury or accident. One medicine man who still knew this chant, recalled something about it:

"Sometimes a man breaks an arm or leg and may have a broken bone sticking out of the flesh. You can't go in and set it without preparations. You have to use the ceremony. You have to have herbs to bathe the injury. While you or your assistant sings the songs you begin to set the bone. You have to do it properly, it's a delicate thing to do."

For most other chants the indications are based on more mythological ideas of etiology. Animals such as the bear, deer, coyote, porcupine, eagle, and snake may cause disease by contact, or infection, from the power they carry. Dreams, lightning, thunder, wind, and other striking phenomena of nature may also be etiological agents. In another class, ghosts and witches, associated with darkness and foreigners, are dangerous. Improper behavior during a ceremony, violation of the taboo against careless handling of a corpse or sexual misconduct (incestuous or with foreigners) causes disease. A pregnant woman subject to any of these influences may pass it on to her fetus, causing illness later in its life.

Natani Tso said: "Several things may affect a person, a very bad headache, maybe crippled or paralyzed limbs. His mouth may be twisted up, or his eyes crossed. These things might happen if a chant gets violated. I look at his eyesight, his breathing, his mouth movements. From these things I can tell if a man needs the ceremony." From such remarks I gained the impression that most of the patients treated in recent times are suffering from psychiatric or psychosomatic types of ailments. Most of the strictly physical illnesses, including broken bones, are likely at present to be sent to the clinic or hospital, even by the medicine men themselves. Denet Tsosi said: "Sometimes Navaho people need treatment in a hospital. In your practice of medicine, there you operate, you cut him with a knife. When he comes back he feels he should have a Life Way to heal the wound. We Navaho would like to have cooperation with white men to help preserve the Navaho traditions. If we hold together, the white man and the Navaho, that is the best for the Navaho people."

Fee setting is discussed ahead of time with the patient and his relatives and is usually a hard-headed, realistic process. No good results can be expected from the ceremony if the fee is not right. Natani Tso said: "There is no standard rate for the Big Star

Chant. If someone comes to me who I know is wealthy, he will offer more than a poor person might. A wealthy person might pay me forty or fifty dollars when a poor person will give beads or a sheep. I'll do the ceremony anyway." Over and above the fee of the medicine man, there is great expense in collecting all the special gifts for those involved in the performance and furnishing food for the entire assembly during the whole period of the chant. The longer chants might involve expenditures of well over a thousand dollars, which is extremely high given the extremely low income of the Navaho. The family and kin of the patient are expected to pitch in and help with the cost as well as the preparation of the food. Great expense, effort, and careful planning are involved, so a ceremony is not undertaken lightly.

When asked if their efforts are successful, the medicine men would often respond with an anecdotal example of a cure they performed (like doctors anywhere). Natani Tso said: "There was a woman from Red Mesa who was in the hospital in Albuquerque. She had a gall bladder operation. After she came home she still wasn't feeling well, but after I did Blessingway for her she felt all right."

Dreams are not part of the ceremony proper, but they are used in a simple, straightforward way as an omen or diagnostic aid. Alan George said: "Dreams are very important, they tell you something that's ahead of you, something that will happen. You whites don't do that, but we Navahos think it's important. For example, if you have a relative or close friend that's dead and you dream about him it's a warning that his ghost is coming back to affect you. Then you need prayers." Blessingway is the most recommended cure for bad dreams.

Confession to the medicine man about the breaking of taboos and other infractions of the rules that govern Navaho life is an informal part of the cure, and something held back or left out was often given as a reason for the chant's lack of success. Or it might be that the patient had been directed to the wrong chant, or had in some way failed to follow the medicine man's instructions. The medicine men (again like doctors anywhere) rarely mentioned the inadequacy of their healing methods as a reason for a failure to cure.

Speaking now in general, it is important to recognize that

Navaho medicine men are not true shamans as they are (or were) found in many parts of North and South America, Siberia, and elsewhere. These shamans, as described by Mircea Eliade,[6] operate in the following way: "first an appeal to the auxiliary spirits, which, more often than not, are those of animals and a dialogue with them in a secret language; secondly, drum-playing and a dance, preparatory to the mystic journey; and thirdly, the trance (real or simulated) during which the shaman's soul is believed to have left his body."[7] The Navaho medicine man, except for the drumming on an inverted basket that accompanies his songs, does none of these things. These events—ascending or descending into other worlds; talking to supernaturals, both men and animals, sometimes in a special language; initiation by these supernaturals through many ordeals into secret healing powers; and the return to earth bringing these powers back for the benefit of the people—*are all incorporated in the action of the prayers, rites, myths, and sandpaintings.* The scenario that the true shaman acts out in his person is projected by the Navaho medicine man into the contents of his rituals. He needs no special trance, ecstatic vision, or mystic vocation to enter the role of healer, only the desire and practice to learn the vast amount of symbolic material. He has no guardian spirit or even any special connection with the Holy People, only the ability to manipulate power symbolically and ritually. This symbolic healing complex, fully exemplified by the Navaho, could be called "symbolic shamanism."

There are, on the other hand, several ways in which the Navaho medicine man's professional attitudes and practices are similar to those of a modern psychotherapist. The medicine man puts his reliance on knowledge, not trance phenomena or magical effects. His bearing is restrained and dignified, and for the most part he is a stable, dependable person. He can be fatherly and kind, but he is also shrewd and careful. He must undergo a long period of apprenticeship, and he must pay for his training. He must also be the patient in his chosen chant, preferably four times. He takes a position of surrogate parent toward the patient and often hears his confession and gives him advice. Medicine men do not like to treat their own relatives, although there are instances of it being done. They charge a considerable fee without which the cure cannot be expected to succeed, but the fee is often scaled down to the patient's means. The medicine men seldom refuse to meet an urgent summons. They are held in special regard by the rest of the community, but if they behave in an unexpected or suspicious way, they may be feared and condemned rather than respected and esteemed.

These similarities are not accidental. They define the position of the therapist to the patient in symbolic procedures that will render him vulnerable to intense, inner forces. This is, in effect, a swiftly induced transference situation in which both patient and medicine man are intimately involved. The medicine man must lead, and the patient follow, into a confrontation with dangerous as well as curative imagery. The effect is expected to be forceful, impressive, and transforming.

STRUCTURE OF SYMBOLIC HEALING

How does this effect occur? In the chants, several kinds of healing operate simultaneously. Of these the physical, or physiological, is the least important. There is, as a previous quote from one of the medicine men shows, manipulation of injuries and wounds, and due attention is paid to the physical care of the patient. The herbal remedies used may contain some physiologically active ingredients, and the sweat baths and hot applications have physiotherapeutic effects, but these elements comprise only a minor part of the chant therapy.

There is also a strong psychosocial effect produced by the gathering of friends, relatives, and acquaintances, and even persons barely known to the patient to observe and provide moral support during the chant performance. On the other hand, a chant, especially a shorter one, may be given with only one or two family members present, and very little in the way of social amenity. Nevertheless the chant ceremony is a communal effort, and many persons who know the patient, whether they are present or not, will *expect* that the patient will benefit from it. This vivid expectation (or suggestion) is reiterated again and again in the prayers and songs.

But the most prominent feature of the chant ceremony, the

one given first place by the medicine men, patients, and spectators alike, is the *symbolic form* of the chant ceremony, a complex of songs, prayers, rituals, and sandpaintings (or drypaintings) lasting from two to nine days and nights and centered around detailed myths of the cultural heroes and heroines, who have made mythical journeys to the homes of the gods and acquired there, after many ordeals, healing powers to be brought back for general use. These are regarded as the effective ingredients and are given most attention when the ceremony is being planned. An extra prayer or sandpainting may require a higher fee. In order to understand how these forms enter (or create) the chant structure, it is helpful to consider a sequence of stages through which the chant progresses. These stages blend into one another, and more than one may be operative at the same time, but mostly they are cumulative and provide a basis for comparison with healing rites from other cultures.

The first stage is *purification,* in which the patient and the medicine man are cleansed or exorcized of evil or malignant influences. This is done by fasting, sweating, emesis, sexual continence, bathing and shampooing the hair, and vigil.[8] This produces an open psychic state or condition of emptiness in preparation for the next stages.

The second stage is one of *evocation.* Invocatory rituals such as song sequences sung in a certain fixed order, often to the accompaniment of drumming on an inverted basket, the setting out of painted and ritually prepared prayer sticks, and the offering of jewels (precious stones) and reeds stuffed with wild tobacco are all designed to compel the holy powers to attend the ceremony. Later comes the making and blessing of elaborate sandpaintings and the symbolic use of their power to strengthen and cure the patient. The paintings are made of colored rock and sand collected by the medicine men themselves and released in a carefully controlled trickle from between thumb and forefinger onto the sand-covered floor of the ceremonial hogan (the traditional Navaho six-sided house made of logs and mud mortar, facing east). Sometimes for special ceremonies only organic materials such as pollen, flower petals, and charcoal are used and spread on buckskin. It is a difficult skill that takes much practice to master, but it produces beautiful visual and symbolic designs depicting supernatural animals, heroes and deities from the myths, events in the miraculous history of the Navaho People, powerful forces of nature such as winds, stars, thunders, and much else. After it is completed, which may take from four to eight hours, it is blessed and the power of the gods enters into it. The third and fourth stages, *identification* and *transformation*, now follow close upon one another and are expressed in the songs, prayers, and rites held over the completed sandpaintings (to be described later). In all these ways the patient is brought by the medicine man into psychic union (identification) with the evoked powers. Then the transformation (freedom from disease and disharmony) expected from these powers is described in the prayers and songs in great detail.

The final stage is one of *release,* in which the power built up and used for the patient's benefit must again be disbursed harmlessly to its natural origin. The patient may be given a bead token or head plume for remembrance. For some chants long dances are held on the last night. An all-night sing summarizing and focusing all the events of the preceding days brings the ceremonies to a close. The patient must observe some special restrictions for several days after the sing before he is finally released.

Using Matthews's classic description of the Night Chant[9] (which is often given for diseases of the head—blindness, deafness, or insanity) I will give a brief illustration of how these stages occur in the progress of a specific chant. The first four days and nights (the new day for the Navaho begins at sundown) are devoted largely to stages one and two. On the first night there is a consecration of the hogan; the chanter, moving sunwise around the hogan, rubs sacred cornmeal on the four main supporting timbers. Then a rite of exorcism (purification) is held in which assistants of the medicine man dressed as gods and called god impersonators come into the hogan, touch the patient with closed rings of bent sumac, and then quickly open them. This symbolically releases the patient from his illness, which is thought to be blown away like the wind. The god impersonators utter cries and perform characteristic motions to heighten the effect.

As part of the purification on the first four mornings, a sweat bath ritual is held. Water is thrown on heated stones in a small, specially built sweat lodge. The patient is massaged vigorously by the god impersonators and given cold medicinal infusions to drink. Then he is rubbed with a specially prepared lotion.

On the second night the patient is dressed in evergreen branches symbolizing the constrictions which hold him prisoner. Men impersonating the Navaho warrior twins come in brandishing knives and cut him loose with loud cries. On the fourth night a mask placed over the patient's head is sprung free by the action of a young tree planted in the center of the hogan and bent over to hook under the mask. By the end of the fourth day the purifying rites are nearly complete.

Rites of evocation are going on at the same time. On the first four mornings particular sets of *kethawns*—prayersticks prepared for a certain deity and then set out to invite (or compel) him to attend the ceremony—are made. They are blessed with song and prayer. Painted reeds, called cigarettes, are made and filled with native tobacco. These are sealed with moistened pollen and figuratively lit at one end by sunlight passed through a piece of rock crystal. These sacred objects are placed in the patient's hands and sanctified with long prayers calling the deities' attention to the offering being made for him and describing what is expected of him in return:

> I have made your sacrifice.
> I have prepared a smoke for you.
> My feet restore for me.
> My legs restore for me.
> My body restore for me.
> My mind restore for me.
> My voice restore for me.
> Today take out your spell for me
> Today your spell for me is removed.
> Away from me you have taken it.
> Far off you have done it.
> Today I shall recover.[10]

Then the sacred objects are set out and songs are sung in the hogan that imply the gods have heard and are on the way. On the

fourth night a special evocatory ceremony is held in which masks
of the gods are "brought to life" by feeding them sacred gruel
and shaking them.

Only a small part of the many rites, prayers, and songs of the
Night Chant can even be mentioned here, but as this sample
suggests, by the end of the first four days and nights the patient
has been well purified, or emptied of evil power, and a great concentration of healing power has been made ready for his use. In
a ritual of the first day featuring a representation in sand of the
four sacred mountains, the process of identification is already
begun. As the patient follows the trail around the mountains the
singer intones:

> In a holy place with a god I walk,
> In a holy place with a god I walk,
> On (the sacred mountain) with a god I walk,
> On a chief mountain with a god I walk,
> In old age wandering with a god I walk,
> On a trail of beauty with a god I walk.[11]

Then, on the way to the sweat house, the patient carrying
twelve plumed wands and led by the singer, the identification
grows more definite:

> This I walk with, this I walk with.
> Now Talking God I walk with.
> These are his feet I walk with.
> These are his limbs I walk with.
> This is his body I walk with.
> This is his mind I walk with.
> This is his voice I walk with.
> These are his twelve plumes I walk with.[12]

The most effective devices to facilitate identification are the
sandpaintings made on the afternoons of the last three or four
days of the ceremony. I will describe the one usually made on the
sixth day, the Whirling Log Sandpainting.[13] This painting com-
memorates the visit of the Dreamer, the hero of the Night Chant,
to the Lake of Whirling Waters. There he saw a giant cross made
of spruce logs floating on the water. The gods were sitting on the

arms of the cross and it was whirling in a sunwise direction. The entire figure made a huge sunwise swastika, and in the Night Chant myth it is associated with the secrets of fertility and healing that were later imparted to the hero.

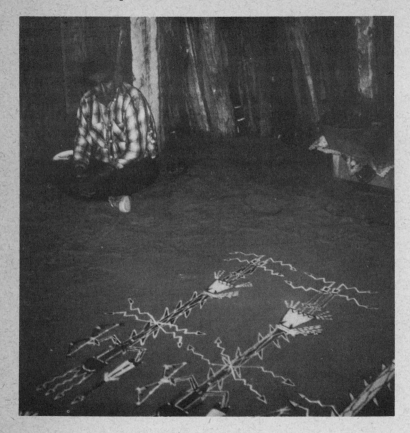

The sandpainting is made on the floor of the hogan, a bowl of water sprinkled with charcoal in the center to symbolize the holy lake. Bars extending in the four cardinal directions are the whirling logs, and on the logs sit eight gods, four male and four female, one pair on each log. Four larger gods standing outside the log circle seem to be whirling the logs around with their wands. Talking God, a kindly guide and benefactor to the

Navaho, is to the east with his white mask, his eagle plume of twelve feathers, and his squirrel-skin pouch. Calling God, a domestic god of fertility and rich harvests, is to the west with his black dress, blue mask, and wand of charcoal. To the north and south, two humpbacked gods dressed as mountain sheep commemorate the first meeting of the Dreamer with the gods. They have blue masks and imitation sheep horns, and their packs are full of seeds. In the semidirections are the four holy plants: white corn, beans, squash, and tobacco. Around the whole is a Rainbow Guardian with an opening to the east.

An event-by-event description of the rite performed on the sandpainting is as follows:

> The sandpainting is finished.
> The medicine man applies cornmeal to the figures on the painting.
> Eight plumed prayer sticks are set up around the painting.
> The medicine man makes a cold, herbal infusion.
> This is placed in between the hands of the Rainbow Guardian.
> He sprinkles pollen on the figures of the gods.
> The patient enters and sprinkles cornmeal on the painting.
> The patient recites a prayer.
> The patient disrobes.
> A god impersonator enters. He sprinkles cold infusion on the painting and offers the patient a sip. He makes a whoop or cry.
> The patient sits on the painting, usually on one of the logs.
> The god impersonator (in other chants it is the medicine man) applies sand from his moistened palms from the body parts of the gods on the painting to the body parts of the patient: feet, hips, chest, shoulders, head. He yells loudly into the patient's ear and leaves.
> The patient gets off the painting and sits elsewhere.

> He is fumigated with water thrown on hot coals.
> The patient leaves.
> The medicine man pulls up the prayer sticks and the
> bowl.
> Spectators trample on the painting, applying sand to
> their bodies.
> The sand is removed and thrown away to the north.[14]

Other sandpaintings made on succeeding afternoons are used in a similar way. The beneficial power is thought to be focused and condensed in the patient; the whole process is brought to a climax on the ninth night. Hundreds of persons may gather for the event. All night long outside the ceremonial hogan, dances are performed by trained teams of singers and dancers. Inside the hogan, songs are sung summarizing and recalling all the preceding rituals.

The public performance of this night begins with the most important ceremony of all, the dance of the Atsalei (or First Dancers). This is performed by Talking God (impersonated) and four male dancers who are identified with thunderbirds. The patient and the medicine man come out of the hogan. The patient sprinkles cornmeal on the dancers, then faces east with the medicine man. They recite the most sacred prayer of invocation. All this time the dancers are swaying from side to side, bending and straightening the left knee. There is perfect silence on the part of everyone present as the medicine man begins the evocation of the dark, male thunderbird. The following is a short excerpt:

> Oh Male God!
> With your moccasins of dark cloud, come to
> us.
> With your leggings of dark cloud, come to us.
> With your shirt of dark cloud, come to us.
> With your head-dress of dark cloud, come to
> us.
> With your mind enveloped in dark cloud,
> come to us.
> With the dark thunder above you, come to us
> soaring.

> With the shaped clouds at your feet, come to
> us soaring.
> With the far darkness of the dark cloud over
> your head, come to us soaring.
> With the far darkness made of the he-rain
> over your head, come to us soaring.
> With the far darkness made of the dark mist
> over your head, come to us soaring.
> With the far darkness made of the she-rain
> over your head, come to us soaring.
> With the zigzag lightning flung on high over
> your head, come to us soaring.
> With the rainbow hanging high over your
> head, come to us soaring.[15]

After further invocation, identification of the patient with the powers of the god, and careful mention of all the sacrifices the patient has made, the desired transformation is described:

> Happily I recover.
> Happily my interior becomes cool.
> Happily my eyes regain their power.
> Happily my head becomes cool.
> Happily my limbs regain their power.
> Happily I hear again.
> Happily for me the spell is taken off.
> Happily I may walk.
> Impervious to pain, I walk.
> Feeling light within, I walk.
> With lively feelings, I walk.

In answer to the outside prayers and dances invoking the gods, the singers within the lodge confirm that the god has heard:

> Above it thunders.
> His thoughts are directed to you,
> He rises toward you.
> Now to your house,
> He approaches for you.
> He arrives for you.

He comes to the door,
He enters for you.
Behind the fireplace
He eats his special dish.
"Your body is strong,
"Your body is holy now," he says.[16]

At the first sign of dawn, the dancers outside the hogan and the singers inside cease their activities. The patient goes outside to inhale the dawn. Special Dawn Songs are sung, and the medicine man gives the benediction. The patient is still overcharged with all the accumulated power, and he must observe special restrictions for at least four more days, also he must not sleep until the next night. The power is gradually released.

BASIC PATTERNS
OF SYMBOLIC HEALING

Within the chant structure, certain basic thematic patterns occur again and again in all of the chants. These are fundamental to the Navaho healing system and may be applicable to other cultures as well. They also make it possible to establish a theoretical connecting link with modern forms of psychotherapy. Four of these basic patterns (there may be others) are as follows: (1) return to the origins, (2) management of evil, (3) death and rebirth, and (4) restoration of a stable universe.

Return to the origins: In Navaho healing, the patient is brought into intimate contact with the orgins of his people and the particular chant being sung for him. As previously mentioned, all of the chants are based on Blessingway, which is concerned with the origin of life on this earth, the placement of the earth, sky, sun and moon, sacred mountains, and vegetation, and the inner forms of all these phenomena. It brings under control the he- and she-rains and establishes the Pollen Path as the Navaho way of blessing and harmony. No disharmony is brought into Blessingway.

One of the drypaintings connected with Blessingway has at its center a black circle symbolizing the hole of Emergence from

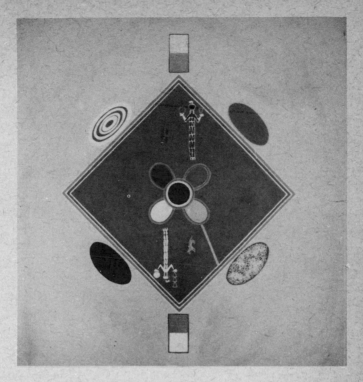

Sandpainting from the Blessingway ceremony
(photo courtesy of the Wheelwright Museum, Santa Fe, New Mexico)

which all gods and creatures entered this world from the lower worlds beneath. Around it are four oval shapes, symbolizing the four underworlds below the present one, positioned as the petals of a flower, each with its characteristic color. These are surrounded by a large blue square indicating the flood that made it necessary to move from one world to the next. A seven-joint reed leading from the yellow oval to the outside indicates the route the people took to escape the flood. There are figures of the Sun and Badger on the eastern part of the painting; Moon and Coyote are on the west. Outside the blue square four oval shapes in the cardinal directions represent the four holy mountains, each with its characteristic color. Also outside the square

are turquoise and white squares symbolizing the houses of Changing Woman and White Shell Woman, two aspects of the great earth mother. When placed in the center of this painting, the patient is brought into relationship with the entire Navaho creation myth.

The body of the chant myths forms an interlocking narrative cycle depicting the evolution of Navaho man. Upward Reaching Way tells the story of his tortuous progress up through the four underworlds; Blessingway tells of the creation of this world and the birth of Changing Woman, who represents the constant renewal of life in nature. The Two Who Came To Their Father tells of the birth and exploits of her sons, Monster Slayer and Child Born of Water. They journey to their father, the Sun, and after surviving terrible ordeals are at last recognized as his sons and given the strength needed to overthrow monsters who are terrorizing the earth. Monster Way tells of the slaying of these monsters and Enemy Way tells of later wars with the neighboring Pueblos. All of the other myths branch off from these and tell how their hero or heroine, after dangerous adventures, visits the homes of the gods and gains from them the myths, rites, and sandpaintings of that particular chant. Through his knowledge of the chant symbolism the medicine man draws the patient into the great, cosmic network of which he is an integral part in body and mind, back to the beginnings of life and consciousness. Through the myths and paintings he becomes a part of the symbolic history of the Navaho people. He has a place in the unity of the whole. Harmony is restored.

Management of evil: The second major principle of Navaho healing is the evocation, manipulation, and banishment of evil, mainly in the form of witchcraft, which is always connected with disease and disharmony. Certain chants specialize in exorcism, but it is found by implication throughout the chant system. The prayers seem to be especially powerful for this purpose. This can be briefly demonstrated by an excerpt from a prayer of exorcism given by Natani Tso, a practitioner of the Big Star Chant to show how he handled evil power. The prayer first evokes the power of Great Snake and all his body parts to form a shield against the power of the witch. Behind that shield the patient and the medicine man are safe, and are then able to direct that power back against the witch himself. Here is a part of that prayer:

> From the bottom of the east the evil thing's power
> [witchcraft] has turned away from me [*repeated*]
> From the bottom of the north the evil thing's power
> [*turned back on him*] has caused him to fall toward
> the north.
> A blood mark is left pointing north. His head points
> north, his eyebrows, eyes, hair, mouth, navel, urine
> stream, hip, knee, and feet point north [the direc-
> tion of evil],
> The earth shakes with his falling; the earth shakes
> with his falling.
> He is taken to the middle of the earth and farther on
> where the earth ends,
> Now he's gone away with the evil power he used him-
> self.
> It has turned on him; it went back inside him.
> It killed him.[17]

The prayer then repeats in several different ways how far away the evil thing and his power have gone. It describes how he is dragged away by red coyote to a dismal underworld place where people don't move. There his evil power is turned to ash and stolen away from him. The medicine man ended this part of the prayer with a loud "Pah!" which symbolized the evil power being blown away. The prayer goes on to tell how the world is restored. It concludes with a prayer of blessing, probably from the Bless-ingway cycle.

In a different prayer published by Gladys Reichard from the Male Shooting Chant[18] the medicine man actually identifies him-self with the evil before he exorcizes it. By carefully controlled incremental repetition, he brings the evil under control and bends it to his will. The Navahos believe that much that is evil can be made good or at least persuaded to cooperate through the use of ritual knowledge, but there is a final, irreducible residue, called *tcindi,* which cannot be accommodated in a harmonious universe and must be banished as rapidly and definitively as possible.

Death and Rebirth: The theme of death and rebirth occurs in the background of nearly all the major chants. In the myth of the Hail Chant,[19] for example, it forms a prominent episode. The hero, Rainboy, is driven away from his home and family because of his excessive gambling. He roams about, living off the countryside until one day he comes upon a house "strung with a rainbow." Upon entering, he finds a beautiful girl who smiles at him enticingly, and finally seduces him. She happens to be the wife of Winter Thunder, one of the most irascible and vindictive of all the forces of nature. Winter Thunder is naturally very angry when he finds out, and he shatters Rainboy with a huge bolt of lightning. After much difficulty he is eventually restored, with the help of Talking God, Calling God, Thunder People, Wind People, ants, bees, Cornbeetle, Pollen Boy, and the great god, Begochidi. The repercussions of this event lead on into the myth and finally, after a great war is waged, results in the taming of Winter Thunder and the ritual control of his power.

The theme of death and rebirth is found not only in the myths. It comes home to the patient in a much more immediate way in the texts of the prayers. In a prayer of invocation and liberation from the Big Star Chant[20] it is the patient, not just the myth hero, who is described as undergoing this transformation. In the beginning of the prayer, Monster Slayer, the great Navaho warrior hero, comes in search of the patient:

> 1. From the center of the earth, Monster Slayer, using his dark staff, comes in search for me;
> With lightning flashing before him, with lightnings flashing behind him, he comes in search for me;
> Using a rock crystal and a talking prayerstick, he comes in search for me.

Further stanzas describe Monster Slayer going down through four layers of mountains, clouds, mists, mosses, and watery domains, past many dangerous guardians, in search of the endangered patient. He finally arrives at the Darkness Hogan:

8. Farther on, he comes in to search for me;
    At that place, in the west corner of the Darkness
        Hogan, behind the Traveler in Darkness,
    Where my feet lie, where my legs lie, where my
        body lies, where my mind lies, where my voice
        lies, where my speech lies, where my power of
        movement lies;
    I came, searching for all these.

Here a part of the patient is identified with Monster Slayer, and "I" is used instead of "he." The rescue continues:

9. "I came searching for you; you and I will begin
        our return, my grandchild.
    We two are now leaving, my grandchild," Monster
        Slayer says to me;
    With the talking prayerstick in his right hand, he
        encircles me with it, in a sunwise direction, and
        places it in my right hand;
    Encircling me, sunwise, with a rainbow, he turns
        me, sunwise, towards himself;
    "We two will now start back, my grandchild," he
        says to me;
    "We two are now leaving, my grandchild," he says
        to me as I return to stand upon the rainbow.

The rescue is brought to completion:

10. From the west corner of the Darkness Hogan,
        Monster Slayer returns with me, whirling his
        dark staff about himself for protection;
    With lightnings flashing behind him, with light-
        nings flashing before him, he returns with me;
    As the rainbow returns with me and the talking
        prayerstick teaches me, Monster Slayer returns
        with me.

The rest of the prayer recounts how the return journey is made, and how the patient is restored to his own land, his own home and his physical body lying there.

Reconstruction of a stable universe: This is one of the main functions of the symbolism of the sandpaintings. Many of them are mandalas, laid out with strict precision, putting the parts of entire Navaho universe in correct relation to one another. The gods, supernaturals, heroes, and powers of nature are pictured in relation to the forces around them. Often the Place of Emergence, or a similar symbol, is in the center, the main healing personages are in the cardinal directions, lesser figures such as the four holy plants are in the semidirections. The four sacred mountains are often set to the outside, and the Rainbow Guardian surrounds the whole. An opening is always left to the east for the gods to come and go, and here two animals are set to guard the entrance. Such would be a typical sandpainting, but there are many exceptions and many variations.

The prayers always end with a restoration of the universe in and around the patient. For instance, at the end of the prayer cited just previously, after the patient has been returned to his hogan, his protector addresses him in the following words:

20. "This is your home, my grandchild!" he says to
me as he sits down beside me;
"I have returned with you to your home, my
grandchild!" he says to me as he sits down be-
side me;
"Upon the pollen figure I have returned to sit
with you, my grandchild!" he says to me as he
sits down beside me;
"Your home is yours again. . . .
"Your fire is yours again. . . .
"Your food is yours again. . . .
"Your resting place is yours again. . . .
"Your feet are yours again. . . .
"Your legs are yours again. . . .
"Your body is yours again. . . .
"Your mind is yours again. . . .
"Your voice is yours again. . . .
"Your speech is yours again. . . .
"Your power of movement is yours again. . . .
"This enables you to live in blessing. . . .

21. "Whatever makes it blessed before me, that shall
      make it blessed before you, my grandchild!" he
      says to me as he sits down beside me;
      "Whatever makes it blessed behind me . . .
      "Whatever makes it blessed below me . . .
      "Whatever makes it blessed above me . . .
      "Whatever makes it blessed all around me . . .
      "Whatever makes my speech blessed, that shall
      make your speech blessed, my grandchild!" he
      says to me as he sits down beside me;
      "Whatever enables me to live long, that shall
      enable you to live long, my grandchild!" he
      says as he sits down beside me;
      "Whatever enables me to live happily, that shall
      enable you to live happily, my grandchild!" he
      says as he sits down beside me;
      "Blessed again it has become, blessed again it has
      become!"

CONCLUSION

To conclude this paper we can entertain, if not answer, an open
question: What can the study of Navaho healing methods mean
to us outside of their general scholarly interest? Their methods
of healing are worlds—or rather, cultures—apart from our own,
and while it may be possible for them to integrate the principles
of scientific medicine into their system, it is not possible for us
to adopt sandpaintings, prayers, and songs into ours. Our medical
profession is not yet ready for that! What we can learn from
their example, however, is the depth and profundity of symbolic
healing and the basic principles of its operation.

Claude Lévi-Strauss,[21] in analyzing the shamanistic practices
of the Cuna Indians of Panama, called a similar process among
them "psychological manipulation," and I have referred to it in
this paper as "symbolic healing." That means healing mediated
almost entirely by the manipulation of culturally accepted sym-

bols acting directly on the patient's unconscious. The theory holds that such a forceful presentation of vivid images causes a transformation in the pattern of psychic energy flow. This can cause fear and sickness, as in witchcraft, or calmness and healing, as in the Navaho ceremonials. Lévi-Strauss said of this type of healing:

The cure would consist, therefore, in making explicit a situation originally existing on the emotional level and in rendering acceptable to the mind pains which the body refused to tolerate. That the mythology of the shaman does not correspond to an objective reality does not matter. The sick woman believes the myth and belongs to a society which believes in it. The tutelary spirits and malevolent spirits, the supernatural monsters and magical animals, are all part of a coherent system on which the native conception of the universe is founded. The sick woman accepts these mythical beings or more accurately, she has never questioned their existence. What she does not accept are the incoherent and arbitrary pains which are an alien element in her system but which the shaman, calling upon the myth, will reintegrate with a whole where everything is meaningful.[22]

Thus the symbolic language given by the medicine man to the patient always works if the patient believes in it. It may actually bring about physical healing (by psychosomatic influence) or it may make inescapable suffering acceptable. As one of the medicine men said: "If the patient really has confidence in me, then he gets cured. If there is no confidence, then that is his problem."

Such symbolic effects cannot be suitably described by such terms as suggestion, persuasion, magical cure, or faith healing, all of which carry pejorative connotations. Symbolic healing *does* use suggestion and persuasion; it *can* be magical and it *does* involve faith. But at its best, as I have tried to show in this paper, it goes beyond these categories and must be judged on its own merits and criticized on its own terms.

This brings me to an important point. It is only by means of cross-cultural studies that the symbolic nature of all medical systems is brought into focus. Behind all methods of nosolgy, etiology, and therapy lies a symbolic view of nature and man that binds medicine and culture in one "symbolic reality." This is particularly evident in the field of psychotherapy, where, without much strain, we can see outlines of the basic patterns of healing I have discussed. Almost all forms of psychotherapy direct the patient back to the beginnings, or origins, of his illness in his childhood. He is encouraged to examine the familial and cultural influences on his condition. Sometimes this is extended even to the experience of birth, the place of emergence for modern psychotherapy. In this way important images are activated in the patient's psyche. What we do with memories, dreams, and fantasies the Navaho medicine men do with prayers, songs, and sandpaintings.

There is also the objectification and attempted resolution of the problem of evil. The designation of evil is always relative to the cultural context in which it occurs; the Navaho idea is not the same as ours. We speak of "shadow complexes," "id contents," and "repressed fantasies" and in doing so we give our idea of evil a definite reality for the patient. It now has a name and a place; he can confront it in the presence of the therapist as the Navaho patient does in the presence of the medicine man. He can integrate some of it and banish the rest to the unconscious, into "outer space" as the Navaho prayer puts it. In spite of the many theoretical differences among modern psychotherapists, I think the process of dealing with evil openly is more important than the specific content or the theoretical constructs used to explain it. They vary with the culture; the basic pattern remains the same.

There is also the theme of death and rebirth, which is found wherever a psychic threshold is reached and crossed. It is not within the scope of this paper to demonstrate it here with fantasies and dream sequences. In *Man and His Symbols*[23] C. G. Jung and his coauthors give several examples of such symbolism in the dreams of modern patients.

Finally, the restoration of a stable universe is a necessary part of any psychotherapeutic process. The regression must be reversed; the transference must be resolved; the patient must be put squarely back into his own life as the Navaho patient in the prayer is brought back to his hogan, restored in mind and body, surrounded by his possessions and familiar cornfields.

There is one more thing we can learn from the Navaho, but

it goes beyond the limits of the healing process. That is his attitude toward nature. He strives not to master nature, but to be at one with it. To do this he relates not to "raw" nature, as the scientist sees it, but to a highly refined, symbolized nature that is intensely alive and imbued with an inner form of superlative beauty. This inner form may be addressed as a kinsman and can be expected to succor the individual as one would a loved child or grandchild.

The ultimate mystery of Navaho religion is said to be the power of rejuvenation obtained by identification with Changing Woman, the archetypal symbol of the natural cycle of birth, death, and rebirth. Contact with her through the chant process can bring a long, blessed life and a state of harmony within and without. Even in death the individual is generally not conceived as going to a *separate* place. The part consonant with the harmony of nature is unified into it. This is nowhere better expressed than in the last song of the hero of Mountain Top Way. He sings it to his brother, after having taught him all his secret knowledge, and then vanishes into the distant cliffs:

> Farewell, my younger brother.
> From the high, holy places
> The gods have come for me.
> You will never see me again.
> But when the showers pass over you,
> And the thunder sounds,
> You will think:
> There is the voice of my elder brother.
> And when the harvests ripen,
> And you hear the voices of small birds of many
>   kinds,
> And the chirping of grasshoppers,
> You will think:
> There is the ordering of my elder brother.
> There is the trail of his mind.[24]

REFERENCES

1   Gladys A. Reichard, *Navaho Medicine Man* (New York: J. J. Augustin, 1939), p. 14.

2   Gladys A. Reichard, in *Ancient Religions*, Vergilius Ferm, ed. (New York: The Citadel Press, 1965), p. 344.

3   Washington Matthews, "The Mountain Chant, A Navaho Ceremony," Fifth Annual Report of the Bureau of American Ethnology to the Secretary of the Smithsonian Institution, Washington, 1887, pp. 379–486.

4   Leland Wyman and Berard Haile, *Blessingway* (Tucson: University of Arizona Press, 1970).

5   Leland C. Wyman, ed., *Beautyway, A Navaho Ceremonial* (New York: Bollingen Foundation and Pantheon Books, 1957), p. 13.

6   Mircea Eliade, *Shamanism, Archaic Techniques of Ecstasy*, Bollingen Series LXXVI (New York: Pantheon Books, 1964).

7   Mircea Eliade, *Myths, Dreams and Mysteries: The Encounter Between Contemporary Faiths and Archaic Realities* (New York: Harper Torchbooks, 1967), p. 61.

8   Reichard, *Navaho Medicine Man*, p. xv.

9   Washington Matthews, "The Night Chant, A Navaho Ceremony," Memoirs of the American Museum of Natural History, New York, Vol. 6, 1902.

10   Ibid., p. 73.

11   Ibid., p. 81.

12   Ibid., p. 76.

13   Ibid., pp. 120–26.

14   Ibid., pp. 123–26.

15   Ibid., p. 143.

16   Ibid., p. 153.

17   From a prayer given by Natani Tso, August, 1969, translated by Albert Sandoval, Jr.

18   Gladys A. Reichard, *Prayer, The Compulsive Word* (New York: J. J. Augustin, 1944).

19   Katherine Spencer, "Mythology and Values, Analysis of Navaho Chantway Myths," *Memoirs of the American Folklore Society* 48 (1957):100.

20   David P. McAllester and Mary Wheelwright, *The Myth and Prayers of the Great Star Chant and the Myth of the Coyote Chant*, Navaho

Religion Series, Vol. 4 (Santa Fe, N.M.: Navaho Museum of Ceremonial Art, 1956), pp. 57–64.

21 Claude Lévi-Strauss, *Structural Anthropology* (New York: Anchor Books, 1967).

22 Ibid., pp. 192–93.

23 C. G. Jung, ed., *Man and His Symbols* (New York: Doubleday and Company, 1964).

24 Matthews, "The Mountain Chant," p. 467.

By Manfred Porkert

Chinese Medicine: A Traditional Healing Science

Improved political contacts between China and the majority of Western governments, the eyewitness account of an American newspaper columnist, and, finally, the informative visits of groups of Western doctors to the Chinese People's Republic have styled into a fashionable topic something that, for quite some time already, ought to have attracted competent scrutiny from universal science—we refer to the means and achievements of traditional Chinese medicine. There are quite a number of reasons to study this healing science and quite a number of obstacles to its proper study and integration into the common pool of human knowledge.

To start with, no single skill or separate discipline of Chinese medicine can be correctly assessed if divorced from the context of the complete theoretical system of that medicine. Couched differently, anyone attempting to bear judgment upon or to improve any single detail of Chinese medicine can succeed only if he has deliberately become familiar at least with the most general criteria of Chinese science.

Therapeutic effectiveness may be a reason to adopt or maintain certain techniques such as acupuncture. But it cannot be the principal let alone the sole criterion for recognizing its scientific validity. An array of techniques of unquestionable therapeutic effectiveness may constitute an eclectic medicine of great practical value; but it cannot aspire to recognition as a scientific system. Hence the dilemma of all those who are convinced that traditional Chinese medicine has great therapeutic potential, but who feel at a loss to plead its case in the court of universal science.

The highly consistent results of Western medicine and the influence it has gradually been able to command throughout the world are due to the highly scientific standards maintained by the majority of its exponents. But it must neither be overlooked that these high standards are confined to the theoretical core of its most successful disciplines and do not extend to the more distant ramifications of everyday health care; nor that a significant number of supposedly minor yet very widespread disorders are entirely beyond the reach of its diagnostic and therapeutic means. In this present situation, the mere existence of Chinese medicine, resting upon rational premises very different from those of scientific Western medicine, confronts us with two apparently equally unsatisfactory alternatives. We may either follow the momentary tendency in the People's Republic of China as well as the example of not a few acupuncturists in the West and pragmatically combine some of its ancient techniques with the procedures of Western medicine. This may produce immediate spot improvements on the practical level; but in the long run, the neglect of achieving the rational reconciliation and integration of empirical data eclectically assembled and made use of will inevitably lead to the disintegration of the theoretical structures and finally entail a downgrading of the whole medicine.

Or we may choose to keep aloof from the legacy of Chinese medicine, an attitude still maintained at this writing by the overwhelming majority of medical faculties outside continental China. Irrespective of whether this attitude is due to ignorance of the essential limitations inherent in the methods of Western medicine or to misinformation on the rational premises of Chinese medicine, the willful or involuntary refusal to draw upon these complementary insights direly needed and already available will lead to an involution of Western medicine similar to that observed for Chinese medicine eight centuries earlier.

A few years ago, a student couple with some knowledge of Chinese spent one year in Taiwan in order to investigate there the present-day situation of traditional Chinese medicine. They questioned traditional healers and their patients, examined the shelves of apothecaries' shops, looked into medical classrooms and into research institutes. The gist of their gloomy findings was this: there is still fairly widespread although vacillating interest in traditional methods, yet the average practitioners have very low professional competence and they seem to be almost ignorant in regard to theoretical considerations. The physicians from Europe and America who, in recent years, have flocked to continental China, to Hong Kong, Japan, and Taiwan in order to get a firsthand impression of Chinese medicine, in remembering the vague and evasive information they gleaned during their trips, will nod their heads in agreement. And yet, although their impressions are very true, the inferences drawn from them are often erroneous.

It is true that the theoretic consciousness of the scientific network of Chinese medicine is at a low ebb, not only at the periphery, in Taiwan, Japan, Hong Kong, but also in the Chinese People's Republic, where, since the fifties, powerful and most impressive efforts have been made to reassess and rebuild traditional medicine. The topnotch acupuncturist in Taipei or Tokyo may be hard-pressed to describe the theoretical foundations of his empirically effective techniques, even more so will this happen with the host of barefoot doctors in China proper who have a mere smattering of medical theory. But it is a grave mistake to believe that the situation was any better, say, at the beginning of the nineteenth century, and yet another mistake to deduce from this that Chinese medicine never produced anything on a par with Western medicine.

HISTORICAL BACKGROUND

To this day, only isolated fragments of Chinese medicine—essentially techniques of acupuncture and of some gymnastic exercises and techniques of massage—have been published in the

West and applied in a *purely empirical manner,* that is, without an understanding of the logical premises of Chinese medicine. By contrast, classical Chinese medicine had emerged from the stage of pure empiricism during the third century B.C. at the latest. During the centuries that followed, it developed into a true healing science, logically stringent in theory, highly effective in practice, a healing science that was at its methodological and technical apogee between the tenth and thirteenth centuries A.D. and then gradually declined. In order to understand the reasons for this decline and the present state of Chinese medicine, we must briefly consider some salient aspects of its history.

Chinese medicine, for almost three millennia, had been fostered and brought to maturity by what, for want of a better term, we may call Taoist consciousness, implying a vivid yet serene awareness of all cosmic phenomena, including the diverse functions of the human personality (we intentionally say "personality," for the Taoists never divorced mental and physical processes).

During the eleventh century, the Confucian administration had definitely taken over the training, examination, and to a large extent even the employment of doctors and pharmacists. At the outset, the results of this change appeared to be quite beneficial: concentration of the most competent physicians and of all the organized training facilities in the provincial centers and at the capital fostered a more intense exchange of ideas as well as wholesome competition among different medical traditions. This in turn led to an extraordinary expansion of medical research and theorizing. The twelfth and thirteenth centuries witnessed a dramatic increase in medical publications. Then, the deleterious influence of Confucian values upon medical thought became evident, an influence that had been latently effective for quite some time. It should be recalled that the salient trait of Confucian thought through more than two millennia consisted in unswerving concentration upon the social phenomena—that is, upon the perception and systematic control of human relations. Its commanding influence on the political evolution of China for nearly two thousand years was the direct result of this singleness of purpose. Unfortunately, the crowning achievement of the neo-Confucian synthesis—namely, the smooth conduct of human relations—led to a self-complacency similar to that engendered in the West by the advances of physical technology: having achieved a decisive breakthrough in one realm of knowledge, people took (and take) it for granted that the generalization of the proven method could not fail to eventually solve all problems of human existence. In comparison to social issues, all other problems, in the eyes of the Confucianists, dwindled to mere trifles, unfit to occupy the mind of any serious scholar. Upon such premises, the integration of medical education and research into the Confucian administrative system gradually yet ineluctably caused humanistic and sociological methods to be applied to the solution of biological and medical problems, a tendency that, in the long run, led to a perversion of theoretical speculation and an erosion of clinical and empirical research.

This degenerative process of medical science in China reached rock bottom during the nineteenth century. In practice, Chinese medicine then consisted only of an odd assortment of proven and fairly crude techniques from which practitioners could hardly grasp, let alone reconstruct, the guiding ideas. Worse still, the widening gaps in what formerly had been a highly consistent scientific system, had been filled with a host of paramedical— that is, magical or exorcist—procedures. Under such conditions, it is little wonder that, since the nineteenth century and until quite recently, Western doctors and their Chinese disciples had a most disparaging view of the indigenous healing methods; and, for the same reason, we clearly perceive the absurdity of founding any judgment or of attempting to assess correctly the scientific standards and potential effectiveness of Chinese medicine upon a survey of its desolate state during the nineteenth century.

Fortunately, this outward decay of scientific method did not obliterate the essence and core of the system: the medical treatises of the first centuries, based upon careful observation and sound reasoning, have all come down to us, sometimes in several parallel versions. And it is to be applauded that, in the course of the revival of the indigenous medical tradition taking place in the People's Republic of China since the fifties, practically all relevant medical texts that had appeared between the third century B.C. and the nineteenth century A.D. have again become available to the entire scientific community in inexpensive editions. The medical classics, moreover, have been published in critical editions, with commentaries and even paraphrased in the modern vernacular. Thus the material obstacles have been removed that, until recently, impeded the reappraisal and reconstruction, as well as the critical investigation, of Chinese medicine, all of which—as has just been pointed out—can only be undertaken by re-establishing contact with the intact scientific system of the eleventh century. On the other hand, this windfall cornucopia of medical literature has to this day stimulated only very modest research despite the quality and quantity of material made available. Quite evidently, it is not the dearth of materials but the absence of adequate heuristic procedures and the lack of qualified research power that today frustrates many noble intentions for the amalgamation of traditional Chinese and modern Western medicines.

THE THEORETICAL FOUNDATIONS
OF CHINESE MEDICINE

The greatest source of misunderstanding concerning the science of Chinese medicine stems from the failure to appreciate the different yet complementary methodological and epistemological bases of Chinese and Western medicines. Chinese medicine, like all Chinese science, reposes upon the inductive and synthetic mode of cognition.* This means that Chinese doctors have at all

* Inductivity corresponds to a logical link between two effective positions existing at the same time in different places in space. (Conversely, causality is the logical link between two effective positions given at different times at the same place in space.) In other words, effects based on positions that are separate in space yet simultaneous in time are mutually inductive and thus are called inductive effects. In Western science prior to the development of electrodynamics and nuclear physics (which are founded essentially on inductivity), the inductive nexus was limited to subordinate uses in proto-sciences such as astrology. Now Western man, as a consequence of two thousand years of intellectual tradition, persists in the habit of making causal connections first and inductive links, if at all, only as an afterthought. This habit must still be considered the biggest obstacle to an adequate appreciation of Chinese science in general and Chinese medicine in particular.

times concentrated their attention, essentially if not exclusively, upon dynamic processes, upon vital dynamics, in other words, upon the biological, psychic, social, and cosmic functions. Western medicine, by contradistinction, as a consequence of its causal and analytical orientation, is interested primarily in the material substratums—that is, in the somatic support of functions—in short, in the concrete body and its components. Further, we should always keep in mind that Western science is not more rational than Chinese science, merely more analytical.

If two observers, quite sympathetic to each other, simultaneously yet from different vantage points (perspectives) attempt to describe a given object, their respective statements will paradoxically be more at variance, the better each observer renders his impressions. The divergence will seem quite irreconcilable, as when the views of an enthusiastic artist on the one hand and a sober scientist on the other are compared. What we intend to underscore is this: different spatial, temporal, cultural, temperamental perspectives condition differences in statements on one and the selfsame object, irrespective of the fact that each of the separate statements must be considered to be positive and pertinent, and regardless of whether differences in attention, acuity of the senses, or intellectual honesty may be invoked. Thus, to revert to our topic, two physicians, the first observing in the pattern of the inductive and synthetic mode, the second oriented by causal analysis, will never succeed in making their positive data converge completely—not in spite of, but precisely because of, their high scientific standards.

At this juncture, some Western doctors versed in the history of ideas will point out that Western medicine, too, for quite some time has paid attention to functional processes but that what matters after all is the exact scientific combination of empirical data, and, to achieve this, causal analysis of substrata offers the only conceivable solution. "Exact scientific combination" applies without reserve also to Chinese medicine; "causal analysis as only solution," however, is a fallacy.

What makes the difference between science and empiricism is that the positive data of science are presented in a systematically integrated and universally accepted form. Classical physics and, in its wake, the majority of Western sciences still operate with numbers and measurements because the criterion that enables us to distinguish similar substrata is their quantity—in other words, their extension, their weight. Yet what endows scientific measurements with their universal significance and at the same time with their universal integrability is not the reference to some fundamental law of nature, no axiomlike causality; it is simply the constant and consistent reference to universally known and accepted standards of measurement, for example, reference to the centimeter-gram-second system (cgs system).

Let us pause for a moment to mull over the term "conventional standards of measurement" just used. A hot fire constitutes an empirical statement highly refractory to stringent integration into a scientific system. Combustion at 380° centigrade, on the other hand, describes the same phenomenon with reference to a conventional standard—the centigrade scale—and thus in such a way as to make the statement directly and unequivocally comparable with all statements on similar observations.

The conventional standards employed in Western science— the cgs system in its multiple applications—are conventional standards of measurement. This is so because the causal and analytical approach of Western science leads to the definition of substrata, and because the criteria permitting the distinction of similar substrata are the dimensions in space of these substrata— in other words, its quantitative data.

By contrast, Chinese medicine, utilizing the inductive and synthetic approach, deals with functions (biological, meteorological, social, and cosmic processes). The criterion that permits us to distinguish similar functions is their relative direction in space or, to use another term, their quality. And of course, qualitative data may be formulated with similar universal significance and integrated with similar precision and stringency as is the case for quantitative data—by consistent reference to *qualitative standards*—in China by reference to yin, yang, the Five Evolutive Phases and their technical derivatives. If we are clearly aware of the key role that the quantitative standards of the cgs system play in the transmission and integration of observational data throughout Western science, then we shall have no difficulty realizing that, similarly, conversancy with the qualitative standards of Chinese science is an essential prerequisite to all serious discussion of the data of Chinese medicine.

Paradoxically, there is ample proof that the majority of people today engaged in one way or another in the study and practice of Chinese medical methods are fairly oblivious of the significance and purpose of these quality standards and hence reluctant to accept and to employ them. An extreme case in point is that of a professor at the renowned Tokyo University who, upon enlisting the aid of a computer, recently spent three years and countless man-hours to prove that the *wu-hsing* (the Five Evolutive Phases) have no foundation whatsoever in reality. Imagine a scholar at London University using the resources of his laboratory for three years to prove the absurdity of the cgs conventions! Still, this is not a matter of facetiousness. For, as we shall presently show, the attempt to judge Chinese medical theory by the utterly alien procedural standards of Western medicine is not the only way in which its highly consistent data are vitiated and obscured.

The principal and basic standards of value used in Chinese medicine and shared by all Chinese sciences are the polar combination yin/yang and the cycle of the Five Evolutive Phases (*wu-hsing*). The terms yin and yang originally designated topographical aspects — the shady and the sunny side of a mountain or the southern and the northern bank of a river respectively. At the constitutive stage of Chinese science, during the second half of the first millennium B.C., they were adopted as designations for the polar aspects of interrelated phenomena. Hence, in modern terms, yang corresponds to all that is active, expansive, centrifugal, aggressive, demanding, negative, and yin implies all that is structive, substantiative, contractive, centripetal, responsive, conservative, positive. Further correspondences include:

YIN	YANG
earth	heaven
moon	sun
autumn, winter	spring, summer
things female	things male
cold, coolness	heat, warmth

YIN	YANG
moisture	dryness
the inside, interior	the outside, surface
darkness	brightness
things small and weak	things big and powerful
the lower part	the upper part
water, rain	fire
quiescence	movement
night	day
the right side	the left side
exhaustion	repletion
the hours between noon and midnight	the hours between midnight and noon
metal, water	wood, fire

For more subtle qualitative graduations, the Chinese have also developed the cycle of the Five Evolutive Phases (*wu-hsing*). This fivefold cycle is often translated as "Five Elements," which is misleading since the term *hsing* means literally "passage" and does not imply a material substratum. The Five Evolutive Phases constitute stretches of time and define conventionally and unequivocally energetic qualities that succeed one another in cyclical order. The Five Evolutive Phases typify these qualities of energy by the use of five concepts (wood, fire, earth, metal, and water) that, because of the richness of their associations, are ideally suited to serve as the crystallizing core for an inductive system of relations and correspondences. There exists an extensive system of correspondences relating the Five Evolutive Phases to the various seasons, cardinal points on the compass, tastes, smells, musical notes, colors, heavenly bodies, emotions, sense organs, orbs, parts of the body, and so on.

In Chinese medicine, the utmost precision in the evaluation of functions is made possible by establishing systems of technical correspondence in the terms of these basic quality standards. Described below are the most widely applied and best known of these technical correspondences: those of *orbisiconography* (*tsang-hsiang*), describing the interaction of the functional orbs of the organism; of *sinarteriology* (*ching-luo*), dealing with the interdependence of physiological signs, pathological symptoms, and therapeutic measures perceptible at or applicable to the body surface; and of *phase energetics* (*yün-chi'i*), postulating criteria for determining the influence of cosmic (that is, meteorological, immunological) functions on the functions of the organisms. These technical correspondences in turn constitute the theoretical framework of all applied and clinical disciplines of Chinese medicine such as pharmacotherapy (*pen-ts'ao*)—the administration of vegetable, animal, and mineral drugs—and acumoxi-therapy (*chen-chiu*)—the application of needles or cauteries to sensitive spots at the body surface.

ORBISICONOGRAPHY

All medical knowledge is centered on the body and its vital manifestations. Naturally, statements bearing on the bodily substratum and its functions constitute, so to speak, the bone and muscle of any medical theory. As with all other disciplines, these medical statements are tinged by the mode of thought of their authors. In anatomy, Western medicine, causal and analytic, describes primarily the aggregate carriers (or substrata) of effects, whereas inductive synthetic Chinese medicine is interested primarily in the fabric of functional manifestations of the different body regions. Consequently, Chinese medicine did not develop any anatomy worth speaking of, has no known histology or biochemistry, and instead has evolved organic energetics, a number of interrelated, highly consistent, physiological subdisciplines. The systematic description of these functional relationships is the Chinese discipline called *tsang-hsiang*, which we translate as orbisiconography, meaning the "imagery of the functional orbs."*
Orbisiconography, dealing almost exclusively with vital func-

---

* The ambiguity of the technical term "orb" (meaning sphere of activity, cyclical functional pattern, cyclical pathway, geometric form) reflects almost exactly that of the Chinese term *tsang*, which refers on one hand to a bodily substratum with ill-defined material and spatial contours, and on the other hand to a physiological function associated with the substratum and qualitatively defined in time with precision and subtlety.

tions, is not a Chinese version of anatomy, but is its very antithesis and complement, a point missed by most modern interpreters of Chinese medicine.

What the Chinese medical literature informs us on coherently, clearly, with rational precision, are the *multiple medically relevant functional relations* (relations often not considered in Western medicine); what Chinese medical literature is silent about or where it contributes nothing of scientific interests are the somatic supports of these functional relations, namely, the bodily substratum.

Having constantly stressed the fundamental difference of outlook at the base of Chinese and Western sciences, we should have no difficulty comprehending that their respective statements can never be completely congruent. This disparity of statements due to differences of perspective acquires critical significance as soon as scientific terminology is involved. Words that, in everyday speech, may be considered perfect equivalents within two languages, can hardly ever be accepted as equivalents as soon as the expression of scientific data gathered from different perspectives is involved. Thus the Chinese words *hsin, kan, shen* ("heart," "liver," "kidneys") correspond to such English terms only if used, say, when buying meat at the butcher's. Their meaning appears to be changed so as to be almost unrecognizable when used in a treatise on Chinese medicine. For, the fact that, as we just pointed out, Chinese scientists had focused their attention on the dynamic aspects of reality—that is, the functions—does not imply that Chinese technical terms preponderantly express such aspects; rather it denotes that literally their whole meaning arises from the perception of functions. In other words, the meaning of a technical term in Chinese medicine is not made up of function-oriented plus substratum-oriented data; it consists practically only of the former.

For instance, when the Chinese medical authors speak of *kan,* we must understand that the term primarily and predominantly designates a specific orb of functions (hepatic orb) that only vaguely relates to most of the ideas someone with a Western education associates with the liver. This is why statements bearing on a certain orb can under no circumstances be made to agree completely with statements bearing on the corresponding organ in Western thought. The better both statements are supported in context by empirical data integrated into their logical systems, the less reconcilable they turn out to be. Given this fundamental divergence, it may happen that for a given orb described by traditional Chinese medicine (for example, the *orbis tricalorii, san-chiao**), Western medicine can define no corresponding physical organ, or inversely, that Chinese medicine does not postulate an orb for an organ (for example, the pancreas) defined by Western medicine.

The persistent refusal of Chinese doctors to perceive and describe anatomical structures will amaze us only if we very much underrate the decisive influence of the perspective modes—inductive versus causal—that produces a complete polarization of reality on the level of empirical description. For, to make the picture complete, Western doctors to this day manage to ignore almost completely a host of quite significant functional changes that they might clearly discern without the aid of any instrument every hour of the day upon their own and their patients' organisms. While the Western medical scientist feels awkward if he has no organ to account for a given vital function, the Chinese medical scientist would have been worried if he failed to tie in properly a newly observed function with the stock of functional observations accumulated by his predecessors. It is these functions and their changes that form the meat and marrow of Chinese medicine, and the description of these functions constitutes the fundamental data coming under the heading of *tsang-hsiang,* orbisiconography.

The description of any orb, its picture (in Chinese: *hsiang,* "image"; in Greek: *eikon,* hence iconography) differs fundamentally in form and content from the apparently comparable de-

---

* There have been numerous futile attempts, both within Chinese medicine itself and by Western interpreters, to identify the anatomical substratum of *san-chiao* ("three heated spaces"). One such theory divides the thorax and abdomen into three spaces; another equates the orb with the endocrine system. However, close and serious study never supports these assumptions, which fail to encompass the entire orb of functions called by the Chinese *san-chiao*.

scriptions of the organ systems in Western anatomy. The description of an orb includes its relation to the basic qualitative standards (yin, yang, and the Five Evolutive Phases and the associated system of correspondences), its interaction with the microcosm (the complementary orb, the associated sinarteries, and specific radial pulse), and the sensuous and substrative projections of the orb (the particular region or body surface, the specific sense organ and body opening, the associated psychic reaction, the secreted fluid, and the dream motifs and anatomical correspondence, if any). The orb is further characterized by its specific functional role in the energetic processes of the human being (note that we did not say "body," for the Chinese did not separate physis and psyche).

If we examine the information laid down in the medical classics on orbisiconography, we rapidly become aware that nearly all the statements bear on the imbricated and interdependent vital functions, on cyclical functional patterns. The selection of "orbs of function" as an equivalent for *tsang* (often translated as "organ" or "viscera") serves us well in making sensible interpretation of the orbisiconographic illustrations and descriptions already alluded to. When the Chinese describe or picture "a *tsang* (orb) called 'heart' connected through the 'lung-pipe' (trachea) with a *tsang* called 'lungs'; the same *tsang* connected by three (or four) separate ducts with other *tsang* called respectively 'liver,' 'spleen,' 'kidneys,' and again 'lungs,' etc.," they are describing functional relationships, not crude anatomical insights. Furthermore, if *tsang* is understood as an "orb of functions," then the pictures of orbisiconography can only represent graphic models similar to those used for example in nuclear physics. No physicist, building a model of some specific atom, will believe that he is simply enlarging a photographic picture of such a structure; and if he represents the electrons by smooth balls, their tracks by metal rings, and the nucleus by a raspberry, he will never pretend that, on a much smaller scale, the real electrons are smooth balls running on metal rails, and the nucleus looks like a raspberry. If his model of the atom incorporates elements more or less resembling known objects, this is merely because he intends to appeal to the imagination and to help the memory of those whom he wants to instruct. Similarly, the medical authors who formerly illustrated the orbisiconographic treatises, did not (and never pretended they meant to) depict what they had observed in an anatomical theatre. The illustrations of orbisiconography were, as a rule, meant primarily as diagrams of function, hence to attempt to view them as anatomical figures is to miss the point. Their unique aim was to facilitate the mnemonic assimilation by the reader of systematized results of positive observation.

SINARTERIOLOGY

In traditional Chinese medical theory, energy is distributed throughout the body along a network of conduits or "sinarteries"* (*ching-luo* or *ching-mo*). These conduits are thought to conduct the different forms of physiological energy between the various orbs and between the interior of the body and its surface. Along the surface portion of these energetic conduits are located hundreds of sensitive points or, "foramina" (*hsüeh*). These sensitive points communicate with a corresponding energetic configuration (an orb) and can be used to induce changes in the functioning of the orb. By inserting needles (acupuncture) or burning small herbal cones (moxibustion) at these sensitive points, the Chinese physician attempts to restore the proper phasing of the energetic flow and restore it to that dynamic balance, which for the Chinese defines health.

Sinarteriology, the theory of energetic conduits and sensitive points, is one of the most original and most important chapters of Chinese medicine. It is important because sinarteriology is an

* The term *ching-mo*, often translated as "meridian," means more precisely "to guide the rhythmic manifestation of energy along definite paths." The Latin term *arteria* (borrowed from the Greek), signifying at the same time "pulse" and "pulsating vein," very closely approximates the meanings of the somewhat ambiguous Chinese term *ching-mo*. In order to avoid any confusion between our term "sinartery" and the word "artery," used in a quite different sense in modern medicine, we have added the prefix "sin-" meaning Chinese.

essential element of Chinese diagnostics, pharmacotherapy, and massage, and the sole foundation of acupuncture and moxibustion. It is original in the sense that the knowledge of hypersensitive points or zones, found in all great civilizations, has nowhere approached the systematic perfection of Chinese sinarteriology.

The origins of the theory of the energetic conduits and sensitive points are lost in the darkness of ancient history. From a study of the ancient literature, however, it may be inferred that stone needles were used for the treatment of disease in the second millennium B.C. and perhaps even toward the end of the Stone Age. At that stage, people must have known of points at the surface of the body through which certain disease symptoms could be influenced. Later, neighboring sensitive points linked with symptoms were connected by lines, the so-called conduits, in an attempt to systematically represent the empirically observed functional relationships. Thus the sensitive points alone provide the positive empirical and historically primary data on which the theory is based; the conduits, on the other hand, are only the result of systematic speculation, and therefore, one would not expect to find a somatic substratum for these conceptual devices. This fact deserves to be underscored, since a considerable number of contemporary physicians in the Soviet Union, in China, and in the West, evidently ignorant of it, vainly strive either to prove that the conduits postulated by Chinese medicine do not really exist or, more frequently, to detect some kind of anatomical substratum corresponding to the conduits. Yet the sole positive phenomenon that Chinese doctors have experienced, and that can be demonstrated by means of modern research apparatus, is the functional distinction between every sensitive point and its neutral surroundings. This dissemblance is defined by measurements of electrical resistance and of thermosensitivity at the surface of the skin.

Consequently the conduits must be conceived in analogy to the lines of force of a magnetic field or to the orbits of planets as defined by gravitation and mass. Like these they can never be demonstrated in the form of substratum but only as effects exercised on substrata. Also analogously, the detailed tracing of the conduits is always subject to slight modification due to new or more precise observations or to individual variations. And the only portion of the conduits that can be plotted is the part of their course that lies at the surface of the body. Their extensions within the body that are devoid of sensitive points—the sections, in other words, closest to the orbs—can be viewed as essentially functional models similar to those of orbisiconography. Their primary purpose is to facilitate the logical and mnemonic association of certain constant physiological and pathological relationships.

PHASE ENERGETICS

It is axiomatic in Chinese thought that all realms of Nature— the macrocosm and all microcosms—are interconnected inductively. The energetic processes of the Cosmos unceasingly modulate the changes that take place in every individual organism. For this reason systematic and qualitatively unequivocal descriptions of temporally variable meteorological, climatological, and immunological influences are needed for diagnosis and therapy of both the exogenous (in Chinese *wai-kan,* literally "induced from without") diseases and of the epidemic and pandemic diseases. The latter are designated by the significant technical term *shih-ping* or *shih-ch'-i-ping,* meaning "diseases dependent on the time," "diseases conditioned by the temporal configuration."

The most basic statement of the macrocosmic variation is the calendar. Since the most ancient times the Chinese have used a combined solar-lunar calendar. To this day, farmers and practitioners of traditional medicine take their cues from it.

Reference to the calendar, common in the medical arts of all cultures, permits only rudimentary prognoses of average probability both in immunology and epidemiology, since certain diseases occur more often in some season than in others; the aggravation of certain symptoms is more frequent at some hours of the day than at others. Although the hours and seasons revolve in endless uniformity, each cycle shows individual meteorological, immunological, and other relevant characteristics. In order to define more precisely the characteristics of each individual interval and incorporate these influences rationally into diagnostics and therapy, Chinese medicine has evolved the qualitative conventions of phase energetics (*yün-chi'i*). Phase energetics aims to define the medical significance of macrocosmic (meteorological, climatic, immunological) influences on microcosmic (physiological) processes.

As an example, the ancient Chinese medical classic *Su-wen* describes the repercussions of energetic deficiency on climate, society, and the microcosm by employing the qualitative standards of the Five Evolutive Phases.

If in a given year Wood is deficient, drought will be rampant; the enlivening energy (ch'i vitale) will lack [sufficient] resonance; the vegetation will be retarded in its development . . . the people will suffer from cold, pains in the flanks and in the abdomen, flatulence, and watery diarrhea . . . If there is a *reversio,* [on the other hand] scorching and sweltering heat will prevail [as an effect of] Fire . . . If in a given year Fire is deficient, cold will be rampant; the regime of growth will not assert itself; plants will bud and then wither . . . the people will suffer from pains in the chest, plethora of the midriff, heaviness of the limbs, ischiatic pains, and sudden aphasia accompanied by pain in the heart. . . . If in a given year Earth is deficient, Wind will be rampant and the energetic configuration required for the ripening [of the crops] will not establish itself; the vegetation may develop luxuriantly . . . yet will only show a splendid appearance, bearing no fruit. . . . The people will suffer from intestinal disease and from cholera, heavy limbs, fatigue, and abdominal pains. . . . If in a given year Metal is deficient, scorching heat and Fire will be rampant; the enlivening energy will assert itself and the energetic configuration favorable to growth will prevail; beings will develop luxuriantly . . . people will suffer from short breath, fatigue of the upper limbs, colds and hematuria. . . . If in a given year Water is deficient, humidity will prevail; the energy favoring growth will assert itself in a perverted manner; maturation will be accelerated . . . the people will suffer from abdominal plethora, fatigue . . . ulcers, and diseases of the joints. . . .

Phase energetics is, however, by far the weakest link in the correspondence system of Chinese medicine. Its methodological defects, both practical and theoretical, are due largely to the inadequacy of its technical foundations. A comprehensive and unequivocal description of the subject matter of phase energetics

—energetic processes of worldwide dimensions—requires adequate astronomical instruments, a far-flung network of precisely coordinated observatories, uniform and exact measurements of time, and calibrated instruments, all of which have become generally available in China only in our century. The authors of the theory of phase energetics, living probably fifteen hundred years before our time, had to rely on very fragmentary empirical data to apply and verify their systematic speculations.

Due to its shortcoming, one may feel tempted to reject the scientific value of phase energetics altogether. Such a categorical rejection would be unjustified, for the basic pattern of phase energetics is worth taking seriously as a paradigm for the further development of modern medicine. Taking into account the complex nature of the phenomena described, phase energetics offers a simple, transparent, and rather consistent mode of explanation for climatic and other macrocosmic influences in physiology. It describes systematically unequivocal relationships, which may be tested by experience, between macrocosmic events on the one hand and physiological, immunological, and pathological conditions on the other.

What phase energetics is deficient in—continuous, precise, and extensive data from meteorological observations—may easily be furnished by modern science. Inversely, for the latter the effective relations between climate and immunology remain almost completely unexplored. Combining what Chinese and Western science have to offer would provide a powerful impulse for the further development of rational therapy.

THE PRACTICAL EFFECTIVENESS
OF CHINESE MEDICINE

Having reviewed the theoretical and methodological background of traditional Chinese medicine, it is possible to reflect on how it meets the practical demands of medicine as we define them today. This discussion, in turn, will furnish support for the thesis that Chinese medicine is not a competitor, but rather a methodical complement to Western therapies. While in China today the disciplines of anatomy, histology, biochemistry, bacteriology, as well as the practice of surgery and hygiene are derived from Western medicine, it is also true that the traditional medical practices of Chinese medicine continue to stand up remarkably well in the diagnosis and treatment of certain types of disease—not only in mainland China, but also in places like Formosa, Singapore, and Hong Kong where economic and political factors are not active in favoring traditional medicine or in impeding the application of Western drugs and instruments. Furthermore, in a notable percentage of diseases encountered in everyday practice, particularly functional diseases, Western medicine has no specific diagnosis or therapy. In some of these diseases Chinese medicine may provide rational diagnoses and specific therapies, which is, after all, the necessary criteria for a scientific medicine.

Chinese medicine is capable of furnishing detailed and rational diagnoses. Western physicians, who disparagingly compare their sophisticated diagnostic procedures and laboratory measurements to the simple procedures used by Chinese physicians, should note that the analytic and causal methodology of Western medicine calls for active intervention in order to identify precisely the antecedent causes of the observed and the somatic substratum involved. The Chinese physician, in contrast, is interested in the present functions and actual symptoms of the patient. *Szu-chen*— his four diagnostic methods: inspection, interrogation, auscultation/olfaction, and palpation of the six radial pulses— are all aimed at a complete appraisal of the momentary functional situation of the patient. The data he looks for are directly open to the senses. Therefore the Chinese diagnostician's job consists of the rational assessment of symptoms by applying the inductive method and its qualitative standards. The fact apparently so difficult to grasp is that because of their epistemological complementarity, Chinese and Western medicines, without one being basically inferior to the other, cannot and do not produce mutually identical results.

The strength of Chinese medicine, primarily attentive to functions, is:

(1) the diagnosis and treatment of diseases manifesting themselves essentially through irregularities of function (as yet) with-

out concomitant alterations in the bodily substratum. Against a vast number of disturbances of good health, Western medicine can only offer nonspecific treatment since no specific organic disorder can be diagnosed; in Chinese medicine, keyed to the observation of functions, such disturbances have differentiated symptoms and a specific therapy.

(2) the diagnosis and treatment of so-called chronodemic diseases or diseases conditioned by the temporal configuration (*shih-ch'i*). A number of diseases (according to Western medicine probably caused by a virus) that flare up simultaneously over vast territories are explained in Chinese medical theory (phase energetics) as deficiencies or redundancies of energy in certain orbs, conditioned by the momentary immunological, meteorological, and climatic situation.

(3) the early diagnosis and prevention of organic disease. There is general agreement that serious organic disease (for example, cardiac failure, diabetes, cancer) is preceded by stages of growing functional disorders. If these are given specific diagnosis and treatment based upon functional assessment, they can be prevented from entering the organic stage, which, in the opinion of Chinese doctors, represents an advanced if not terminal stage of every disease.

By contradistinction, the strength of Western medicine resides in:

(4) the diagnosis and treatment of accidental or sudden organic disease. Organic damage due to sudden accidents or organic disorders with (in the eyes of the traditional Chinese physicians) imprecise diagnostic symptoms (for example, an advanced tubal pregnancy) may be completely corrected by modern surgery.

(5) the causal diagnosis, prevention, and treatment of diseases favored by the physical milieu. The hygiene based on the findings of bacteriology and virology has today, of course, also been accepted by Chinese doctors.

(6) the diagnosis and treatment of serious organic disease. If the diseases mentioned under 3 above, due to negligence of the patient or incompetence of the doctor, have developed into serious manifest organic disease, the more radical therapeutic measures of Western medicine may give better results.

At the outset, we stated that different vantage points, different perspectives, lead to different, mutually exclusive yet equally true views of the same data. But of course, by this statement we did not mean to advocate boundless scientific relativity. Different views, different perspectives, may be equally true, equally legitimate, but they will not, as a rule, be equally adequate. If Western science has produced results of undisputed validity throughout the realm of physics as well as the medical disciplines just enumerated, this is so essentially because its causal and analytic mode— its perspective—was optimally adapted to its objectives of inquiry. And if, on the contrary, such impressive results do not obtain in other realms, this is because the perspective chosen is less adequate for those fields—a situation that can neither be changed by sullen resignation ("Other cultures didn't do any better") nor by stubborn confidence ("It's just a question of time and means"). The situation can be changed only through the adoption of a different perspective, hence by research work in accordance with the different cognitive mode or, quicker still, by the development or integration of data gathered by a more adequate cognitive mode.

This problem of the adequate mode of cognition has been the focus of our research for a number of years. The results arrived at may be summarized thus: If all perceptible effects are arranged according to their degree of differentiation—starting with the elementary particles and advancing through atoms, molecules, cells, lower and higher organisms, human individuals to social, national, cultural communities, celestial bodies, planetary systems and galaxies—viewed from a human perspective, the (apparent) homogeneity of substratums appears to be greatest at the lower end of the scale, and smallest at the upper end. Inversely, the apparent stability of functions is next to insignificant at the lower end, and infinitely large at the upper end. For example, the functions of one single and specific atom, say, the movement of its electrons (hence the functional stability), are so brief in time and so limited in spatial extension as to entirely escape direct and positive observation. However, atoms of a given element, described with respect to their physical properties, resemble each other so closely (apparent homogeneity of the substratum) as to permit the interpretation of data obtained statistically (that is, from the observation of millions of such atoms) to represent the properties of each single atom. Inversely, the physical constituents of a biological organism, say, a human body, are complex to such a degree that any generalization made from the analysis of millions of bodies does not go beyond vague or even tautological generalities: it is utterly without stringency for one particular individual. The functions of the human being, by contrast, evolve over significant lengths of time (apparent stability of functions), may be individually observed with relative ease, precisely described, and compared with the functions of other human beings. Further, the results of such comparisons when integrated into a rational system permit stringent predictions on the evolution of similar functions under the described conditions. The boundary between effects that can be described better by causal analysis and effects that can be more clearly registered by inductive synthesis runs right through the center of the realm of biology—the field of medical endeavor. This boundary coincides with the dividing line between methodologic superiority of Western and Chinese medicines respectively.

THE SYNTHESIS OF CHINESE AND WESTERN MEDICINE

This leads us right up to our final question: If the amalgamation of Western and Chinese medicines is a necessity, how can it be accomplished? To make any headway in this direction presupposes, to start with, general familiarity with medical problems. Hence, almost all publications on Chinese medicine in Western languages had been written by medical doctors. On the other hand, there is no denying that physicians in the contemporary sense—physicians trained and licensed to practice Western medicine—lack essential qualifications to accomplish any rational interpretations of Chinese medicine. It is notorious that, after thorough training and years of practical experience, the average physician devoted to healing his patients only very rarely attains a reflected and clear consciousness of the epistemological premises of the kind of Western science that he believes to practice. And even for professors at medical schools to have such a clear grasp of the methodological premises of their discipline is the exception, not the rule. If that is so, how can we expect someone who knows how to employ but not how to articulately describe his science to give pertinent and germane information on a system of science diametrically opposed to his own?

Can we then look to the East Asians for a comprehensive and modern interpretation of Chinese medicine? It is a worldwide myth that any Chinese or Japanese with a fair education has simply to put out his hand in order to seize the essentials of the science of his forebears. On the contrary, the graduated M.D.s of East Asia have been trained exclusively in Western medicine and have adopted Western scientific theory, which is at complete variance with the intellectual heritage of their own culture. The result is that most of them take a supercilious or derogative attitude to traditional medical theory, and those who do not are, because of their split intellectual loyalties, rarely able to attain any degree of distant appraisal of either system. Since the "modern M.D.s" are practically inarticulate with regard to traditional Chinese medicine, and since, on the other hand, the few remaining traditional practitioners who were trained in the last days of the Empire have no real grasp of the fundamental premises of modern sciences, we find when we look to the East conservative and diffident interpretations at best, forced and haphazard modernizations at worst.

Ample proof of this reserved assessment is available in the experience made in the People's Republic of China. There, facilities for the clinical application of traditional medicine are provided in all fairly large cities, and medical assistance and the so-called barefoot doctors carry proven remedies to the remotest village. Theoretical and basic research, however, is limited to a comparatively small number of institutions. For even in China proper, highly qualified experts on traditional Chinese medicine are rare. The best known of these research institutions, usually called "academies of Chinese medicine," are those of Peking, Nanking, Chengtu, Canton, Shanghai. Their assignments comprise the publication of new editions of the medical classics and, more important, the collective compilation of modern textbooks. Among the latter, mention should be made of the *General Compendium of Chinese Medicine* first brought out in 1958, revised and enlarged in 1959, and of which, up to now, probably some two million copies have been distributed; also of the series "Revised Tentative Teaching Materials of Chinese Medicine for Medical Academies," the publication of which got under way after a conference held in Shanghai in 1963, and in which, up to now, some seventeen titles have appeared; finally of the *Compendium of Chinese Medicine (for Doctors of Western Medicine)* that came out in 1972 with an initial printing of a million copies. As far as authoritativeness, clarity, and completeness are concerned, these publications represent the best of what has appeared on the subject of traditional Chinese medicine in recent times. But they contribute practically nothing to the amalgamation of Chinese and Western medical theory. In the *General Compendium of Chinese Medicine* and in most texts of the series "Revised Tentative Teaching Materials," the theorems of Chinese medicine are expounded from the classics quite as if no other medicine existed; in a few titles of the series and in the *Compendium of Chinese Medicine (for Doctors of Western Medicine)*, the gap between Chinese and Western medical theory is factitiously bridged by "interpreting" Chinese theory through Western terminology.

The goal of understanding the essence of Chinese thought about nature in the light of modern science can only be attained if on the one hand we abstain from substituting analytical Western equivalents for Chinese synthetic terms (which would destroy their integral significance); and if on the other hand we define and circumscribe these same Chinese terms analytically. Only thus will the scientist, who moves in a radically different sphere of ideas than the Sinologist, be able to assimilate and reconstruct the notions expressed by these terms.

Surely, on the practical and empirical level compromise is possible at all times. The ethnologist observing the habits of a tribe of indigenes may put on a loincloth, paint his face, and at the same time manipulate tape-recorders and cameras; the East Asian medium may carry a Swiss-made chronometer on his wrist when executing his hoary ceremonies; the surgeon a la mode may induce local anesthesia in his patients by means of acupuncture. On the level of rational science, however, only such data may be combined, integrated, amalgamated that have been logically perceived in all their extent. Consequently, if the system of classical Chinese medicine at the present juncture is to be assessed and described in a scientific way, thorough knowledge of the philology involved in dealing with Chinese medical texts as well as something better than a smattering of epistemology is indispensable. It is hard to conceive where else than at research and teaching institutions in the West such a combination of skills can be produced, refined, and passed on to coming generations of scholars and practicing physicians.

If we are to achieve the rational appreciation and integration of Chinese medicine into the pool of universal science, then we must acknowledge the fundamental methodological difference and mutual complementarity of Chinese and Western medicines. We have attempted to show here some of the problems associated with the modern study of Chinese medicine and give a brief glimpse of the vast increment of knowledge that can result from the amalgamation of Chinese and Western medicines.

BIBLIOGRAPHY

Needham, Joseph. *History of Scientific Thought.* Science and Civilization in China, Vol. 2. Cambridge: Cambridge University Press, 1956.

Porkert, Manfred. *The Theoretical Foundations of Chinese Medicine: Systems of Correspondence.* Cambridge, Mass.: MIT Press, 1974.

————. "On the Dilemma of Present-day Interpretations of Chinese Medicine and on the Way to Overcome This Dilemma." In *Medicine in Chinese Cultures,* ed. A. Kleinman, et al. Washington, D.C.: John E. Fogarty International Center, 1975.

————. "The Intellectual and Social Impulses Behind the Evolution of Traditional Chinese Medicine." In *Asian Medical Systems,* ed. Charles Leslie, Burg Wartenstein Symposium No. 53, Berkeley: University of California Press, 1976.

Sivin, Nathan. "An Introductory Bibliography of Traditional Chinese Science: Books and Articles in Western Languages." In S. Nakayama and N. Sivin (editors), *Chinese Science: Explorations of an Ancient Tradition.* (Cambridge, Mass.: MIT Press, 1973.)

Translated by Ilza Veith

From *The Yellow Emperor's Classic of Internal Medicine*

TREATISE ON THE NATURAL TRUTH IN ANCIENT TIMES

The Yellow Emperor once addressed T'ien Shih, the divinely inspired teacher: "I have heard that in ancient times the people lived [through the years] to be over a hundred years, and yet they remained active and did not become decrepit in their activities. But nowadays people reach only half of that age and yet become decrepit and failing. Is it because the world changes from generation to generation? Or is it that mankind is becoming negligent [of the laws of nature]?"

Ch'i Po answered: "In ancient times those people who understood Tao [the way of self-cultivation] patterned themselves upon the Yin and the Yang [the two principles in nature] and they lived in harmony with the arts of divination.

"There was temperance in eating and drinking. Their hours of rising and retiring were regular and not disorderly and wild. By these means the ancients kept their bodies united with their souls, so as to fulfill their allotted span completely, measuring unto a hundred years before they passed away.

"Nowadays people are not like this; they use wine as beverage and they adopt recklessness as usual behavior. They enter the chamber [of love] in an intoxicated condition; their passions exhaust their vital forces; their cravings dissipate their true [essence]; they do not know how to find contentment within themselves; they are not skilled in the control of their spirits. They devote all their attention to the amusement of their minds, thus cutting themselves off from the joys of long [life]. Their rising and retiring is without regularity. For these reasons they reach only one half of the hundred years and then they degenerate.

"In the most ancient times the teachings of the sages were followed by those beneath them; they said that weakness and noxious influences and injurious winds should be avoided at specific times. They [the sages] were tranquilly content in nothingness and the true vital force accompanied them always; their vital [original] spirit was preserved within; thus, how could illness come to them?

"They exercised restraint of their wills and reduced their desires; their hearts were at peace and without any fear; their bodies toiled and yet did not become weary.

"Their spirit followed in harmony and obedience; everything was satisfactory to their wishes and they could achieve whatever they wished. Any kind of food was beautiful [to them]; and any kind of clothing was satisfactory. They felt happy under any condition. To them it did not matter whether a man held a high or a low position in life. These men can be called pure at heart. No kind of desire can tempt the eyes of those pure people and their mind cannot be misled by excessiveness and evil.

"[In such a society] no matter whether men are wise or foolish, virtuous or bad, they are without fear of anything; they are in harmony with Tao, the Right Way. Thus they could live more than one hundred years and remain active without becoming decrepit, because their virtue was perfect and never imperiled" (pp. 97–98).

Thus the interaction of the four seasons and the interaction of Yin and Yang [the two principles in nature] is the foundation of everything in creation. Hence the sages conceived and developed their Yang in Spring and Summer, and conceived and developed their Yin in Fall and Winter in order to follow the rule of rules; and thus [the sages], together with everything in creation, maintained themselves at the gate of life and development.

Those who rebel against the basic rules of the universe sever their own roots and ruin their true selves. Yin and Yang, the two principles in nature, and the four seasons are the beginning and the end of everything and they are also the cause of life and death. Those who disobey the laws of the universe will give rise to calamities and visitations, while those who follow the laws of the universe remain free from dangerous illness, for they are the ones who have obtained Tao, the Right Way.

Tao was practiced by the sages and admired by the ignorant people. Obedience to the laws of Yin and Yang means life; disobedience means death. The obedient ones will rule while the rebels will be in disorder and confusion. Anything contrary to harmony [with nature] is disobedience and means rebellion to nature.

Hence the sages did not treat those who were already ill; they instructed those who were not yet ill. They did not want to rule those who were already rebellious; they guided those who were not yet rebellious. This is the meaning of the entire preceding discussion. To administer medicines to diseases which have already developed and to suppress revolts which have already developed is comparable to the behavior of those persons who begin to dig a well after they have become thirsty, and of those who begin to cast weapons after they have already engaged in battle. Would these actions not be too late? (pp. 104–05).

MICROCOSM-MACROCOSM

The Yellow Emperor said: "I desire to hear how it is possible that the twelve viscera send each other that which is precious and that which is worthless."

Ch'i Po answered: "How can I best answer this question? May I ask you to follow these words: the heart is like the minister of the monarch who excels through insight and understanding; the lungs are the symbols of the interpretation and conduct of the official jurisdiction and regulation; the liver has the functions of a military leader who excels in his strategic planning; the gall bladder occupies the position of an important and upright official who excels through his decisions and judgment; the middle of the thorax [the part between the breasts] is like the official of the center who guides the subjects in their joys and pleasures; the stomach acts as the official of the public granaries and grants the five tastes; the lower intestines are like the officials who propagate the Right Way of Living, and they generate evolution and change; the small intestines are like the officials who are trusted with riches, and they create changes of the physical substance; the kidneys are like the officials who do energetic work, and they excel through their ability and cleverness; the burning spaces are like the officials who plan the construction of ditches and sluices, and they create waterways; the groins and the bladder are like the magistrates of a region or a district, they store the overflow and the fluid secretions which serve to regulate vaporization. These twelve officials should not fail to assist one another.

"When the monarch is intelligent and enlightened, there is peace and contentment among his subjects; they can thus beget offspring, bring up their children, earn a living and lead a long and happy life. And because there are no more dangers and perils, the earth is considered glorious and prosperous.

"But when the monarch is not intelligent and enlightened, the twelve officials become dangerous and perilous; the use of Tao [the Right Way] is obstructed and blocked, and Tao no longer circulates warnings against physical excesses. When one attains Tao [the Right Way], even in small and trifling matters, the change will not exhaust and impoverish the people, for they know how to search for themselves" (pp. 133–34).

The east wind arises in Spring; its sickness is located in the liver and there are disturbances in the throat and neck. The south wind arises in Summer; its sickness is located in the heart and there are disturbances in the chest and ribs. The west arises in Fall; its sickness is located in the lungs and disturbances arise at the shoulders and at the back. The north wind arises in Winter; its sickness is located in the kidneys and disturbances arise in the loins and thighs. In the center there is the earth; its sickness is located in the spleen and disturbances arise in the spine (p. 110).

The heavenly climate circulates within the lungs; the climate of the earth circulates within the throat; the wind circulates within the liver, thunder penetrates the heart; the air of a ravine penetrates the stomach; the rain penetrates the kidneys. The six arteries generate streams; the bowels and the stomach generate the oceans; the nine orifices generate flowing water; and Heaven and Earth generate Yin and Yang [the two opposing principles] (p. 123).

Huang Ti asked: "Since the five viscera correspond with the four seasons, does each of the viscera receive some influence?"

Ch'i Po replied: "Yes. Green is the color of the East, it pervades the liver and lays open the eyes and retains the essential substances within the liver. Its sickness is a nervous disease, its taste is sour; its kind [element] is grass and trees [wood]; its animal is the chicken; its grain is wheat; it conforms to the four seasons and corresponds to the plant Jupiter, the year star. Thus the breath of Spring is located in the head. Its sound is chio; its number is eight; and thus it becomes known that its diseases are located in the muscles; its smell is offensive and fetid.

"Red is the color of the South, it pervades the heart and lays open the ears and retains the essential substances within the heart. Its sickness is located in the five viscera; its taste is bitter; its kind [element] is fire; its animal are sheep; its grain is glutinous panicled millet; it conforms to the four seasons and corresponds to the planet Mars. And thus it becomes known that its diseases are located in the pulse; its sound is chih; its number is seven; and its smell is scorched" (p. 112).

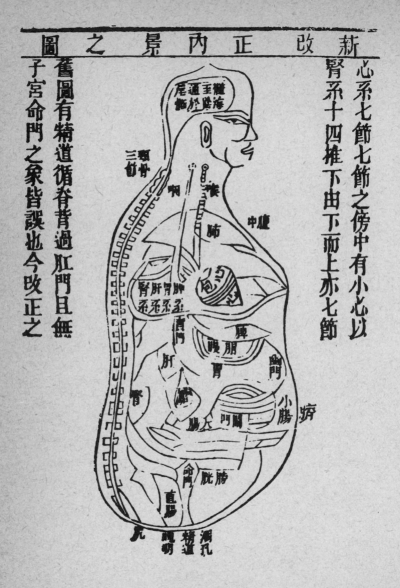

The internal organs

(from *I Tsung Pi Tu*, compiled c. 1575 A.D.)

"What is meant by *hsing*, the body [the visible form], and what is meant by shên, the spirit? I desire to hear it all."

Ch'i Po replied: "Let me discuss *hsing*, the body [the visible form]. What is the body? The body is regarded as holding that which is subtle and minute, and it is held responsible and investigated for its diseases. By searching into it and pondering over its regular conduct, much will become apparent; but to place the hand in front of it does not reveal the facts [details] of the case. Therefore it is called *hsing*, the body, the physical appearance."

The Emperor asked: "And what is meant by *shên*, the spirit?"

Ch'i Po answered: "Let me discuss *shên*, the spirit. What is the spirit? The spirit cannot be heard with the ear. The eye must be brilliant of perception and the heart must be open and attentive, and then the spirit is suddenly revealed through one's own consciousness. It cannot be expressed through the mouth; only the heart can express all that can be looked upon. If one pays close attention one may suddenly know it but one can just as suddenly lose this knowledge. But shên, the spirit, becomes clear to man as though the wind has blown away the cloud. Therefore one speaks of it as the spirit" (p. 222).

TREATISE ON THE IMPORTANCE OF THE PULSE AND THE SUBTLE SKILL OF ITS EXAMINATION

If it were not for excellent technique and the subtlety of the pulse one would not be able to examine it. But the examination must be done according to a plan, and the system of Yin and Yang [the two principles of nature] serves as basis for examination. When this basis is established one can investigate the twelve main vessels and the five elements that generate life. Life itself follows a pattern that was set by the four seasons.

In order to effect a cure and relief one must not err towards the laws of Heaven nor towards those of the Earth, for they form a unit. When this feeling for Heaven and Earth as one unit has been attained, then one is able to know death as well as life (p. 162).

One should feel whether the pulse is in motion or whether it is still and one should observe attentively and with skill. One should examine the five colors and the five viscera, whether they suffer from excess or whether they show an insufficiency, and one should examine the six bowels whether they are strong or weak. One should investigate the appearance of the body whether it is flourishing or deteriorating. One should use all these five examinations and combine their results, and then one will be able to decide upon the share of life and death (p. 159).

When the pulse beats in accord with Yin and Yang, the disease changes for the better and comes to an end; but when the pulse beats in opposition to Yin and Yang the disease becomes worse. When the pulse obediently follows the four seasons there will be no disease; but when the pulse does not beat in consonance with the four seasons it will not extend to the regions between the five viscera and the resulting disease will be a difficult one to cure (p. 171).

All those who excel in the art of feeling the pulse find that when it is fine, slow, and short, there is an excess of Yang and when the pulse is slippery, like pebbles rolling in a basin, there is an excess of Yin (p. 167).

[The experts in the art of examination] take into consideration whether the day is cold or warm, whether the moon is empty or full, they consider the four seasons and whether the atmosphere is light or heavy; and they consider how these factors associate with each other, their mutual affinity and their blending and harmony (p. 219).

The Yellow Emperor said: "Man's place of residence, his motion and rest [his circumstances of life], his courage and cowardice—do they not also cause change within the vascular system [pulse]?"

Ch'i Po answered: "Yes, in general man's fear and apprehension, his passion [anger] and his suffering, his motion and his rest, they all cause changes.

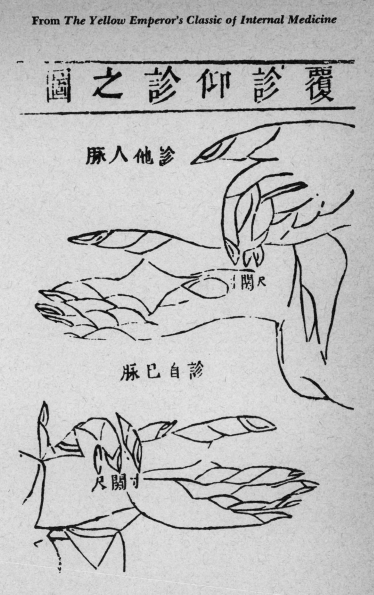

The pulses

(from *T'u Chu Mo Chüeh*, by Chang Shih-hsien of the Ming period, published in 1510)

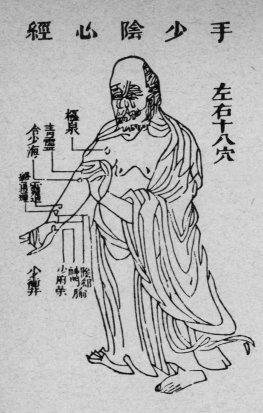

The heart vessel of the lesser Yin showing
acupuncture spots
(from *Ling Shu Su Wên Chieh Yao*)

"Those who are about at night have difficulties in breathing emanating from the kidneys. Those whose demeanor is dissolute and licentious get a disease of the lungs. Those who are lazy and full of apprehension and fear have difficulties in breathing, emanating from the lungs. Those whose deportment is licentious and excessive will injure their spleen. Those whose demeanor is immoral and dissolute will injure their hearts.

"Therefore it is said: In order to examine the course of a

disease one must investigate whether man is courageous or nervous and cowardly, and one must examine his bones, flesh, and skin and then one can know the facts of the case which are necessary for the methods of treatment" (p. 195).

By observing myself I know about others and their diseases are revealed to me, and by observing the external symptoms one gathers knowledge about internal disturbances. One should watch beyond the ordinary limits for rules which are unfit and inadequate; one should observe minute and trifling things as if they were of normal size, and when they are thus treated they cannot become dangerous (p. 124).

THE DIFFERENT METHODS OF TREATMENT AND THE APPROPRIATE PRESCRIPTIONS

The Yellow Emperor asked: "When the physicians treat diseases, do they treat each disease differently from the others and can they all be healed?"

Ch'i Po answered: "Yes, they can all be healed according to the physical features of the place where one lives.

"Beginning and creation come from the East. Fish and salt are the products of water and ocean and of the shores near the water. The people of the regions of the East eat fish and crave salt; their living is tranquil and their food delicious. Fish causes people to burn within [thirst], and the eating of salt injures [defeats] the blood. Therefore the people of these regions are all of dark complexion and careless and lax in their principles. Their diseases are ulcers, which are most properly treated with acupuncture by means of a needle of flint. Thus the treatment with acupuncture with a needle of flint has its origin in the regions of the East.

"Precious metals and jade come from the regions of the West. The dwellings in the West are built of pebbles and sandstone. Nature [Heaven and Earth] exerts itself to bring a good harvest. The people of these regions live on hills and, because of the great amount of wind, water, and soil, become robust and energetic. The people of these regions wear no clothes other than those of coarse woolen stuff or coarse matting. They eat good and variegated food and therefore they are flourishing and fertile. Hence evil cannot injure their external bodies, and if they get diseases they strike at the inner body. These diseases are most successfully cured with poison medicines. Thus the treatment with poison medicines comes from the West.

"The North is the region of storing and laying by. The country is hilly and mountainous, there are biting cold winds, frost and ice. The people of these regions find pleasure in living in this wilderness, and they live on milk products. The extreme cold causes many diseases. These diseases are most fittingly treated with cauterization by burning the dried tinder of the artemisia [moxa]. Hence the treatment with cauterization has its origin in the regions of the North.

"Nourishment and growth come from the South. The Sun makes the life of those who live in the regions of the South plentiful and nourishing. Although there is water beneath the earth, the soil is deficient, [but] it collects dew and mist. The people who live in the regions of the South crave sour food and curd. They are secretive and soft in their ways and attached to the red color. Their diseases are bent and contracted muscles and numbness. These diseases are most fittingly treated with acupuncture with fine needles. Hence the treatment with the fine needles comes from the South.

"The region of the center, the Earth, is level and moist. Everything that is created by the Universe meets in the center and is absorbed by the Earth. The people of the regions of the center eat mixed food and do not [suffer or weary at their] toil. Their diseases are many: they suffer from complete paralysis and chills and fever. These diseases are most fittingly treated with breathing exercises, massage of skin and flesh, and exercises of hands and feet. Hence the treatment with breathing exercises, massage and exercises of the limbs has its origin in the center regions.

"The ancient sages combined these various treatments for the purpose of cure, and each patient received the treatment that was most fitting for him. These treatments were so extraordinary and so different in each case that all diseases were healed. Thus the circumstances and the needs of each disease were ascertained and the principle of the art of healing became known" (pp. 147–48).

The superior physician helps before the early budding of the disease. He must first examine the three regions of the body and define the atmosphere of the nine subdivisions so that they are entirely in harmony, and nothing can be destroyed, and then his help sets in. Therefore he is called the superior physician.

The inferior physician begins to help when [the disease] has already developed; he helps when destruction has already set in. And since his help comes when the disease has already developed it is said of him that he is ignorant (p. 220).

TREATISE ON THE TRANSMITTAL OF THE ESSENCE AND THE TRANSFORMATION OF THE LIFE-GIVING PRINCIPLE

The Yellow Emperor asked: "I understand that in olden times the treatment of diseases consisted merely of the transmittal of the Essence and the transformation of the life-giving principle. One could invoke the gods and this was the way to treat. The present generation treats internal diseases with the [5] poison medicines and they treat external diseases with acupuncture, and sometimes the patients are healed and sometimes the patients are not healed. How can you explain this?"

Ch'i Po answered: "In former times man lived among birds, beasts and reptiles; he worked, moved and stirred in order to avoid and to escape the cold and the darkness, and he sought a dwelling into which he could flee from the heat. Within him there were no family ties which bound him with love; on the outside there were no officials who could guide out and correct his physical appearance. Into this tranquil and peaceful era evil influences could not penetrate deeply. Therefore poison medicines were not needed for the treatment of internal diseases, and acupuncture was not needed for the cure of external diseases. Hence it was sufficient to transmit the Essence and to invoke the gods; and this was the way to treat.

"But the present world is a different one. Grief, calamity, and evil cause inner bitterness, while the body receives wounds from the outside; moreover there is neglect against the laws of the four seasons, there is disobedience and rebellion and there are those who violate the customs of what is proper during the cold of Winter and the heat of Summer. Reprimands are in vain. Evil influences strike from early morning until late at night; they injure the five viscera, the bones and the marrow within the body, and externally they injure the mind and reduce its intelligence and they also injure the muscles and the flesh. Hence the minor illnesses are bound to become grave and the serious diseases are bound to result in death. Therefore the invocation of the gods is no longer the way to cure" (pp. 148–49).

The treatment in this past age was quite different. It was not based upon the four seasons, there was no knowledge of sun and moon, there was no examination as to obedience or disobedience [towards the laws of nature]. In order to terminate physical illnesses and to bring health, external diseases were treated with acupuncture and internal diseases with hot water or soups, and liquid medicines (p. 150).

The method of the needle [acupuncture] is available to all the people; but the people know only how to live, they do not understand how to apply the five methods in order to get well from their diseases. The first method cures the spirit; the second gives knowledge of how to nourish the body; the third gives knowledge of the true effects of poisons and medicines; the fourth explains acupuncture and the use of the small and the large needle; the fifth tells how to examine and to treat the intestines and the viscera, the blood and the breath. These five methods are drawn up together so that each has one that precedes it.

Nowadays, in this latest period, acupuncture is applied in

order to supply what is lacking and in order to drain off excessive fullness. All those who work [in these fields] share this knowledge.

Since these methods are those of Heaven, the Earth follows and adjusts its action. Those who are in harmony are like an echo; those who are in accord with these methods are like shadows; they follow [their way] Tao, and need neither demons nor gods, for they are free and independent (p. 215).

The Emperor asked: "When the body is worn out and the blood is exhausted, is it still possible to achieve good results?" Ch'i Po replied: "No, because there is no more energy left." The Emperor inquired: "What does it mean, there is no more energy left?"

Ch'i Po answered: "This is the way of acupuncture: if man's vitality and energy do not propel his own will his disease cannot be cured.

"Nowadays vitality and energy are considered the foundation of life; in order to keep them flourishing they must be protected and the life-giving force must rule. When this force does not support life, its foundation will dissolve, and how can a disease be cured when there is no spiritual energy within the body?" The Emperor said: "Thus life itself is really the beginning of illness!" (p. 152).

The Emperor said: "I should like to be informed about the essential doctrines [of healing]." Ch'i Po answered: "The utmost in the art of healing can be achieved when there is unity." The Emperor inquired: "What is meant by unity?" Ch'i Po answered: "When the minds of the people are closed and wisdom is locked out they remain tied to disease. Yet their feelings and desires should be investigated and made known, their wishes and ideas should be followed; and then it becomes apparent that those who have attained spirit and energy are flourishing and prosperous, while those perish who lose their spirit and energy." The Emperor exclaimed: "Excellent, indeed!" (pp. 150–51).

Translated by W. H. S. Jones

≈⁓

From *The Works of Hippocrates*

I declare, however, that we ought not to reject the ancient art as non-existent, or on the ground that its method of inquiry is faulty, just because it has not attained exactness in every detail, but much rather, because it has been able by reasoning to rise from deep ignorance to approximately perfect accuracy, I think we ought to admire the discoveries as the work, not of chance, but of inquiry rightly and correctly conducted.

Ancient Medicine, Chapter XII[1]

ENVIRONMENTAL MEDICINE

Airs, Waters, and Places

Whoever wishes to pursue properly the science of medicine must proceed thus. First he ought to consider what effects each season of the year can produce; for the seasons are not at all alike, but differ widely both in themselves and at their changes. The next point is the hot winds and the cold, especially those that are universal, but also those that are peculiar to each par-

From *Hippocrates,* translated by W. H. S. Jones (Cambridge, Mass.: Harvard University Press, 1923 and 1931). Reprinted by permission of the publishers and The Loeb Classical Library.

ticular region. He must also consider the properties of the waters; for as these differ in taste and in weight, so the property of each is far different from that of any other. Therefore, on arrival at a town with which he is unfamiliar, a physician should examine its position with respect to the winds and to the risings of the sun. For a northern, a southern, an eastern, and a western aspect has each its own individual property. He must consider with the greatest care both these things and how the natives are off for water, whether they use marshy, soft waters, or such as are hard and come from rocky heights, or brackish and harsh. The soil too, whether bare and dry or wooded and watered, hollow and hot or high and cold. The mode of life also of the inhabitants that is pleasing to them, whether they are heavy drinkers, taking lunch, and inactive, or athletic, industrious, eating much and drinking little . . .

As time and the year passes he will be able to tell what epidemic diseases will attack the city either in summer or in winter as well as those peculiar to the individual which are likely to occur through change in mode of life. For knowing the changes of the seasons, and the risings and settings of the stars, with the circumstances of each of these phenomena, he will know beforehand the nature of the year that is coming. Through these considerations and by learning the times beforehand, he will have full knowledge of each particular case, will succeed best in securing health, and will achieve the greatest triumphs in the practice of his art. If it be thought that all this belongs to meteorology, he will find out, on second thoughts, that the contribution of astronomy to medicine is not a very small one but a very great one indeed. For with the seasons men's diseases, like their digestive organs, suffer change.

Airs Waters Places, Chapter I–II[2]

Inhabitants of a region which is mountainous, rugged, high, and watered, where the changes of the seasons exhibit sharp contrasts, are likely to be of big physique, with a nature well adapted for endurance and courage, and such possess not a little wildness and ferocity. The inhabitants of hollow regions that are meadowy, stifling, with more hot than cool winds, and where the water used is hot, will be neither tall nor well-made, but inclined to be broad, fleshy, and dark-haired; they themselves are dark rather than fair, less subject to phlegm than to bile. Similar bravery and endurance are not by nature part of their character, but the imposition of law can produce them artificially. Should there be rivers in the land, which drain off from the ground the stagnant water and the rain water, these will be healthy and bright. But if there be no rivers, and the water that the people drink be marshy, stagnant, and fenny, the physique of the people must show protruding bellies and enlarged spleens. Such as dwell in a high land that is level, windy, and watered, will be tall in physique and similar to one another, but rather unmanly and tame in character. As to those that dwell on thin, dry, and bare soil, and where the changes of the seasons exhibit sharp contrasts, it is likely that in such country the people will be hard in physique and well-braced, fair rather than dark, stubborn and independent in character and in temper. For where the changes of the seasons are most frequent and most sharply contrasted, there you will find the greatest diversity in physique, in character, and in constitution.

These are the most important factors that create differences in men's constitutions; next come the land in which a man is reared, and the water. For in general you will find assimilated to the nature of the land both the physique and the characteristics of the inhabitants. For where the land is rich, soft, and well-watered, and the water is very near the surface, so as to be hot in summer and cold in winter, and if the situation be favourable as regards the seasons, there the inhabitants are fleshy, ill-articulated, moist, lazy, and generally cowardly in character. Slackness and sleepiness can be observed in them, and as far as the arts are concerned they are thick-witted, and neither subtle nor sharp. But where the land is bare, waterless, rough, oppressed by winter's storms and burnt by the sun, there you will see men who are hard, lean, well-articulated, well-braced, and hairy; such natures will be found energetic, vigilant, stubborn and independent in character and in temper, wild rather than tame, of more than average sharpness and intelligence in the arts, and in war of more than average courage. The things also that grow in the earth all assimilate themselves to the earth.

Airs Waters Places, Chapter XXIV[3]

Constitution of the Seasons

What the character of a season's diseases and constitutions will be you must foretell from the following signs. If the seasons proceed normally and regularly, they produce diseases that come easily to a crisis. The diseases that are peculiar to the seasons are clear as to their fashions. According to the alterations in a season, the diseases such as arise in this season will be either like or unlike their usual nature. If the season proceeds normally, similar or somewhat similar to the normal will be the diseases, as, for example, autumnal jaundice; for cold spells succeed to hot spells and heat to cold. If the summer prove bilious, and if the increased bile be left behind, there will also be diseases of the spleen. So when spring too has had a bilious constitution, there occur cases of jaundice in spring also. For this motion is very closely akin to the season when it has this nature. When summer turns out like to spring, sweats occur in fevers; these are mild, not acute, and do not parch the tongue. When the spring turns out wintry, with after-winter storms, the diseases too are wintry, with coughs, pneumonia or angina. So in autumn, should there be sudden and unseasonable wintry weather, symptoms are not continuously autumnal, because they began in their wrong season, but irregularities occur. So seasons, like diseases, can fail to show crisis or to remain true to type, should they break out suddenly, or be determined too soon, or be left behind. For seasons, too, suffer from relapses, and so cause diseases. Accordingly, account must also be taken of the condition of a body when the seasons come upon it.

Humours, Chapter XIII[4]

Constitutions and Predispositions

The constitutions of men are well or ill adapted to the seasons, some to summer, some to winter; others again to districts, to periods of life, to modes of living, to the various constitutions of diseases. Periods of life too are well or ill adapted to districts, seasons, modes of living and constitutions of diseases. So with the seasons vary modes of living, foods and drinks.

Humours, Chapter XVI[5]

Know in what seasons the humours break out, what diseases they cause in each, and what symptoms they cause in each disease. As to the body generally, know to what disease the physical constitution most inclines. For example, a swollen spleen produces a certain effect, to which the constitution contributes something.

Humours, Chapter VIII[6]

Changes

It is changes that are chiefly responsible for diseases, especially the greatest changes, the violent alterations both in the seasons and in other things. But seasons which come on gradually are the safest, as are gradual changes of regimen and temperature, and gradual changes from one period of life to another.

Humours, Chapter XV[7]

Excess and suddenness in evacuating the body, or in replenishing, warming, cooling, or in any other way disturbing it, is dangerous; in fact all excess is hostile to nature. But "little by little" is a safe rule, especially in cases of change from one thing to another.

Aphorisms, Section II, Chapter LI[8]

Things to which one has been used a long time, even though they be more severe than unaccustomed things, usually cause less distress. Nevertheless, change to unaccustomed things may be necessary.

Aphorisms, Section II, Chapter L[9]

HEALTH AND DISEASE

Vis Medicatrix Naturae

Nature [*physis*] heals disease. Inherent mechanisms act automatically as reflexes, much as the reflexes that we use in winking the eyelids or moving the tongue, for nature is active without training and without schooling in these essentials.

Epidemics VI, Chapter 5[10]

All Things in Sympathy

The nature of the body must be regarded as a whole, in every consideration of the medical art.

Places in the Body, Chapter 2[11]

According to my concept of the body there is no beginning, everything is beginning and everything is end, as in a circle. This is true of disease and of the body as a whole ... When disease is localized in one part it is apt to involve other parts ... If one injures the smallest part of the body, the whole body actually would experience the disturbance for the very simple reason that the very smallest part actually is composed of the same things as the whole and the single part transmits even the smallest impulse, good or bad, to all other parts that are associated; this because the entire body is integrated with the small parts in pain as well as in pleasure, for the smallest parts transmit to related parts and these again pass on the impulse.

De Locis in Homine, Chapter 1[12]

Conflux one, conspiration one, all things in sympathy; all parts forming a whole, and severally the parts in each part, with reference to the work.

Nutriment, Chapter XXIII[13]

Balance of the Humours

The body of man has in itself blood, phlegm, yellow bile and black bile; these make up the nature of his body, and through these he feels pain or enjoys health. Now he enjoys the most perfect health when these elements are duly proportioned to one another in respect of compounding, power, and bulk, and when they are perfectly mingled. Pain is felt when one of these elements is in defect or excess, or is isolated in the body without being compounded with all the others. For when an element is isolated and stands by itself, not only must the place which it left become diseased, but the place where it stands in a flood must, because of the excess, cause pain and distress.

Nature of Man, Chapter IV[14]

Health

For the healthy condition of a human being is a nature that has naturally attained a movement, not alien but perfectly adapted, having produced it by means of breath, warmth and coction of humours, in every way, by complete regimen and by everything combined, unless there be some congenital or early deficiency.

Precepts, Chapter IX[15]

THE ART OF MEDICINE

Aphorism

Life is short, the Art long, opportunity fleeting, experiment treacherous, judgment difficult. The physician himself must be ready, not only to do his duty himself, but also to secure the co-operation of the patient, of the attendants and of externals... So one ought to have an eye to season, district, age and disease, to see if the treatment is, or is not, proper in the circumstance.

Aphorisms, Section I, Chapters I and II[16]

Individuation

There is no demonstrable beginning of treatment which is properly a beginning of medicine generally, nor is there a second point, nor a middle, nor an end; rather, we begin treatment sometimes by speaking, sometimes by acting, and finish in the same way; and in speaking, we do not begin from the same statements, not even if we are speaking of the same objects, nor do we end with the same statements; and likewise, in acting, we neither begin treatment nor end it with the same actions.

Diseases, Book I, Chapter 9[17]

To Help or at Least to Do No Harm

Declare the past, diagnose the present, foretell the future; practice these acts. As to diseases, make a habit of two things—to help or at least to do no harm. The art has three factors, the disease, the patient, and the physician. The physician is the servant of the art. The patient must co-operate with the physician in combating the disease.

Epidemics I, Chapter XI[18]

It is only when the art sees its way that it thinks it right to give treatment, considering how it may give it, not by daring but by judgment, not by violence but by gentleness.

The Art, Chapter XI[19]

Analysis and Synthesis

The following were the circumstances attending the diseases, from which I framed my judgment, learning from the common nature of all and the particular nature of the individual, from the disease, the patient, the regimen prescribed and the prescriber—for these make a diagnosis more favourable or less; from the constitution, both as a whole and with respect to the parts, of the weather and of each region; from the custom, mode of life, practices and ages of each patient; from talk, manner, silence, thoughts, sleep or absence of sleep, the nature and time of dreams, pluckings, scratchings, tears; from the exacerbations, stools, urine, sputa, vomit, the antecedents and consequents of each member in the successions of diseases, and the abscessions to a fatal issue or a crisis, sweat, rigor, chill, cough, sneezes, hiccoughs, breathing, belchings, flatulence, silent or noisy, hemorrhages, and hemorrhoids. From these things must we consider what their consequents also will be.

Epidemics I, Chapter XXIII[20]

For so I think the whole art has been set forth, by observing some part of the final end in each of many particulars, and then combining all into a single whole. So one must pay attention to generalities in incidents, with help and quietness rather than with professions and the excuses that accompany ill-success.

Precepts, Chapter II[21]

To Teach

It is particularly necessary, in my opinion, for one who discusses this art to discuss things familiar to ordinary folk. For the subject of inquiry and discussion is simply and solely the sufferings of these same ordinary folk when they are sick or in pain. Now to learn by themselves how their own sufferings come about and cease, and the reasons why they get worse or better, is not an easy task for ordinary folk; but when these things have been discovered and are set forth by another, it is simple. For merely an effort of memory is required of each man when he listens to a statement of his experiences. But if you miss being understood by laymen, and fail to put your hearers in this condition, you will miss reality.

Ancient Medicine, Chapter II[22]

Love of Man, Love of the Art

I urge you not to be too unkind, but to consider carefully your patient's superabundance or means. Sometimes give your services for nothing, calling to mind a previous benefaction or present satisfaction. And if there be an opportunity of serving one who is a stranger in financial straits, give full assistance to all such. For where there is love of man, there is also love of the art. For some patients, though conscious that their condition is perilous, recover their health simply through their contentment with the goodness of the physician. And it is well to superintend the sick to make them well, to care for the healthy to keep them well, but also to care for one's own self, so as to observe what is seemly.

Precepts, Chapter VI[23]

Wisdom and Medicine

Transplant wisdom into medicine and medicine into wisdom. For a physician who is a lover of wisdom is the equal of a god. Between wisdom and medicine there is no gulf fixed.

Decorum, Chapter V[24]

REGIMEN IN HEALTH

Ways of Health

A physician's studies should include a consideration of what is beneficial in a patient's regimen while he is yet in health.

Regimen in Acute Diseases, Chapter XXVIII[25]

I maintain that he who aspires to treat correctly of human regimen must first acquire knowledge and discernment of the nature of man in general—knowledge of its primary constituents and discernment of the components by which it is controlled. For if he be ignorant of the primary constitution, he will be unable to gain knowledge of their effects; if he be ignorant of the controlling thing in the body he will not be capable of administering to a patient suitable treatment. These things therefore the author must know, and further the power possessed severally by all the foods and drinks of our regimen, both the power each of them possessed by nature and the power given them by the constraint of human art. For it is necessary to know both how one ought to lessen the power of these when they are strong by nature, and when they are weak to add by art strength to them, seizing each opportunity as it occurs. Even when all this is known, the care of a man is not yet complete, because eating alone will not keep a man well; he must also take exercise. For food and exercise, while possessing opposite qualities, yet work together to produce health. For it is the nature of exercise to use up material, but of food and drink to make good deficiencies. And it is necessary, as it appears, to discern the power of the various exercises, both natural exercises and artificial, to know which of them tends to increase flesh and which to lessen it; and not only this, but also to proportion exercise to bulk of food, to the constitution of the patient, to the age of the individual, to the season of the year, to the changes of the winds, to the situation of the region in which the patient resides, and to the constitution of the year. A man must observe the risings and settings of stars, that he may know how to watch for change and excess in food, drink, wind and the whole universe, from which diseases exist among men.

Regimen I, Chapter II[26]

Diet and Exercise

The normal ordinary person ought to order his regimen in the following way. In winter eat as much as possible and drink as little as possible; drink should be wine as undiluted as possible, and food should be bread, with all meats roasted; during this season take as few vegetables as possible, for so will the body be most dry and hot. When spring comes, increase drink and make it very diluted, taking a little at a time; use softer foods and less in quantity; substitute for bread barley-cake; on the same principle diminish meats, taking them all boiled instead of roasted, and eating when spring comes a few vegetables, in order that a man may be prepared for summer by taking all foods soft, meats boiled, and vegetables raw or boiled. Drinks should be as diluted and as copious as possible, the change to be slight, gradual and not sudden. In summer the barley-cake to be soft, the drink diluted and copious, and the meats in all cases boiled. For one must use these, when it is summer, that the body may become cold and soft. For the season is hot and dry, and makes bodies burning and parched. Accordingly these conditions must be counteracted by way of living. On the same principle the change from spring to summer will be prepared for in like manner to that from winter to spring, by lessening food and increasing drink. Similarly, by opposing opposites prepare for the change from summer to winter. In autumn make food more abundant and drier, and meats too similar, while drinks should be smaller and less diluted, so that the winter may be healthy and a man may take his drink neat and scanty and his food as abundant and as dry as possible. For in this way he will be most healthy and least chilly, as the season is cold and wet.

Those with physiques that are fleshy, soft and red, find it beneficial to adopt a rather dry regimen for the greater part of the year. For the nature of these physiques is moist. Those that are lean and sinewy, whether ruddy or dark, should adopt a moister regimen for the greater part of the time, for the bodies of such are constitutionally dry. Young people also do well to adopt a softer and moister regimen, for this age is dry, and young bodies are firm. Older people should have a drier kind of diet for the greater part of the time, for bodies at this age are moist and soft and cold. So in fixing regimen pay attention to age, season, habit, land, and physique, and counteract the prevailing heat or cold. For in this way will the best health be enjoyed.

Regimen in Health, Chapters I–II[27]

Prevention

Such is my advice to the great mass of mankind, who of necessity live a haphazard life without the chance of neglecting everything to concentrate on taking care of their health. But when a man is thus favourably situated, and is convinced that neither wealth nor anything else is of any value without health, I can add to his blessings a regimen that I have discovered, one that approximates to the truth as closely as is possible. . . . It comprises prognosis before illness and diagnosis of what is the matter with the body, whether exercise overpowers food, or whether the two are duly proportioned. For it is from the overpowering of one or the other that diseases arise, while from their being evenly balanced comes good health. Now these different conditions I will set forth, and explain their nature and their arising in men who appear to be in health, eat with an appetite, can take their exercise, and are in good condition and of a healthy complexion.

Regimen III, Chapter LXIX[28]

I have discovered these things, as well as the forecasting of an illness before the patient falls sick, based upon the direction in which is the excess. For diseases do not arise among men all at once; they gather themselves together gradually before appearing with a sudden spring. So I have discovered the symptoms shown in a patient before health is mastered by disease, and how these are to be replaced by a state of health.

Regimen I, Chapter II[29]

In some other cases appear the following symptoms. The stools that pass are undigested, and the body wastes away, getting no profit from the food. In course of time such people fall ill. In these cases the bowels are cold and dry. So when they take neither suitable food nor suitable exercises, their symptoms are those I have said. This kind of person is benefited by taking bread of bolted meal, oven-baked, boiled fish in sauce, boiled pork, extremities thoroughly boiled, fat meats roasted, of acrid, salt foods such as are moistening, and also piquant sauces. Wines to be dark and soft. Some grapes and some figs to be taken with food. A little luncheon too should be eaten. Exercises should be above the average, double-track running should be gradually increased, while the last running should be on the circular track; after the running should come wrestling with the body oiled. After the exercises there should be short walks, after dinner mere strolls, but in the early morning longer walks. Let the bath be warm. Unguents should be used. Let sleep be plentiful and on a soft bed. Some sexual intercourse is necessary. Reduce food by one-third. Take twelve days to bring food back to normal.

Regimen III, Chapter LXXX[30]

Furthermore, one must know that diseases due to repletion are cured by evacuation, and those due to evacuation are cured by repletion; those due to exercise are cured by rest, and those due to idleness are cured by exercise. To know the whole matter, the physician must set himself against the established character of diseases, of constitutions, of seasons and of ages; he must relax what is tense and make tense what is relaxed. For in this way the diseased part would rest most, and this, in my opinion, constitutes treatment.

Nature of Man, Chapter IX[31]

What is necessary is to exercise forethought before the diseases attack. . . . The wise man should not let things drift, but as soon as he recognizes the first signs should carry out a cure.

Regimen III, Chapters LXXI, LXXII[32]

A wise man should consider that health is the greatest of human blessings, and learn how by his own thought to derive benefit in his illness.

Regimen in Health, Chapter IX[33]

Prayer

Prayer indeed is good, but while calling on the gods a man should himself lend a hand.

Regimen IV, Chapter LXXXVII[34]

REFERENCES

1   W. H. S. Jones, trans., *Hippocrates,* vol. 1, The Loeb Classical Library (Cambridge: Harvard University Press, 1923), p. 33.
2   Ibid., 1:71, 73.
3   Ibid., 1:133, 135, 137.
4   Ibid., 4:85, 87.
5   Ibid., 4:89, 91.
6   Ibid., 4:79.
7   Ibid., 4:89.
8   Ibid., 4:121.
9   Ibid.
10 William F. Peterson, *Hippocratic Wisdom: For Him Who Wishes to Pursue Properly the Science of Medicine* (Springfield, Illinois: Charles C. Thomas, 1946), p. 137.
11 Ibid., p. 138.
12 Ibid., p. 185.

13 Jones, *Hippocrates,* 1:351.
14 Ibid., 4:11–13.
15 Ibid., 1:325, 327.
16 Ibid., 4:99.
17 Edwin Burton Levine, *Hippocrates* (New York: Twayne, 1971), p. 93.
18 Jones, *Hippocrates,* 1:165.
19 Ibid., 2:211.
20 Ibid., 1:181.
21 Ibid., 1:315.
22 Ibid., 1:15, 17.
23 Ibid., 1:319.
24 Ibid., 2:287.
25 Ibid., 2:85.
26 Ibid., 4:227, 229.
27 Ibid., 4:45, 47, 49.
28 Ibid., 4:381, 383.
29 Ibid., 4:231.
30 Ibid., 4:407, 409.
31 Ibid., 4:25.
32 Ibid., 4:389, 391.
33 Ibid., 4:59.
34 Ibid., 4:423.

By René Dubos

Hippocrates
in Modern Dress

Fifty years ago, the specialists in infectious disease, nutrition, and metabolism were still the scientific heroes of the medical world. Their disciplines had yielded rich harvests of practical results, and had enlarged man's understanding of his relation to the environment. The intellectual atmosphere in medical schools, however, was even then beginning to change. In 1920, the development of a practical method for the production of insulin made it obvious that medicine had entered a new phase; emphasis had shifted from the external to the internal agents of disease. Today the focus of attention is shifting even further away from the preoccupations of the early 1900's. More and more scientific medicine is identified with the esoteric knowledge of molecular biology or biological electronics, and with the spectacular performances of medical engineering in the lungs, the brain, the heart or the kidneys.

. . . As a representative of one of the downgraded scientific disciplines, medical microbiology, I should therefore feel embarrassed at speaking for the future. But instead, I feel gently amused because I am convinced that the glamorous achievements of today will appear old fashioned fifty years hence. . . .

As there is no good prospective without retrospective, I shall

From *The Proceedings of the Institute of Medicine of Chicago* 25, no. 9 (May 1965): 242–51. Reprinted by permission of René Dubos and The Institute of Medicine of Chicago.

first try to review briefly the forces which have been at work during the past 2,500 years to prepare the forthcoming change in direction of medical effort. I shall first say a few words on Hippocratic medicine, which came to an end one hundred years ago. Then I shall define the two complementary medical philosophies which, in succession, have dominated post-Hippocratic medicine during the past century. Finally I shall announce, with tongue in cheek, the advent of neo-Hippocratic medicine based on a new science dedicated to the interplay between whole man and his environment.

HIPPOCRATES AND THE
BIRTH OF ENVIRONMENTAL MEDICINE

The Hippocratic tradition remained a living force in Western medicine until the last two decades of the 19th century. Surprising as it may seem to us, the treatise on "Airs, Waters, and Places" was reprinted for use in medical schools as late as 1874. ... The 19th century physicians recognized, of course, that the Hippocratic writings were not directly applicable to the clinical problems of their time; they went to Hippocrates for general medical wisdom rather than for practical information. I shall limit my remarks to a discussion of one aspect of this wisdom, namely the role of the external environment on the characteristics of man in health and in disease.

The treatise on "Airs, Waters, and Places" did more than relate the types and frequency of diseases to environmental conditions. It boldly suggested that climate, topography, soil, food, and water affect not only the physical stature, health, and temperament of different national groups, but also their military prowess and social institutions. The relevance of environmental forces to the problems of human biology, medicine, and sociology has never been formulated with greater breadth and sharper vision than it was at the dawn of scientific history! The intellectual basis of Hippocratic medicine was thus the belief that many important physiological and behavioral characteristics are conditioned, and to a large extent, determined by the environmental conditions under which man is born and develops. This generalization is probably unpalatable to those of our contemporaries who have been brainwashed—either by political or scientific propaganda—into believing that nothing biological is of much importance except the genetic endowment. But, in fact, recent experiments in animals, and observations in human children, have established beyond doubt that early environmental influences affect the whole of human life— even more profoundly and lastingly than Hippocrates had anticipated.

If the development of man is an expression of his responses to environmental factors, it follows that there must exist at any given time some kind of equilibrium between his physical and mental attributes and the forces which have shaped them. The Greek concept of health as harmony between man's nature and external nature thus derives its philosophical validity from biological facts. Hence also the emphasis throughout the Hippocratic writings on the role played by sudden changes in weather, in food, or in the ways of life, in the causation of disease. The doctrine of the four humours also finds its place in this medical philosophy. The Hippocratic writings admittedly fail to provide explanations for environmental effects. But they clearly state that health depends upon the maintenance of a state of equilibrium between the various forces of the body and the mind (the humours and the passions) and between them and the external world. For this reason, the Hippocratic Corpus has always been the Bible of those who hold to the thesis that medicine must never lose sight of the whole man in his total environment.

The treatise on "Airs, Water, and Places" ceased being used as a guide to physicians at the end of the 19th century for the obvious reason that the natural sciences had by then undermined its authority. Many of the medical problems associated with topography and with seasonal changes became explainable in the precise terms of the germ theory of disease and of the nutritional sciences; the doctrine of specific etiology displaced in the mind of physicians and of medical scientists the theories based on the role of climate, the qualities of the water, the layout of the land, and other environmental factors. At the same time precise knowledge began to accumulate concerning the structures of the body fabric as well as the forces which hold them together and make them function. Even more importantly, the doctrine of the balance of the humours was restated in the form of the chemical and hormonal processes which tend to assure the fixity of the milieu intérieur.

The past hundred years can thus be regarded as having introduced into scientific medicine two components which made Hippocratic medicine obsolete, namely the doctrine of specific etiology, and the description of the organism in terms of elementary structures and mechanisms. The theoretical and practical achievements of post-Hippocratic medicine during the century which has just elapsed are so spectacular, that it would seem that modern medicine need only continue along the road on which it is now traveling, to bring the world to medical Utopia. Yet, I believe that a change of direction is imperative, and indeed is about to be made. My purpose [here] is to examine the reasons which make it necessary for medicine to move from its present post-Hippocratic phase to a neo-Hippocratic era. First, however, I shall attempt to define the main trends of scientific medicine during the past 100 years.

POST-HIPPOCRATIC MEDICINE

Man in his environment was one of the main themes of European culture during the second half of the 19th century. Political theorists, novelists, and art critics were then prone to trace social, ethical, and cultural problems to the responses made by man and his societies to physical, economic, and historical forces. Similarly, Lamarck and Darwin, each in his own way, regarded organic evolution as the outcome of the interplay between living organisms and their environment. Claude Bernard formulated the view that disease was the result of faulty attempts of the organism to adapt to environmental insults. And Virchow proclaimed that disease was life under changed conditions.

The reformers of the 19th century proceeded on the assumption that most disease problems originate from poverty and filth, and therefore could be solved by improving living conditions. Indeed, great triumphs over disease were achieved during that period by the sanitary crusade based on the motto "Pure Air, Pure Water, Pure Food." During the last quarter of the 19th century, the crusade against poverty, malnutrition, and filth received scientific support from the doctrine of specific etiology. Whereas social betterment and "biological purity" had been the goals of sanitarians and reformers, the war against microbes and malnutrition became the dominant activity of physicians and medical scientists during the post-Hippocratic era.

Whether based on the vague concepts of the sanitary crusade, or on the more precise information derived from experimental science, the campaign against environmental agents of disease remained the main approach to disease control until a few decades ago. The dramatic fall in mortality rates all over the Western world leaves no doubt as to the efficacy of this approach against the infectious and nutritional diseases which dominated the medical picture after the first Industrial Revolution.

Needless to say, environmental control remains as important today as it was a century ago and its future potentialities are far from being exhausted. But there is no doubt that sanitation and other orthodox aspects of public health are now regarded as routine and of little intellectual interest. Around the turn of the century the focus of medical interest shifted from the environment to the intimate structures and mechanisms of living organisms. This shift occurred simultaneously in medicine and in the various fields of general biology. For example, the Darwinian approach to evolution was replaced by studies focused first on chromosomes, then on genes, finally on molecular genetics. In experimental medicine studies on the spread of infection or on the quality of foodstuffs lost ground to the chemical analysis of immunological processes, of intermediary metabolism or of endocrine control. Even the environmental determinants of Pavlovian reflexes or of Freudian complexes are beginning to appear old fashioned when compared with the detailed analysis of neural mechanisms or of memory storage and retrieval.

The shift of interest from the environmental factors that affect human life to the elementary structures and functions of the body machine naturally had a profound influence on the selection of experimental models both for investigation and for teaching. Since all living things have so many characteristics in common and indeed are often almost indistinguishable at the subcellular level, there has been a natural tendency to focus attention on the organisms which are easiest to manipulate in the laboratory. This tendency is based on the widespread though unproven assumption that complete understanding of man's problems will eventually emerge from the detailed knowledge of the structures and functions which are common to all living things. There is no doubt, indeed, that the most spectacular achievements of the biomedical sciences during recent decades have come from the study of simple laboratory models.

Whereas the greatest contribution to health during the 19th century have been in the prevention of disease through manipulation of the environment, the most brilliant successes of 20th century medicine have been in the treatment of disease through action on the intimate mechanisms of the body.[1] The use of insulin and other hormones, the dietary control of phenylketonuria, the maintenance of normal physiological processes during surgical interventions, the operation of artificial kidneys or of cardiac pace setters, are but a few examples of therapeutic procedures which could not have been developed without a detailed knowledge of body components and functions. There

---

[1] The 20th century can of course boast of spectacular feats in the prevention of disease, but these achievements have come in all cases from the direct application of 19th century concepts. For example, the development of new vaccines against bacterial and viral infections did not depend on knowledge of body structures or functions. The 20th century achievements in immunization were the fruits of theoretical concepts developed and successfully used by 19th century immunologists. Similarly, the virtual elimination of deficiency diseases was achieved through nutritional improvements which were little influenced by knowledge of the precise role played by vitamins or amino acids in metabolic, synthetic, or regulatory processes.

is even hope that some of the mental disorders can be managed through this approach.

NEO-HIPPOCRATIC SCIENCE

Medicine and the Humanities

Paradoxically the phenomenal growth of scientific medicine has been accompanied by a parallel increase in the popularity of what has been called "fringe medicine." The various forms of faith-healing and of semimystical oriental practices, the drugs and treatments based on folklore remedies, and the perennial attempts to solve the problems of modern man by a return to the ways of nature, are but a few of the countless manifestations of fringe medicine which prosper in all industrialized Western societies, yet are not derived from Western medical science and are often incompatible with its teachings. To a large extent, the success of fringe medicine reflects of course the credulity of the public and its pathetic longing for miraculous cures, or at least for easy solutions to the problems of disease. But this is not the whole story. Whether fringe medicine is pure deceit, or whether some of its forms have therapeutic merit is irrelevant here. The point of importance is that its popularity points to the failure of the present biomedical sciences to satisfy some large human needs.

Dissatisfaction with scientific medicine as presently conceived extends beyond the uneducated public. It reaches into the most sophisticated classes of society and indeed into many strata of the medical profession. The complaint that the doctor treats the disease but is not interested in the patient or that medicine loses contact with the human condition when it becomes "too" scientific is voiced almost as loudly and frequently by physicians as it is by the general public. The uneasy feeling of the medical profession in this regard expresses itself in many forms, for example: the assertion that the science of medicine must be complemented by the "art" of medicine; the plea for more emphasis on "the whole man" in clinical teaching; the wide-spread practice of urging prospective medical students to cultivate the "humanities" rather than purely scientific disciplines during their college years. I shall discuss together these various symptoms of uneasiness because they all have the same origin and the same implications. In particular, I shall emphasize that the solution to the difficulty is not to make medicine less scientific, but rather to broaden its scientific basis.

Interestingly enough, emphasis on the "whole man" in medical schools became fashionable at the same time that schools of technology began to find it advisable to introduce humanistic disciplines on their campuses. Engineering and architecture, just like medicine, present of course technical problems which are interesting per se and which can be studied for their own sake. But engineers and architects just like physicians can successfully relate their work to human welfare only if they are guided by the knowledge of man's fundamental needs and aspirations. Applicants to schools of medicine or technology are urged to cultivate humanistic studies, because it is assumed that acquaintance with philosophy, literature, and the arts will help them gain a better understanding of the human condition. There is something ironical in the fact that the humanities, long regarded by many scientists as little more than entertaining ornaments of life are now being thought to be essential to the human success of technological civilization!

Like other human beings, physicians and technologists of course derive benefits from exposure to the broad atmosphere provided by courses in philosophy, literature, and the arts. But it is questionable that their professional achievements can be significantly improved by exposure to these disciplines. While humanists and artists have dealt with the universal and eternal aspects of human life, they should not be expected to throw much light on the new problems encountered by man in the modern world. These problems come from challenges for which there is no precedent because the human environment and ways of life are endlessly changing.

Man feels threatened and *is* threatened by the constant and unavoidable exposure to the stimuli of urban and industrial civilization; by the varied aspects of environmental pollution;

by the physiological disturbances associated with sudden changes in the ways of life; by his estrangement from the conditions and natural cycles under which human evolution has occurred; by the emotional trauma and the paradoxical solitude in congested cities; by the monotony, the boredom, indeed the compulsory leisure ensuing from automated work. These are the very influences which are now at the origin of most medical problems. To a very large extent, the disorders of the body and the mind are but the expression of inadequate responses to environmental influences. Physicians and technologists can deal effectively with the needs and problems of man in the modern world only if they can base their action on a knowledge of his nature to supplement the age-old wisdom transmitted through the humanities.

For several thousand years, there has grown a broad and subtle understanding of the human condition, in happiness and in despair; during the past three hundred years, the biomedical sciences have accumulated an immense number of precise facts concerning the human body and the human mind, in health and in disease. The physician, it would seem at first sight, need only synthesize existing humanistic and scientific knowledge to apprehend all the attributes, needs, and urges which make up total man. But imposing as these two aspects of knowledge are, and complementary as they appear to be, they do not constitute together a true science of man. They do not form a coherent structure, because there is hardly any contact between the aspects of human biology most extensively studied by scientists, and the experiences of the human condition which humanists try to understand and artists to express.

One often hears that scientists, humanists, and creative artists all deal with the same world, even though they use such different techniques to recognize and describe reality. In practice, however, scientists and humanists are concerned with entirely different problems even when they look at the same living organism. The difference in outlook comes from the fact that scientists deal with the *stuff and mechanics* of life, whereas humanists (and creative artists) are concerned with the *experience* of life. Scientists focus their attention on the structures and mechanisms through which living organisms function, and on a few environmental factors which can be measured and manipulated; as a result, they tend to equate unicellular organism and man; they regard as most scientific and "fundamental" those studies which deal with the elemental structures and reactions common to all forms of life. Humanists and artists, in contrast, are little if at all concerned with the so-called fundamental structures and mechanisms through which living things operate; they deal with the experiences of throbbing men and women, responding in all their complexity to the stimuli and challenges of their total environment.

Western medicine occupies a peculiar place between science and the humanities, because it partakes of both activities. On the one hand, it utilizes sophisticated scientific methods to carry out a reductionist analysis of man's attributes. On the other hand, it has learned from practical experience that scientific findings can contribute to man's welfare only if the physician applies them with a kind of skill akin to art.

The art of medicine demands of the physician a holistic attitude very different from the typical scientific approach. It involves the ability to select, intuitively as it were, those aspects of the total medical situation in all its complexity which can be manipulated not only by scientific medical technologies but also by any other kind of influence which promises to be useful. Seen in this light, the art of medicine appears so complex and personal as to be outside the scope of the scientific method, just as is artistic creation. Nevertheless, there is reason to hope that the art of medicine could become more scientific if a vigorous effort were made to study man's responses to the various forces which affect his well-being. A few examples will show that the knowledge needed here must deal with man as a whole, rather than with the reductionist analysis of his constituent parts.

The humanness of man creates problems not definable in exact scientific terms. Nevertheless, many of his responses are amenable to objective study. The task is naturally easiest for the responses which are the direct results of the effects exerted by environmental forces on the components of the body machine. Physiochemical reactions and simple reflex mechanisms are manifestations of this direct impact which constitute favorite topics of study because they lend themselves to precise analysis by orthodox scientific methods. It is obvious, however, that such simple phenomena account for only a very small proportion, and probably the least important, of the experiences and responses which make up human life.

Man responds not as a mechanical assemblage of parts, but as an integrated organism with a complex history. Any physiochemical or psychic stimulus which impinges on him sets in motion a host of secondary processes with very indirect and often delayed effects. Seeing an object which recalls an article of food may stimulate appetite or cause nausea; smelling an artificial perfume may evoke the heat of a summer day, or the chill of a fall evening; hearing a faint but unexpected noise at night may cause either a rise or fall in blood pressure. In other words, the ultimate physiological or mental expression of stimuli commonly has little bearing on their primary direct effects.

Fortunately, knowledge relevant to even the most complex and indirect of man's responses can be derived from the study of animal life, because models for almost any particular human problem can be found occurring naturally or be created experimentally in one or another animal species. The effects on man of isolation or crowding, of overstimulation or understimulation, of disturbances in behavior patterns or in social organization, are but a few of the human problems for which counterparts exist in the animal world. These problems can be studied experimentally in animal models just as certainly as the effects of physical stimuli or of environmental pollutants. A day will certainly come when the study of "life situations" in the form of animal models will have as much glamour in sophisticated medical schools as that now possessed by models derived from molecular biology or electronic systems.

The Living Past

The magnitude of the indirect effects exerted by the ordinary events of life on man is in large part the consequence of his propensity to symbolize events and to react to the symbols as if they were the real stimuli. Furthermore, and perhaps most importantly, ~~his responses to almost any situation are conditioned by his past.~~ His evolutionary development and his personal experiences are inscribed in his flesh and bone; the traditions of ~~his social group condition his beliefs, attitudes, and tastes.~~ Each person incorporates, one could almost say incarnates, his history in his own total being. The persistence of the past plays such an immense role in human life that it bids fair to constitute one of the most important medical aspects of the science of man, and therefore deserves some emphasis here.

~~Most physiological functions exhibit diurnal, seasonal,~~ and ~~lunar rhythms which persist even when the person is shielded from awareness of the passage of time or of the movements of celestial bodies.~~ It is clear that biological rhythms were inscribed in man's genetic makeup during evolutionary development when human life was closely linked to the natural events determined by the movements of the earth around the sun and of the moon around the earth. Biological rhythms are important for the understanding of modern man because they persist even though he now lives in an artificial environment. He may intellectually forget diurnal, lunar, and seasonal influences, but he cannot escape their physiological and mental effects.

~~Ancient man also developed a series of automatic physiological and mental mechanisms which increased his chances of survival or of biological success, when he encountered a threat~~ such as coming from a wild beast or from a human stranger. These mechanisms rapidly mobilized in his body the hormonal and chemical reactions which facilitated fight or flight. As is well known, the so-called fight and flight response, in its many forms, still occurs when modern man finds himself in social situations which he interprets as threatening, even though the need for expenditure of physical energy rarely arises under the conditions of civilized life.

These two classical examples illustrate how much the art of medicine could be enriched by more precise knowledge of man's evolutionary endowment. For it is certain that just as modern man has retained from his evolutionary past useless and often annoying anatomical vestiges, similarly he has retained many unrecognized physiological and mental attributes which are ill suited to civilized life. In other words, he must meet the challenges of today with an anachronistic biological equipment. Many peculiarities in his responses, and many forms of organic and mental disease, originate from the paleolithic biological equipment with which he must face the conditions of modern life.

All human beings have fundamentally the same anatomical structure, function through the same chemical activities, exhibit the same physiological manifestations, and are driven by the same biological urges; yet no two human beings are alike. Clearly, knowledge of the attributes which are common to mankind as a whole is not sufficient to account for the manner in which each individual person behaves as he does, develops his own peculiarities, in brief, becomes different from all other human beings. Individual persons differ, of course, by reason of the fact that they do not have the same genetic makeup; only identical twins are alike genetically. But at least equally important is the fact that the individual characteristics of human beings are constantly being shaped and modified by environmental factors which endlessly vary with time, differ from one place to the other, and therefore are never the same for two different persons, even though they be idential twins.

Recent studies have confirmed the ancient awareness of the fact that many characteristics of the adult result from the effects of so-called early influences, namely of those environmental factors which impinge on the organism during early life, while he is still developing. Such formative effects can take place even *in utero*. Prenatal and early postnatal influences can affect almost every trait—from nutritional needs and rates of growth, to learning ability and emotional attitudes. Moreover, the effects of early influences are so deeply rooted in the biological structure of the person involved that they often and perhaps always persist throughout his whole life span. One of the greatest contributions of the Hippocratic school, and in our own times of Freud, has been to emphasize the importance of taking a "history" in the examination of the patient. History-taking will certainly become an even more important aspect of medical care in the future, when more is known of the extent to which the experiential past can affect all aspects of life.

The biological and psychological processes set in motion by

the interplay between human beings provide other examples of the lasting and profound influence which the past exerts on modern man. Because he evolved as a social animal, man cannot develop well physically and mentally, or even long remain normal, unless in association with other human beings. But on the other hand, crowding and excess of social stimuli may over-stimulate certain of his hormonal activities and thereby have undesirable consequences. The threshold of safety with regard to the type and intensity of social contacts is ill defined and indeed differs according to the history of the person concerned and of his group. Qualitatively and quantitatively, man's responses to the social environment are conditioned not only by his genetic endowment and his early experiences, but also by the traditional conventions and values of the group within which he developed and in which he functions. Man's nature is conditioned by his social past, whether he rebels against its traditions, or passively accepts it as embodying the truth.

Medicine and the Science of Man

Human life being so profoundly influenced by the evolutionary, experiential, and social past, it is certain that the science of man cannot possibly be based exclusively on knowledge of the reactions exhibited by components isolated from the body. The past, like the mind, disappears when the organism is taken apart. The statement that most responses involve the whole organism functioning as an integrated unit is so obvious as to seem trivial. But it has large implications for medical teaching and medical research.

The time has come to give to the study of the responses that the living organism makes to its total environment the same dignity and support which is being given at present to the science of parts and reactions isolated from the organism. Exclusive emphasis on the reductionist approach will otherwise lead medicine into blind alleys. Unless a program of organismic and environmental research is vigorously prosecuted, medicine will be unable to support the loads placed on it by the health problems arising from the new environmental forces created by modern life.

A great difficulty in developing the science of man is that the life of each individual person is made up of situations which are unique and therefore appear incompatible with the generalizations of which science is made. In reality, however, all human beings have in common many fundamental traits; furthermore, most members of any given culture share a number of experiences, values, and modes of thought which make their responses statistically predictable. It should be possible, therefore, to base the science of man on a large body of working assumptions and thus to assess the effect of certain environmental conditions on health and performance.

Since all important responses have multiple determinants, new scientific methods will have to be developed to investigate complex systems in which various factors act simultaneously. Here again the difficulties, while very great, are not insuperable as indicated by recent experiences. The training of men for operation in the arctic, in the tropics, or in space vehicles; the study of brainwashing and of various forms of sensory deprivation as caused, for example, by confinement or by automated work, are but a few examples where practical demands have compelled the development of methods for a multifactorial approach to human problems. I am convinced that if medical scientists would set their minds to it, organismic and environmental medicine would soon become a sophisticated and productive field of science.

The study of the complex problems posed by the human responses to new environments will require of course the participation of many scientific specialties other than medicine. But medicine seems best suited nevertheless to preside in an architectonic way over the development of a new science of man. Granted the inescapable limitations of their initial training in the various specialized sciences, physicians have the overwhelming advantage that bedside experience gives them an awareness of the fundamental needs and potentialities of the human condition. One of the fruits of medical training is a concrete awareness of the complexity and plasticity of man's nature, and of the creative way in which most human beings respond to environmental challenges.

The development of methods for studying the responses of the whole integrated organism would complement the reductionist analysis of structures and mechanisms, and thereby enlarge enormously the scope of biomedical sciences. In fact, the study of responses is medical biology *par excellence*, because it provides information bearing directly on the well-being of man. The role of medicine is to help man function well, as long as possible, and if possible happily in all his endeavors—whether he is toiling for his daily bread, creating urban civilization, writng a poem, or attempting to reach the moon. These examples are not taken at random. I have selected them to symbolize that medicine relates to all human activities, to the responses of man in the worlds of nature, of thought, of feeling, and of technology.

Medicine was at the beginning of civilization the mother of sciences and played a large role in the integration of early cultures. Then it constituted for a long time the bridge over which science and humanism maintained some contact. Today it has once more the opportunity of becoming a catalytic force in civilization by pointing to the need, and providing the leadership, for the development of a science of man. The continued growth of technological civilization, indeed its very survival, requires an enlargement of our understanding of man's nature. Man can function well only when his external environment is compatible with the needs created by the traits which he retains from his evolutionary, experiential, and social past, and also by his aspirations for the future. In its highest form, medicine remains potentially the richest expression of science because it is concerned with all the various aspects of man's humanness.

PART THREE

UNORTHODOX
MEDICINE

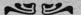

Introduction

One day Nasrudin found a weary falcon sitting on his window sill.

He had never seen a bird of this kind before.

"You poor thing," he said, "how ever were you allowed to get into this state?"

He clipped the falcon's talons and cut its beak straight, and trimmed its feathers.

"There, now you look more like a bird," said Nasrudin.

Idries Shah, *The Exploits of the Incomparable Mulla Nasrudin*

Unorthodox, unconventional, alternative, marginal, boundary, fringe, irregular, sectarian, cult, and quack are a few of the terms used to describe certain health beliefs, practices, and practitioners that lie outside the medical orthodoxy. The relativity of such terms is immediately apparent. While primitive healing ceremonies are regarded as unorthodox in modern Western societies, scientific medicine is similarly held to violate the conventions and legitimated practices of most non-Western cultures. Practices such as bloodletting and purging, once regarded as orthodox treatments, are now viewed as unconventional. Similarly, many of the medical beliefs and practices now accepted and vigorously defended in the mainstream may soon find themselves in the ranks of unorthodoxy. The point is that "orthodox" is not synonymous with "true" or "efficacious." Conversely, "unorthodox" does not mean "untrue" or "ineffective"; it only describes a position that does not conform with the usual or established conventions, conventions that themselves may or may not be true.

Although we may wish to think that contemporary scientific medicine represents the objective accumulation of effective therapies, familiarity with the history and politics of medicine reveals the intense political, economic, cultural, and personal forces that have shaped and, at times, distorted the development of contemporary medicine. Competition and ethnocentrism have often prevailed over any real concern with the relative value or efficacy of different therapies.

At the outset, unorthodox medicine should be distinguished from quackery, in which patients are deliberately deceived. There is no evidence to suggest that charlatanry, profiteering, or exploitation occur any more frequently among unorthodox practitioners than among the orthodox. For the most part, unconventional practitioners, no matter what their practices or doctrines, sincerely believe in the efficacy of what they do.

The types of practices and practitioners labeled as unorthodox in Western societies are extremely diverse. Some have ancient roots, others are of rather recent vintage. Some systems originated and flourished in proximity, and often in opposition, to Western scientific medicine, while others have developed in areas where orthodox medicine was not available or accessible. Some unorthodox practitioners, known as the "straights," reject any attempt to integrate or interact with the orthodox mainstream, while the so-called mixers draw freely from other unorthodox systems as well as orthodox medicine. Some unorthodox systems have formal schools and elaborate training programs; others depend upon apprenticeships or, in certain cases, divine inspiration and revelation. Some offer distinct, even competitive, alternatives to orthodox medicine, while others stress the supplementary and complementary aspects of their activities. Whatever their differences, the distinguishing feature of the unorthodox systems of medicine is that they are based on concepts of disease, forms of treatment, and criteria for evaluating efficacy that are divergent from the contemporary mainstream of Western medicine.

The extent of unorthodox medicine in our society has not

been adequately assessed. It is known that the vast majority of diagnosis and treatment of ill-health takes place outside of the formal medical system, mostly in the family and popular health culture where health beliefs and practices may differ considerably from prevailing professional views. Judging from the proliferation of popular health books and health food stores, the recent resurgence of interest in folk practitioners, faith healers, herbalists, acupuncturists, chiropractors, and nutritionists as well as the elaboration of health-related spin-offs from the "counter-culture" and "human potential movement," one could conclude that the interest in unconventional medicine is extensive and growing. One recent survey estimated that nearly a third of individuals in this culture may consult marginal practitioners of one sort or another; if the use of home remedies and folk medical practices were included in this estimate, the proportion would be considerably greater. As another indicator of the scope of unorthodox medicine, an international conference held in Italy several years ago featured over fifty different presentations on the "other" medicine.

The phenomenon of unorthodox medicine cannot be ignored or dismissed as only another example of human gullibility and superstitiousness. Medicine is a practical endeavor. Patients will seek alternative therapies and practitioners if their needs, ranging from relief of symptoms to hope in the face of life-threatening disease, are not adequately met by orthodox practitioners.

Unorthodox practitioners tend to flourish at the borders of orthodox medicine, dealing with illnesses and concerns where modern medicine is not very successful. Some unorthodox practitioners offer services that are not readily, if at all, available from the medical care system—for example, counseling in self-care, diet, exercise, relaxation and health promotion. Many people go to unorthodox practitioners because of the financial, geographic, or cultural barriers to regular medical care. Many patients with psychosomatic complaints, chronic and degenerative diseases, or terminal illnesses turn to unorthodox practitioners for a sense of hope, personal attention, physical contact, or a regard for the whole person which seems to be overlooked in the technical concerns of the Western physician. For even when nothing can be done in a technical sense to alter the biological course of a disease, there is still much that can be done in a caring sense to help make the human experience of disease personally more meaningful and understandable. Many unorthodox practitioners seem better able to communicate with patients, relating more closely to the world view of the patient, which is often at some disance from the impersonal and technical domain of modern medicine.

The plurality of our medical care system may in fact be one of its greatest strengths. Besides meeting the diverse needs of a diverse population, the existence of unorthodox systems allows for alternative channels for therapeutic innovation. The orthodoxy is conservative by nature, encouraging research only within an accepted ideology. Unorthodox systems may provide the stimulus for research into approaches not developed or even considered in the mainstream. For example, the interest in psychic healing highlights our lack of understanding of the role of psychological factors in health and healing. Similarly, traditional healing ceremonies call attention to cultural factors in healing, while chiropractic and its kindred practices urge us to reconsider the importance of body mechanics. Unorthodox medicine may also serve as a corrective to the therapeutic exuberance of contemporary medicine, as homeopathy did in the nineteenth century when extreme and often fatal treatments were the accepted practices.

There are substantial barriers to a serious and dispassionate evaluation of unorthodox medicine, not the least of which are posed by economic and political forces as mentioned above. However, the unorthodox systems themselves present problems that make their study difficult. Many present-day practices represent a degeneration of original therapies and philosophies and therefore offer little opportunity for understanding the insights that initially gave rise to the system. This degeneration is particularly true of the ancient healing systems as we have seen with Chinese medicine, but it also applies to the unorthodox systems that depend on oral transmission and apprenticeship training.

Another obstacle is the paucity of scientific evidence supporting most of the unorthodox practices. The lack of careful investigation exists, in part, because most unconventional practitioners are either uninterested or untrained in the methods of scientific research. For the most part, they and their patients are completely convinced by clinical experience that their practices are effective and therefore do not need to be proved. Unfortunately the lack of controlled studies and the reliance on anecdotal evidence and clinical testimony are generally regarded by orthodox medicine as a sign of the falsity of the practices, not as an invitation for more investigation. This situation is not helped by the defensiveness and paranoia that further insulates unorthodox medicine. Interchange is also hampered by the outlandish claims and faulty rationalizations advanced by many unorthodox practitioners. Techniques are all too often represented as panaceas and theories as dogma or sometimes divinely inspired law. The reaction by orthodox health professionals is predictable. The therapeutic claims and empirical observations of unconventional practitioners are either disregarded completely or quickly dismissed by invoking such poorly understood concepts as placebo effect, suggestion, and spontaneous remission. The result is that little objective research is available on which to evaluate unorthodox medicine.

The theories and packaging of unorthodox medicine commonly includes strange and invented terminology either because the existing body of scientific knowledge was unfamiliar to the unconventional practitioner or inadequate to explain the practices. It is tempting to dismiss these divergent theories out of hand or to try to clean them up, make them look more familiar, as Nasrudin did to the falcon. This brings us to the most troubling and, at the same time, intriguing aspect of unorthodox medicine, namely, that unorthodox medicine is often not in accord with the existing scientific paradigm. It may not be possible to completely rationalize these systems within the physiochemical explanatory framework of Western medicine without distortion and loss. The unorthodox systems are rather strange, but this strangeness may offer us the opportunity to learn if we resist the temptation to clip the falcon's talons to make it look more like a familiar bird.

Of course, it is not possible to seriously consider all the forms of unorthodox medicine. For the purposes of discussion, I have selected three articles that illustrate not only three different unconventional ways of healing but also three different approaches —comparative, experimental, and descriptive—to studying these healing systems.

Jerome Frank, a psychiatrist and psychologist, takes a penetrating look at the psychosocial factors involved in healing. He presents a comparison of the healing process in primitive societies, at the Western Shrine of Lourdes, and among various secular and religious healers. Underlying these diverse practices are common therapeutic features that include mobilizing the patient's natural healing powers, arousing hope and expectancy of cure, and reinforcing ties with the social group and the cultural world view. These healing techniques serve to underline the importance of emotional and cognitive states in illness as well as in healing. A similar demonstration of this crucial mind-body interaction can be found in the later section on techniques of self-regulation. While unorthodox healers tend to maximize these powerful psychological factors, Western medicine tends to underestimate their importance. In concluding his psychological analysis of nonmedical healing, Frank states that while "the healing power of faith resides in the patient's state of mind, not the validity of its object . . . [nevertheless] some individuals . . . may have a gift for healing that defies scientific explanation. . . . Nor can one rule out the possibility—indeed the evidence for it is quite persuasive—that some healers serve as a kind of conduit for a healing force in the universe, often called the life force."

Frank's conclusion is Bernard Grad's starting point as he describes his experimental investigation of healing by the laying on of hands. It is somewhat remarkable that although the laying on of hands has been used for thousands of years and the scientific methodology to explore it has existed for many years, there have been few attempts to test the efficacy or biological effects of this technique. The discussion of the laying on of hands has, for the most part, been in the form of an impassioned argument between believers and disbelievers, between anecdotal evidence and theoretical impossibility. Usually the effects of the laying on of hands are attributed solely to suggestion (whatever that means) or to divine intervention (whatever that means). Most agree, at the very least, that a certain sense of comfort and solace can be conveyed to the sick through the human touch, although this simple act has become increasingly rare in orthodox medical practice

Bernard Grad, a research biologist, became interested in the possibility of scientifically testing the claims made by a certain healer. Grad devised a series of double-blind controlled experiments to evaluate the laying on of hands in terms of its effects on experimentally induced injuries in mice and plants. In one series, the healer treated sealed bottles of water with the laying on of hands. The water was then transferred to the plants and the growth rate was measured and compared with control plants. The results indicated small but statistically significant positive effects on the treated plants, biological effects that could not be accounted for solely in terms of suggestion or any known physical or chemical forces. These results, however, must be viewed with caution; the experiments are by no means conclusive and will require careful and independent replication. Nevertheless, they do demonstrate that this form of healing can be scientifically investigated much as other therapeutic modalities can be evaluated. The preliminary findings also suggest that there may be important, unexplored factors in healing, which, because of their subtlety, their association with the unorthodox and occult, and their "impossibility" in terms of the current scientific paradigm, have been systematically ignored. Clearly this subject demands further investigation.

In the concluding essay on unorthodox medicine, Harris Coulter, an historian, describes the basic principles and practices of homeopathic medicine. Homeopathy was developed in Germany in the early 1800s by Dr. Samuel Hahnemann as an alternative to the heroic practices of bloodletting, purging, and harsh cathartics. Homeopathy spread to America in the 1820s and flourished until the early 1900s. At its peak there were numerous homeopathic medical schools and as many as one in ten physicians in some parts of America practiced homeopathy. Today, it continues to be practiced in such countries as England, France, Germany, Greece, and India, but its use in America has all but died out. The reasons for this decline are numerous and include political and economic factors as much as the failure to produce sufficient evidence of clinical efficacy that is acceptable to the medical profession and the public.

In his essay, Coulter contrasts the principles and practices of homeopathy with those of orthodox, or allopathic, medicine. According to Coulter, the essentially materialistic approach of orthodox medicine attempts to identify and counteract the specific agents and symptoms of disease. Homeopathy, in contrast, takes a vitalistic approach in which symptoms are viewed as part of the curative process and are, therefore, supported, not counteracted. In homeopathy, attention is directed toward the changing subjective symptom reports of the patient (both bodily and mental) rather than the objective physiological and pathological reports from the laboratory. In this sense, homeopathy is not unlike traditional Chinese medicine in its focus on functional changes rather than pathological and organic alterations. In homeopathy, the appropriate drug remedy is selected by matching the symptoms reported by the patient with the symptoms produced by the same drug when given to a healthy person; that is, the remedy is selected to support and reinforce the curative symptom response of the patient. This therapeutic principle, known as the Law of Similars, or "like cures like," is reflected in the term homeopathy from the Greek *homoion*, meaning similar, and *pathos*, meaning suffering. The closest orthodox medicine comes to this practice is in immunization, where small, attenuated doses of a pathogenic agent are given to stimulate the defenses of the body. Homeopathy also relies upon extremely attenuated doses of drugs, diluted at times to the point where, according to prevailing Western medical science, no physiological effect is theoretically possible. Coulter introduces us to the difficult, if not "impossible," principles of homeopathy.

Clearly the topics discussed here will disturb some readers; I have not attempted not to trim the falcon's talons. It is hoped that these essays will provoke inquiry and investigation, not necessarily agreement. At least, unorthodox medicine may challenge us to examine our assumptions; at best, we may find new and complementary approaches to health and healing.

By Jerome D. Frank

❧ ☙

Nonmedical Healing: Religious and Secular

"I can't believe *that*," said Alice. "Can't you?" the Queen
said in a pitying tone. "Try again; draw a long breath,
and shut your eyes."

Lewis Carroll, *Through the Looking Glass*

Western industrial societies view illness essentially as a malfunctioning of the body, to be corrected by appropriate medical and
surgical interventions. Many believe, not without reason, that
the causes of even so-called mental illnesses will be discovered to
be subtle derangements of the brain. In this view, which gains
strong support from the triumphs of scientific medicine, the
physician is a highly skilled scientist-technician, whose job is to
diagnose the bodily disturbance and correct it, much as a good
auto mechanic would deal with a poorly running automobile.

While this approach to illness has scored notable successes and
will undoubtedly score many more, it is seriously deficient in a
crucial respect. It fails to acknowledge that psychological and
bodily processes can profoundly affect each other. High among
the former are the meanings of illness emerging from the inter-

From *Persuasion and Healing*, pp. 46–77 (Baltimore: The Johns Hopkins
University Press, 1973). Copyright © 1973 by The Johns Hopkins University
Press. Reprinted by permission.

play of the sick person with his family and his culture. All ill-nesses, whatever their bodily components, have implications that may give rise to noxious emotions, raise difficult moral issues, damage the patient's self-esteem, and estrange him from his compatriots. Chronic illness, especially, causes demoralization. Constant misery, forced relinquishment of the activities and roles that supported the patient's self-esteem and gave his life signif-icance, the threat of suffering and death—all may generate feel-ings of anxiety and despair, which, in turn, may be intensified by reactions of anxiety, impatience, and progressive withdrawal in those close to him, especially when his illness threatens their security as well as his own. Thus illness often creates a vicious circle by evoking emotions that aggravate it.

The insensitivity of scientific medicine to the noxious effects of these emotions probably accounts for many of its failures and also impels the ill to seek out forms of healing which operate on a different premise. "People do not visit a fringe practitioner be-cause they are gullible, stupid or superstitious, though they may be; they go to him because they think, or hope, they can get some-thing from him that their doctor no longer gives. They are right; often the doctor does not pretend to be able to give it."[1]

All practitioners of nonmedical healing, who, incidentally, minister to many more sufferers throughout the world than do physicians, see illness as a disorder of the total person, involving not only his body but his image of himself and his relations to his group; instead of emphasizing conquest of the disease, they focus on stimulating or strengthening the patient's natural heal-ing powers. They believe that this can be done by the ministra-tions of a healer who, whatever his methods, enters into an in-tense relationship with the patient. In contrast with scientific medicine which, while paying copious lip service to the doctor-patient relationship, in actuality largely ignores it, all nonmed-

[1] Inglis (1965), pp. 53–54. He classifies nonmedical healing into three cate-gories, progressively more distant from scientific medicine: those emphasizing the body, such as herbalism, homeopathy, chiropractic, and osteopathy; those emphasizing the mind, such as psychotherapy, hypnotherapy, and autosuggestion; and those stressing the spirit, such as Christian Science and spiritual healing.

ical healing methods attach great importance to it. Those operating in a religious context, which includes all forms of healing in primitive societies and faith healing in industrial ones, also see themselves as bringing supernatural forces to bear on the patient, with the healer acting primarily as a conduit for them.

This chapter focuses on healing in primitive societies, considers one Western healing shrine, and takes a brief glance at secular forms of nonmedical healing in the West.[2]

Examination of religious healing in so-called primitive societies and in Western society illuminates certain aspects of human functioning that are relevant to psychotherapy. Methods of supernatural healing highlight the close interplay of assumptive systems and emotional states and the intimate relation of both to health and illness. They also bring out the parallel between inner disorganization and disturbed relations with one's group, and indicate how patterned interaction of patient, healer, and group within the framework of a self-consistent assumptive world can promote healing. Certain properties of healing rituals in primitive societies, finally, show interesting resemblances to naturalistic psychotherapeutic methods that may serve to increase understanding of both.

The view that illness can be caused and cured by the intervention of supernatural forces stretches back to furthest antiquity and continues to be important, though often in attenuated form, in most modern cultures. Patients who come from ethnic groups that harbor beliefs in supernaturalism may attribute their illness to supernatural forces more often than they are willing to admit to the physician. Three patients recently seen in the psychiatric clinic of a teaching hospital, a veritable citadel of scientific medicine, come to mind. None was in any sense psychotic. One, born in Sicily, sheepishly confessed that he believed his nervousness and restlessness were caused by the evil eye, incurred because he had flirted with someone else's girl. Another, raised in Appalachia, attributed her severe anxiety to a fortuneteller's prophecy that her father was about to die. She believed firmly in vampires

---

[2] For a comprehensive review of psychotherapy and religious healing, see Torrey (1972).

and was convinced that her grandmother was a witch. A third, a devout Catholic, was more than half convinced that her two miscarriages were God's punishment for having divorced her husband and married a Protestant.

Belief in supernatural forces, moreover, is not confined to the uneducated. A highly respected Negro physician once confided to me that, having failed to gain relief from foot pain from physicians, she finally was cured by a voodoo practitioner. The growing interest in astrology, targot cards, I-Ching, and the like among the educated, as well as the widespread use of consciousness-altering drugs to produce transcendental experiences, all point to a resurgence of supernaturalism.

It is possible to make all kinds of distinctions in regard to the type of supernatural theories invoked, as to whether they dominate a society or are believed only by deviant groups, and in regard to the social acceptance and status of the healers. We shall consider primarily those theories that are integral parts of the religion of the total society or of a respectable and numerous portion of it, and in which the healing rituals are public and socially sanctioned. Thus the term "religious" seems applicable to them, even though few readers of this book would accept the validity of the religious beliefs on which most of these forms of healing are based.

Religious healing in primitive societies, as in the Western world, tends to exist side by side with naturalistic treatment by medicines, manipulations, and surgery. Its sphere of influence tends to shrink in the face of secularization and the introduction of scientific medicine.[3] In all cultures its chief realm is the treatment of illnesses with important emotional components—that is, the conditions for which naturalistically based psychotherapies are also used. It therefore is not surprising that, although their theoretical foundations differ profoundly, religious and naturalistic healing methods have much in common. Furthermore, both

---

[3] But religious healing still maintains a very strong hold, especially among members of a society not exposed to Western ideas (see, for example, Jahoda, 1961). In addition, as indicated below, healing cults based on theories that are scientifically bizarre continue to flourish in the United States.

types of healing have persisted through the ages, suggesting that their efficacy may lie partly in their common features. In this chapter we shall search for these features in religious healing methods of primitive societies and note to what extent they are also found in a great contemporary shrine of miraculous healing.

To avoid the necessity of qualifying every statement, let it be said at the start that although the characteristics to be discussed are widespread, they are not universal. The diversity of healing methods in primitive societies is very great and exceptions can be found to any generalization.[4] Moreover, the examples are not offered to prove a line of argument (which would require consideration of negative instances) but simply to support and illustrate it.

ILLNESSES IN PRIMITIVE SOCIETIES

Primitive societies regard illness as a misfortune involving the entire person, directly affecting his relationships with the spirit world and with other members of his group. Although they recognize different kinds of illness, their classifications often bear no relation to those of Western medicine. In particular, they may not distinguish sharply between mental and bodily illness, or between that due to natural and that due to supernatural causes.

Illnesses tend to be viewed as symbolic expressions of internal conflicts or of disturbed relationships to others, or both. Thus they may be attributed to soul loss, possession by an evil spirit, the magical insertion of a harmful body by a sorcerer, or the machinations of offended or malicious ancestral ghosts. It is usually assumed that the patient laid himself open to these calamities through some witting or unwitting transgression against the supernatural world, or through incurring the enmity of a sorcerer or someone who has employed a sorcerer to wreak revenge. The transgression need not have been committed by the patient himself. He may fall ill through the sin of a kinsman.

Although many societies recognize that certain illnesses have natural causes, this does not exclude the simultaneous role of

---

[4] Kiev (1964) provides an excellent sampling.

supernatural ones. A broken leg may be recognized as caused by a fall from a tree, but the cause of the fall may have been an evil thought or a witch's curse.

Because of the high mortality rates among primitive peoples, many diseases represent a great threat to the patient, and the longer the illness lasts, the greater the threat becomes. In societies subsisting on a marginal level, illness is a threat to the group as well as to the invalid. It prevents the invalid from making his full contribution to the group's support and diverts the energies of those who must care for him from group purposes. Therefore, it seems likely that every illness has overtones of anxiety, despair and similar emotions, mounting as cure is delayed. That is, persons for whom healing rituals are performed probably are experiencing emotions that aggravate their distress and disability, whatever the underlying pathological condition. The invalid is in conflict within himself and out of harmony with his group. The group is faced with the choice of abandoning him to his fate by completing the process of extrusion, or of making strenuous efforts to heal him, thereby restoring him to useful membership in his community.

These considerations may be exemplified by a personal disaster that can befall members of certain groups and that may have a counterpart in civilized societies. This is the so-called taboo death, which apparently results from noxious emotional states related to certain individual and group assumptive systems about supernatural forces and which also involve the victim's relationships with his group.

Anthropological literature contains anecdotes of savages who, on learning that they have inadvertently broken a taboo, go into a state of panic and excitement leading to death in a few hours.[5] Unfortunately in none of these cases can more mundane causes of rapid death, such as overwhelming infection, be entirely excluded.[6] The evidence that members of certain tribes may pine away and die within a brief period after learning that they have

5 For examples see Webster (1942).
6 Since patients who believe themselves cursed also may refuse food and drink, dehydration and starvation may be contributory causes to taboo deaths (Barber, 1961).

been cursed is more fully documented and more convincing. The *post hoc* nature of the explanations must not be overlooked, especially since in groups where this type of death occurs, practically all illness and death is attributed to the invalid having been cursed. Nevertheless, the process has been observed in sufficient detail in different tribes to make the explanation highly plausible.

The most convincing examples are those in which a native at the point of death from a curse rapidly recovers when the spell is broken by a more powerful one, as in the following anecdote, which can be multiplied many times:

Some years ago my father, who lived in Kenya, employed a Kikuyu garden "boy," of whom we were all fond. Njombo was gay, cheerful and in the prime of life. He was paying goats to purchase a wife and looking forward to marriage and a bit of land of his own. One day we noticed he was beginning to lose weight and looked pinched and miserable. We dosed him with all the usual medicines to no avail. Then we persuaded him, much against his will, to go into a hospital. Three weeks later he was back with a note from the doctor: "There is nothing wrong with this man except that he has made up his mind to die."

After that Njombo took to his bed, a heap of skins, and refused all food and drink. He shrank to nothing and at last went into a coma. Nothing we could do or say would strike a spark, and all seemed to be up with him.

As a last resort, my father went to the local chief and threatened him with all sorts of dreadful penalties if he did not take action to save Njombo's life. This was largely bluff, but the chief fell for it. That evening we saw a man with a bag of stoppered gourds entering Njombo's hut. We did not interfere, and no doubt a goat was slaughtered. Next morning, Njombo allowed us to feed him a little beef tea. From that moment he started to rally—the will to live was restored. We asked no questions, but learned some time later that Njombo had had a serious quarrel over the girl and that his rival had cursed him. Only when the curse was removed could he hope to survive.[7]

In certain societies, the victim's expectation of death may be powerfully reinforced by the attitudes of his group. For example,

---

[7] Elspeth Huxley (1959), p. 19. Presumably Njombo was aware of the ministrations of the shaman, although he appeared comatose to his employers.

in the Murngin, a North Australian tribe, when the theft of a man's soul becomes general knowledge, he and his tribe collaborate in hastening his demise.[8] Having lost his soul, he is already "half dead." Since his soul is in neither this world nor the next, he is a danger to himself as a spiritual entity and also to his tribe because his soul, not having been properly laid away, is likely to cause illness and death among his kin. All normal social activity with him therefore ceases and he is left alone. Then, shortly before he dies, the group returns to him under the guidance of a ceremonial leader to perform mourning rites, the purpose of which is "to cut him off entirely from the ordinary world and ultimately place him . . . in . . . the . . . world . . . of the dead." The victim, concomitantly, recognizes his change of status: ". . . the wounded feudist killed by magic dances his totem dance to . . . insure his immediate passage to the totem well. . . . His effort is not to live but to die." The writer concludes: "If all a man's near kin . . . business associates, friends, and all other members of the society, should suddenly withdraw themselves because of some dramatic circumstance . . . looking at the man as one already dead, and then after some little time perform over him a sacred ceremony believed with certainty to guide him out of the land of the living . . . the enormous suggestive power of this twofold movement of the community . . . can be somewhat understood by ourselves."

Although this account stresses the role of group influences, the major source of the victim's decline is probably the emotional state induced by his conviction—grounded in his belief system—that he has lost his soul. In this example the group's withdrawal reinforces this conviction. It is conceivable, however, that the victim would have died even if surrounded by their loving care if his conviction that the situation was hopeless were sufficiently strong. Calling attention to the interpersonal forces involved in the process should not be taken as minimizing the importance of intrapersonal ones.

Plausible speculations based on work with animals have been offered to explain the physiological mechanism of death in these cases. One hypothesis is that it might be due to prolonged adrenal

8 Warner (1941). The quotes are from pp. 241 and 242.

overexcitation caused by terror, leading to a state analogous to surgical shock.[9] Another, based on studies of physiological changes in wild rats who give up and die when placed in a stressful situation after their whiskers have been clipped, suggests that the emotional state is more one of despair than terror, and that the mechanism of death is stoppage of the heart resulting from overactivity of the vagus nerve.[10] This view is supported by fascinating and suggestive parallels between this phenomenon in wild rats and taboo deaths in primitive peoples—for example, prompt recovery even at the point of death if the stress is suddenly removed. Both hypotheses are plausible, and each may account for a particular variety of emotionally caused death—the first for the rapid form, if it occurs, and the second for the slower variety.

In civilized as well as primitive societies a person's conviction that his predicament is hopeless may cause or hasten his disintegration and death. For example, the death rate of the aged shortly after admission to state mental hospitals is unduly high, and with these and other age groups often no adequate cause of death is found at autopsy, raising the possibility that some of these deaths are caused by hopelessness, aggravated by abandonment by the patient's group. Similarly, some young schizophrenics may go into overactive panic states in which they exhaust themselves and die. This fortunately rare reaction usually occurs in conjunction with the patient's admission to the hospital—that is, at the moment when his family withdraws and he feels abandoned. Sometimes it can be successfully interrupted if a member of the treatment staff succeeds in making contact with the patient and getting across to him, by one means or another, that some still care about him.[11]

---

[9] Cannon (1957).

[10] Richter (1957).

[11] Will (1959) cites two examples of deaths of schizophrenics possibly precipitated by their sense of "unrelatedness." Adland (1947) reviews the literature on "acute exhaustive psychoses" up to that time and cites a case in which the process was successfully interrupted when the psychiatrist succeeded in making contact with the patient. Rosen (1946) describes his successful interruption of three acute catatonic excitements by playing the role of the patient's protector, in terms of the patient's delusional system. The less dramatic but careful studies of Lesse (1958) demonstrate that anxiety is a forerunner of many psychopathological symptoms and parallels them in severity.

Descriptions of the "give-up-itis" reaction of American prisoners of war of the Japanese and Koreans suggest a similar interaction of hopelessness and group isolation to produce death. A former prisoner of war well describes this reaction.[12] He lists the major factors that had to be dealt with in order to survive as: "the initial shock and subsequent depression induced by being taken prisoner by Oriental people; the feeling of being deserted and abandoned by one's own people; the severe deprivation of food, warmth, clothes, living comforts, and sense of respectability; the constant intimidation and physical beatings from the captors; loss of self-respect and the respect of others; the day-to-day uncertainty of livelihood and the vague indeterminable unknown future date of deliverance." It will be noted that physical and psychological threats are placed on the same footing. Under these circumstances: "Occasionally an individual would . . . lose interest in himself and his future, which was reflected in quiet or sullen withdrawal from the group, filth of body and clothes, trading of food for cigarettes, slowing of work rate . . . and an expressed attitude of not giving a damn. . . . If this attitude were not met with firm resistance . . . death inevitably resulted."

This is clearly a description of hopelessness. It could be successfully combatted by "forced hot soap-and-water bathing, shaving and delousing, special appetizing food, obtaining a few days rest in camp . . . a mixture of kindly sympathetic interest and anger-inducing attitudes. Victory was assured with the first sign of a smile or evidence of pique." It is of interest that successful measures may include anger-arousing as well as nurturant behavior. As another observer reports: "One of the best ways to get a man on his feet initially was to make him so mad, by goading, prodding, or blows, that he tried to get up and beat you. If you could manage this, the man invariably got well."[13] Thus it may be that any kind of emotional stimulus, whether pleasant or not, may successfully counteract lethal despair if it succeeds in breaking through the victim's isolation, demonstrates that others care

---

[12] Nardini (1952). The quotes are from pp. 244 and 245.
[13] Major Clarence L. Anderson, quoted in Kinkead (1959), p. 149. Strassman *et al.* (1956) present an interesting discussion of apathy as a reaction to severe stress in war prisoners.

about him, and implies that there are things he can do to help himself.

To descend to less spectacular examples of the harmful effects of emotional states, a study of forty-two patients hospitalized with medical illnesses concluded that "psychic states of helplessness or hopelessness may be related to increased biological vulnerability."[14] The findings of [another] study . . . suggested that emotions such as anxiety, depression, and resentment were associated with delayed convalescence from a fluke infestation.[15] A series of elegantly designed investigations has produced convincing evidence that depression, which could not be attributed to the illness itself, is associated with delayed convalescence from both undulant fever and influenza.[16]

THE ROLE OF THE SHAMAN IN PRIMITIVE SOCIETIES

Having considered how certain emotional states activated by personal assumptive systems interacting with group forces may contribute to disintegration and death, let us turn now to the role of these factors in healing, as illustrated by religious healing rituals in primitive societies.[17] These rituals, which grow directly out of the tribe's world view, are usually conducted by a shaman[18] and involve participation of the patient and usually members of his family and tribe.

14 Schmale (1958), p. 271. Although methodologically flawed, the study gains plausibility from accounts of a similar relationship of illness to noxious emotional states in primitives and prisoners.

15 Frank (1946).

16 Imboden *et al.* (1959, 1961).

17 The discussion of primitive healing is based primarily on the following sources: Deren (1953); Gillin (1948); Leighton (1968); Lévi-Strauss (1958); Opler (1963); Sachs (1947); and Spiro (1967).

18 Although anthropologists draw distinctions between terms such as "shaman," "witch doctor," and "medicine man," "shaman" seems to be gaining acceptance as the generic designation for primitive healers of all types and is so used in the text.

The powers of the shaman are explained in terms of the society's assumptive world and are unquestioningly accepted as genuine by it. The routes for acquiring shamanistic powers vary greatly. In some societies the shaman acquires them, sometimes against his will, through personal and private mystical experiences, and he is regarded as a deviant person with little status except when his powers are invoked. In others, shamans are drawn from the ranks of cured patients.[19] And in others, as in the Kwakiutl, they undergo an elaborate training course, analogous to medical training in our culture, and enjoy a high prestige.

Shamans usually are adept at distinguishing illnesses they can treat successfully from those that are beyond their powers, and they manage to reject patients with whom they are likely to fail. This enables them to maintain a reputation for success which, by arousing favorable expectancies in the patient and the group, undoubtedly enhances their healing power.

The importance of the group's attitudes in determining not only the shaman's effectiveness but also his self-evaluation is well illustrated by the remarkable autobiography of Quesalid, a Kwakiutl shaman.[20] He entered training motivated by skepticism concerning the shaman's powers and by the desire to expose them. (Perhaps, like many converts, he exaggerated his former skepticism.) The training included learning to master various arts of deception, and especially how to spit out of one's mouth at the right moment a bit of down covered with blood, representing the foreign body that had made the patient ill and had been magically extracted from him.

[19] See Field (1955). According to Spiro (1967), Burmese healers may be shamans, recruited from those with pathogenic symptoms, who can only propitiate harmful supernatural spirits, and exorcists or members of magico-religious sects who can control them. The Burmese example points to at least two sources of a healer's ability to inspire a patient's confidence: having successfully overcome similar problems (which should also strengthen rapport) and being a member of a culturally-valued healing sect. The analysed psychoanalyst partakes of both. See Prince (1968). Henry (1966) considers parallels between life histories of shamans and American psychotherapists. Another way of acquiring shamanistic powers is through inheritance, calling to mind the frequency of physician dynasties in all societies (Sachs, 1947).

[20] Lévi-Strauss (1958). Quotes are from pp. 193, 194, and 196. Translation is by Elizabeth K. Frank.

Knowing that he was in training, a family called him in to treat a patient, and he was brilliantly successful. He attributed the cure to psychological factors: "... because the patient believed strongly in his dream about me." What shook his skepticism was a visit to a neighboring Koskimo tribe, in which the shamans simply spit a little saliva into their hands and dared to pretend that this was the illness. In order to find out "what is the power of these shamans, if it is real or if they only pretend to be shamans," he asked and received permission to try his method since theirs had failed. Again the patient said she was cured. Apparently some forms of healing were more fraudulent than others. This presented Quesalid with a problem "not without parallel in the development of modern science: two systems, both known to be inadequate, nevertheless, compared with each other appear to differ in value both logically and experimentally. In what frame of reference should they be judged?"

The Koskimo shamans, "covered with shame" because they had been discredited in the eyes of their countrymen, and thrown into self-doubts, tried very hard to ferret out his secrets, but to no avail. Finally one of the most eminent challenged him to a healing duel, and Quesalid again succeeded where the other failed. Two interesting consequences followed. The old shaman, fearing to die of shame and unable to get Quesalid to reveal his secret, vanished the same night with all his relatives "sick at heart," returned after a year insane, and died three years later. Quesalid, although he continues to expose imposters and is full of scorn for the profession, remains uncertain about whether there are real shamans or not: "only once have I seen a shaman who treated patients by suction and I was never able to find out if he was a real shaman or a faker. For this reason only, I believe that he was a shaman. He did not allow those he had cured to pay him. And truly I never once saw him laugh." At the end it is unclear whether he considers himself to be a real shaman: "... he pursues his calling with conscience ... is proud of his successes and ... defends heatedly against all rival schools the technique of the bloodstained down whose deceptive nature he seems completely to have lost sight of, and which he had scoffed at so much in the beginning." Quesalid's skepticism is not able to withstand his own successes and the belief of his group in his powers.

THE HEALING CEREMONY IN
PRIMITIVE SOCIETIES

Healing in primitive societies utilizes both individual and group methods. It may be conducted by the shaman with the patient alone, analogous to the pattern of Western medicine. The shaman makes a diagnosis by performing certain acts and then offers a remedy, which may be a medication or the performance of suitable incantations as in the example cited above.[21] The healing power of these procedures probably lies in the patient's expectation of help, based on his perception of the shaman as possessing special healing powers, derived from his ability to communicate with the spirit world.

Other forms of primitive healing involve a long-term two-person relationship between shaman and patient, which seems analogous in some ways to long-term psychotherapy.[22] The only available descriptions, however, are too sketchy to warrant consideration here.

This section considers a third type of primitive healing which has been adequately described by anthropologists and which bears on psychotherapy—the group healing ceremonial. These rituals may involve ancestral or other spirits, for example, and are intensive, time-limited efforts aimed at curing specific illness and involving members of the patient's family. As a result, they cast little, if any, light on certain features that may be of central importance in long-term individual psychotherapy, such as the development and examination of transference reactions between patient and therapist. On the other hand, they throw certain aspects of long-term therapy into relief, as it were, by compressing them into a brief time span, and highlight the healing role of group and cultural forces, which may be underestimated in individual therapy because they are present only implicitly. With these considerations in mind, it may be instruc-

---

21 See also Sachs (1947).
22 Field (1955) gives sketchy examples of long-term individual therapy in the African Gold Coast, and Lederer (1959) adds a consideration of exorcism in the Middle Ages and in Zen Buddhism. Both writers discuss parallels with Western psychotherapy.

tive to consider a healing ceremony in some detail—the treatment of "espanto" in a sixty-three-year-old Guatemalan Indian woman.[23] This was her eighth attack. Her symptoms seem similar to those that would lead an American psychiatrist to diagnose an agitated depression. The Indians attribute it to soul loss.

The treatment began with a diagnostic session attended not only by the patient but by her husband, a male friend, and two anthropologists. The healer felt her pulse for a while, while looking her in the eye, then confirmed that she was suffering from "espanto." He then told her in a calm, authoritative manner that it had happened near the river when she saw her husband foolishly lose her money to a loose woman, and he urged her to tell the whole story. After a brief period of reluctance, the patient "loosed a flood of words telling of her life frustrations and anxieties. . . . During the recital . . . the curer . . . nodded noncommitally, but permissively, keeping his eyes fixed on her face. Then he said that it was good that she should tell him of her life." Finally they went over the precipitating incident of the present attack in detail. In essence, she and her husband were passing near the spot where he had been deceived by the loose woman She upbraided him, and he struck her with a rock.

The curer then told her he was confident she could be cured and outlined in detail the preparations that she would have to make for the curing session four days later. She was responsible for these preparations, which involved procuring and preparing certain medications, preparing a feast, persuading a woman friend or kinsman to be her "servant" during the preparatory period and healing session, and persuading one of the six chiefs of the village to participate with the medicine man in the ceremony.

The ceremony itself began at four in the afternoon and lasted until five the next morning. Before the healer arrived, the house and the house altar[24] had been decorated with pine boughs, and

23 Gillin (1948). Quotes are from pp. 389, 391, and 394.
24 The altars are Christian. In Christianized societies embarrassing problems may be created by incompatibilities between the assumptive systems underlying healing rituals and Christian beliefs. As a result, a considerable part of the healing rite may be devoted to arranging a truce between them, as in the example.

numerous invited guests and participants had assembled. After they were all present, the healer made his entrance, shook hands all around, and checked the preparations carefully. Then there was a period of light refreshment and social chitchat, which apparently helped to organize a social group around the patient and to relax tension.

After dusk the healer, chief, and others of the group went off to church, apparently to appease the Christian deities in advance, since "recovery of a soul involves dealing with renegade saints and familiar spirits certainly not approved of by God Almighty." When they returned, a large meal was served. The patient did not eat, but was complimented by all present on her food. Then the healer carried out a long series of rituals involving such activities as making wax dolls of the chief of evil spirits and his wife, to whom the healer appealed for return of the patient's soul, and elaborate massage of the patient with whole eggs, which were believed to absorb some of the sickness from the patient's body.[25] The curer, the chief, two male helpers, and the ever-present anthropologists next took the eggs and a variety of paraphernalia, including gifts for the evil spirits, to the place where the patient had lost her soul, and the healer pleaded with various spirits to restore her soul to her.

On their return they were met at the door by the patient, who showed an intense desire to know whether the mission had been successful. The curer spoke noncommittal but comforting words. This was followed by much praying by the healer and the chief before the house altar and a special ground altar set up outside, and by rites to purify and sanctify the house. Some of these activities were devoted to explaining to the household patron

---

[25] With a few notable exceptions, such as Wilhelm Reich and J. L. Moreno, Western psychotherapists have eschewed bodily contact, relying solely on words as means of communication. This probably reflects a culturally induced suspicion that all bodily contacts are erotic. As a result, psychotherapists have deprived themselves of a powerful means of relieving tension and strengthening rapport, widely used in other cultures (Torrey, 1972). The appeal of chiropractors and osteopaths may lie partly in their free use of massage and manipulation. The encouragement of members to indulge in a wide variety of bodily contacts may also help to account for the attraction of sensitivity training and encounter groups.

saint why it was necessary to deal with evil spirits. About 2 A.M., the ceremony came to a climax. The patient, naked except for a small loin cloth, went outside. Before the audience, the healer sprayed her entire body with a magic fluid that had been prepared during the ritual and that had a high alcoholic content. Then she had to sit, naked and shivering, in the cold air for about ten minutes. Finally she drank about a pint of the fluid. Then they returned indoors, the patient lay down in front of the altar, and the healer massaged her vigorously and systematically with the eggs, then with one of his sandals. She then arose, put on her clothes, lay down on the rustic platform bed, and was covered with blankets. By this time she was thoroughly relaxed.

Finally, the healer broke the six eggs used in the massage into a bowl of water one by one, and as he watched their swirling whites he reviewed the history of the patient's eight "espantos," pointing out the "proofs" in the eggs. The sinking of the eggs to the bottom of the bowl showed that all the previous "espantos" had been cured and that the present symptoms would shortly disappear. The healer "pronounced the cure finished. The patient roused herself briefly on the bed and shouted hoarsely, 'That is right.' Then she sank back into a deep snoring sleep." This ended the ceremony and everyone left but the patient's immediate family.

The patient had a high fever for the following few days. This did not concern the healer, whose position was that everyone died sooner or later anyway, and if the patient died, it was better for her to die with her soul than without it. He refused to see her again, as his work was done. The anthropologist treated her with antibiotics, and she made a good recovery from the fever and the depression. The author notes that for the four weeks he was able to observe her "she seemed to have developed a new personality. . . . The hypochondriacal complaints, nagging of her husband and relatives, withdrawal from her social contacts, and anxiety symptoms all disappeared."

This example illustrates certain generalizations about religious healing which, if not universal, are at least widely applicable. It should be noted that healing rituals are not undertaken lightly. Usually they are resorted to only after simpler healing methods have failed. The analogy springs to mind that in America patients are often referred for psychiatric treatment only after all other forms of treatment have failed to relieve their suffering. In any case, this suggests that the state of mind of a patient receiving a healing ritual and that of one receiving psychotherapy often resemble each other in some respects. Both types of patient are apt to be discouraged and apprehensive about their condition, while at the same time hopeful for relief from the treatment.

The theory of illness and healing, and the healing method itself, are integral parts of the culture's assumptive world. They supply the patient with a conceptual framework for making sense out of his chaotic and mysterious feelings, and suggest a plan of action, thus helping him to gain a sense of direction and mastery and to resolve his inner conflicts. As has been said about another magical cure:

That the mythology of the shaman does not correspond to objective reality does not matter. The patient believes in it and belongs to a society that believes in it. The protecting spirits, the evil spirits, the supernatural monsters and magical monsters are elements of a coherent system which are the basis of the natives' concept of the universe. The patient accepts them, or rather she has never doubted them. What she does not accept are the incomprehensible and arbitrary pains which represent an element foreign to her system but which the shaman, by invoking the myth, will replace in a whole in which everything has its proper place.[26]

The shaman's activities validate his supernatural powers. In this example his manner in the diagnostic interview and especially his revelation to the patient of an event that she did not know he knew, and that he therefore presumably learned about through magic, must have had this effect. In other rituals the shaman may start by reciting how he got his "call" or citing examples of the previous cures, to which others present may add confirmation. He may resort to legerdemain, as in the Kwakiutl, but most authorities agree that this is not regarded as trickery, even when the audience knows how it is done. They seem to give emotional assent to the proposition that the bloody bit of cotton

26 Lévi-Strauss (1958), p. 217. See also Leighton (1968) on the functions of the "dramatic myth" underlying all primitive healing rituals.

is the patient's illness and has been extracted from his body, while at another level they know perfectly well that it is only a piece of cotton. Perhaps their state of mind is analogous to that of partakers of communion, for whom in one sense the bread and wine are the body and blood of Christ while in another they are just bread and wine. In any case, the healing ritual reinforces the image of the shaman as a powerful ally in the patient's struggle with the malign forces that have made him ill.

In his struggle with the forces of evil, the shaman may risk his own soul.[27] Heightening the emotional intensity of the ritual may increase its therapeutic power in several ways. It implies that the shaman has sufficient confidence in his own powers to risk the danger; this not only increases the patient's confidence in him, but conveys the message that the shaman cares enough about the patient and considers him important enough to risk his own safety on his behalf.

The conceptual scheme is validated and reinforced by the rituals that it prescribes. In the above example, this reinforcement occurred especially when the healer examined the eggs swirling in the water and pointed out to the assembled group the "proofs" of the patient's previous illnesses. The scheme, moreover, cannot be shaken by failure of the ritual to cure the patient. If this one had died, the ceremony would still have been regarded as successful in restoring her soul.[28]

Rituals often involve a preparatory period, which represents a dramatic break in the usual routine of daily activities. In the case of "espanto," the preparation for the ritual served to jolt the patient out of her usual routines, heighten her sense of personal importance by letting her have a "servant," and start the process of rallying family and group forces to her aid. In addition, like the rest of the ritual, it gave her something to do to combat her

27 Fox (1964, p. 185) describes titantic battles between doctors and evil spirits in Cochiti therapy, during which, according to a doctor, "we are more scared than [the lay participants] are. The witches are out to get us." See also Spiro (1967), p. 200.

28 As in Western medicine, the criterion of the success of a healing procedure is not always the patient's recovery. The old surgical quip comes to mind: "The operation was successful but the patient died."

illness, in itself a powerful allayer of anxiety and a boost to hopes of cure. The patient's family, as well as respected representatives of the tribe, convey their concern for him by their participation. Since they represent a healthy group, the patient's associates are not likely to reinforce his pathological trends, as may occur, for example, in a mental hospital.[29]

Aspects of the healing ritual heighten the patient's sense of self-worth, and, in fact, increase the merit of all participants. The patient is the focus of the group's attention and, by implication, worthy of the invocation of supernatural forces on his behalf. Important, also, is the altruistic quality of the activities. The group tries to help the patient by performing parts of the ritual, interceding for him with the powers he has presumably offended, or defending the patient to them. Sometimes the patient also performs services for the group. In our example, the patient was responsible for preparing the feast. Mutual performance of services cements the tie between patient and group. The patient's activities may also help to counteract his morbid self-absorption and enhance his sense of self-worth by demonstrating that he can still be of use to others.

In those ceremonies that involve confession, atonement, and forgiveness, the gaining of merit is especially apparent.[30] The fact that confession is required for cure implies a close link between illness and transgression, as discussed earlier. Impersonal forms of confession and repentance, as in some Christian liturgies, serve the purpose of general purification.

Some healing rituals elicit confessions of specific personal transgressions based on detailed review of the patient's past history with special emphasis on the events surrounding his illness. These events are expressed or interpreted in terms of the tribe's assumptive world. In addition to its confessional aspect, this procedure brings the patient's vague, chaotic, conflicting, and mysterious feelings to the center of his attention and places them in a self-consistent conceptual system. Thus they are "realized

---

29 Cf. "network therapy" in Speck and Rueveni (1969).
30 See LaBarre (1964) for many examples of confessional rituals in North and South American Indian tribes. Rasmussen (1929) offers an excellent account of a confessional ritual.

in an order and on a level which permits them to unfold freely and leads to their resolution."[31]

Naming something is the first step toward controlling it, for "naming a sin is to recall it, to give it form and substance, so that the officiating medicine man can deal with it in the prescribed manner. No vague announcement of sinfulness suffices; each sin that has been committed must be specified. Sometimes when the patient can think of nothing serious done by him he will confess imaginary sins."[32]

As in the example cited, the shaman's technique of eliciting this type of confession may be a way of demonstrating his powers. That is, he warns the patient that the spirits have already told him what the true facts are and that they cannot be hidden. As the patient confesses, the shaman confirms that this is what he already knew and urges the patient to confess further. Often the other participants jog the patient's memory or bring up episodes with the patient in which they too trangressed, or even crimes ostensibly unrelated to the patient's illness. Thus the process further cements the group, and participants other than the patient may gain virtue from it. The confession may be followed by intercession with the spirit world on behalf of the patient by the whole group as well as by the shaman, heightening the patient's hope that forgiveness will be forthcoming.

Thus confession may have many implications. It helps the patient to make sense of his condition, counteracts his consciousness of sin, brings him into closer relationship with his group, impresses him with the shaman's powers, and improves the relationship of all concerned with the spirit world. In these ways it counteracts his anxiety, strengthens his self-esteem, and helps him to resolve his conflicts.

Healing ceremonies are highly charged emotionally.[33] As mentioned above, a shaman may act out a life-and-death struggle be-

---

[31] Lévi-Strauss (1958), p. 219.

[32] Webster (1942), p. 311. Labeling is common to all forms of psychotherapy, as we shall see. The confessions of prisoners undergoing thought reform frequently contained fabrications as did the "memories" of Freud's early patients.

[33] Deren (1953) gives a fascinating account of the emotional exaltation of a Haitian voodoo ceremony that she experienced.

tween his spirit and the evil spirit that has possessed the patient. The patient may vividly reenact past experiences or act out the struggles of spirit forces within himself. The emotional excitement may be intensified by rhythmic music, chanting, and dancing. It frequently mounts to the point of exhausting the patient and not infrequently is enhanced by some strong physical shock. In our example, it will be recalled, the patient was sprayed by an alcoholic liquid, which gave her a bad chill.

Finally, many rituals make a strong aesthetic appeal. The setting may be especially decorated for the occasion, and participants may costume themselves elaborately, perform stylized dances, draw sand paintings, and the like. Since these trappings and activities have symbolic meanings, they not only are soothing and inspiring aesthetically but also represent tangible reinforcements of the conceptual organization that the ritual endeavors to impose on the patient's inchoate sufferings. Participation of the whole group either actively or as attentive spectators fosters group solidarity.

In short, methods of primitive healing involve an interplay between patient, healer, group and the world of the supernatural; this serves to raise the patient's expectancy of cure, help him to harmonize his inner conflicts, reintegrate him with his group and the spirit world, supply a conceptual framework to aid this, and stir him emotionally. The total process combats his demoralization and strengthens his sense of self-worth.

LOURDES AND RELIGIOUS HEALING
IN THE WESTERN WORLD

From its inception, Christianity has included the notion of healing through divine intervention. Starting with the healing miracles of Christ, this form of curing has persisted through the centuries. Today healing sects (like Christian Science) and shrines of miraculous healing have millions of devotees. Since the rituals of these groups and places parallel religious healing in primitive societies in many ways, it may be of interest to take a look at one of them. The great modern shrine of Lourdes is particularly suitable because it has been well described and because the cures of severe illness that have occurred there are exceptionally well documented and have received careful critical scrutiny.[34]

The history of Lourdes, starting with the visions of Bernadette Soubirous in 1858, is too well known to require retelling here. It is perhaps odd, in view of subsequent developments, that the apparition that appeared to Bernadette and told her where to dig for the spring said nothing about its healing powers. Be that as it may, miraculous cures following immersion in the spring were soon reported, and today over two million pilgrims visit Lourdes every year, including over thirty thousand sick.

The world view supporting Lourdes, like those on which religious healing in primitive tribes is based, is all-inclusive and is shared by almost all the pilgrims to the shrine. While cures are regarded as validating it, failures cannot shake it. Those who seek help at Lourdes have usually been sick a long time and have failed to respond to medical remedies. Like the primitives who undergo a healing ritual, most are close to despair. Being chronic invalids, they have had to withdraw from most or all of their community activities and have become burdens to their families. Their activities have become routinized and constricted, their lives bleak and monotonous, and they have nothing to anticipate but further suffering and death.

The decision to make the pilgrimage to Lourdes changes all this. The preparatory period is a dramatic break in routine. Collecting funds for the journey, arranging for medical examinations, and making the travel plans requires the cooperative effort of members of the patient's family and the wider community. Often the congregation contributes financial aid. Prayers and masses are offered for the invalid. Members of the family, and often the patient's physician or a priest, accompany him to Lourdes and serve as tangible evidence of the interest of the family and larger group in his welfare. Often pilgrims from many communities travel together, and there are religious ceremonies while the train is en route and at every stop. In short, the

[34] The account of Lourdes is drawn mainly from Cranston (1955). The quotes are from pp. 31, 36–37, and 127, respectively. See also Janet (1925), vol. 1, chap. 1.

preparatory period is emotionally stirring, brings the patient from the periphery of his group to its center, and enhances his expectation of help. It is interesting in this connection that, except for the original cures, Lourdes has failed to heal those who live in its vicinity. This suggests that the emotional excitement connected with the preparatory period and journey to the shrine may be essential for healing to occur.

On arrival at Lourdes after an exhausting, even life-endangering journey, the sufferer's expectation of help is further strengthened. He is plunged into "a city of pilgrims, and they are everywhere; people who have come from the four corners of the earth with but one purpose: prayer, and healing for themselves or for their loved ones. . . . One is surrounded by them, and steeped in their atmosphere every moment of existence in Lourdes." Everyone hopes to witness or experience a miraculous cure. Accounts of previous cures are on every tongue, and the pilgrim sees the votive offerings and the piles of discarded crutches of those who have been healed. Thus the ritual may be said to begin with a validation of the shrine's power, analogous to the shaman's review of his cures in primitive healing rites.

The pilgrims' days are filled with religious services and trips to the Grotto, where they are immersed in the ice-cold spring. Every afternoon all the pilgrims and invalids who are at Lourdes at the time—usually forty or fifty thousand—gather at the Esplanade in front of the shrine for the procession that is the climax of each day's activities. The bedridden are placed nearest the shrine, those who can sit up are behind them, the ambulatory invalids behind them, while the hordes of visitors fill the rest of the space. The enormous emotional and aesthetic impact of the procession is well conveyed by the following quotation:

At four the bells begin to peal—the Procession begins to form. The priests in their various robes assemble at the Grotto. . . . The bishop appears with the monstrance under the sacred canopy. The loud-speakers open up. A great hymn rolls out, the huge crowd joining in unison, magnificently. The Procession begins its long, impressive way down one side and up the other of the sunny Esplanade. First the Children of Mary, young girls in blue capes, white veils . . . then forty or fifty priests in black cassocks . . . other priests in white surplices . . .

then come the Bishops in purple . . . and finally the officiating Archbishop in his white and gold robes under the golden canopy. Bringing up the rear large numbers of men and women of the different pilgrimages, Sisters, Nurses, members of various religious organizations; last of all the doctors. . . . Hymns, prayers, fervent, unceasing. In the Square the sick line up in two rows. . . . Every few feet, in front of them, kneeling priests with arms outstretched praying earnestly, leading the responses. Nurses and orderlies on their knees, praying too. . . . Ardor mounts as the Blessed Sacrament approaches. Prayers gather intensity. . . . The Bishop leaves the shelter of the canopy, carrying the monstrance. The Sacred Host is raised above each sick one. The great crowd falls to its knees. All arms are outstretched in one vast cry to Heaven. As far as one can see in any direction, people are on their knees, praying. . . .

What are the results of the tremendous outpouring of emotion and faith? The great majority of the sick do not experience a cure. However, most of the pilgrims seem to derive some psychological benefit from the experience. Like participation in healing rituals in primitive societies, the pilgrimage is regarded as conferring merit in itself and the whole atmosphere of Lourdes is spiritually uplifting. In this connection, the altruism of all involved is especially worthy of note. Physicians, brancardiers (who serve the sick), and helpers of all sorts give their time and effort freely, and throughout the ceremonies the emphasis is on self-forgetfulness and devotion to the welfare of others. The pilgrims pray for the sick and the sick for each other, not themselves. Therefore, the words attributed to an old pilgrim may well be largely true: "Of the uncured none despair. All go away filled with hope and a new feeling of strength. The trip to Lourdes is never made in vain."

The evidence that an occasional cure of advanced organic disease does occur at Lourdes is as strong as that for any other phenomenon accepted as true. The reported frequency of such cures varies widely depending on the criteria used. The piles of crutches attest to the fact that many achieve improved functioning, at least temporarily. In many of these cases, however, improvement is probably attributable to heightened morale, enabling the patient to function better in the face of an unchanged organic handicap. Fully documented cures of unquestionable and gross organic disease are extremely infrequent—probably no more frequent than similar ones occurring in secular settings.

In the century of the shrine's existence, less than a hundred cures have passed the stringent test leading the Church to declare them miraculous. This figure may be much too low, as many convincing cases fail to qualify because they lack the extensive documentary support required. But even several thousand cures of organic diseases would represent only a small fraction of 1 percent of those who have made the pilgrimage. As a sympathetic student of spiritual healing writes: ". . . there is probably no stream in Britain which could not boast of as high a proportion of cures as the stream at Lourdes if patients came in the same numbers and in the same psychological state of expectant excitement."[35]

The processes by which cures at Lourdes occur do not seem to differ in kind from those involved in normal healing, although they are remarkably strengthened and accelerated. Careful reading of the reports reveals that healing is not instantaneous, as is often claimed, but that, like normal healing, it requires time. It is true that the consciousness of cure is often (not always) sudden and may be accompanied by immediate improvement in function—the paralyzed walk, the blind see, and those who had been unable to retain food suddenly regain their appetites. But actual tissue healing takes hours, days, or weeks, and persons who have lost much weight require the usual period of time to regain it, as would be expected if healing occurred by the usual processes. Moreover, gaps of specialized tissues such as skin are not restored but are filled by scar formation as in normal healing. No one has regrown an amputated limb at Lourdes.

It should be added that cures at Lourdes involve the person's total personality, not merely his body. The healed, whatever they were like before their recovery, all are said to be possessed of a remarkable serenity and a desire to be of service to others.

Rivers of ink have been spilled in controversy over whether or not the cures at Lourdes are genuine, based on the erroneous assumption that one's acceptance or rejection of them is necessarily linked to belief or disbelief in miracles or in the Catholic

[35] Weatherhead (1951), p. 153.

faith. Actually, it is perfectly possible to accept some Lourdes cures as genuine while maintaining skepticism about miraculous causation, or to be a devout Catholic while rejecting modern miracles. The world is full of phenomena that cannot be explained by our present cosmologies.

Inexplicable cures of serious organic disease occur in everyday medical practice. Every physician has either personally treated or heard about patients who mysteriously recovered from a seemingly fatal illness. Two surgeons have assembled from the literature 176 cases of unquestionable cancer that regressed without adequate treatment.[36] Had these remissions occurred after a visit to Lourdes, many would have regarded them as miraculous. Since no physician sees enough of these phenomena to acquire sufficient sample for scientific study, and since they cannot be explained by current medical theories, the fascinating questions they raise have been neglected. Depending on one's theoretical predilections, one may choose to believe that all, none, or a certain class of spontaneous recoveries from what appear to be fatal illnesses are miraculous. The mere fact of their occurrence leaves the question of their cause completely open.

A not implausible assumption, in the light of our review of primitive healing, is that Lourdes cures are in some way related to the sufferer's emotional state. This view is supported by the conditions under which the cures occur, and the type of person who seems most apt to experience them. Although they may occur en route to Lourdes, on the return journey, or even months later, most cures occur at the shrine and at the moments of greatest emotional intensity and spiritual fervor—while taking communion, or during immersion in the spring or when the host is raised over the sick at the passing of the sacrament during the procession. The persons who have been cured include the deserving and the sinful, believers and apparent skeptics, but they tend to have one common characteristic: they are "almost invariably simple people—the poor and the humble; people who

---

[36] Everson and Cole (1966). The authors stress that regression does not necessarily imply cure, but about half their cases were well two years or more after cancer was diagnosed, and about one-eighth had been followed ten years or more without recurrence. Unfortunately, the possible role of psychological factors is not even mentioned, much less considered.

do not interpose a strong intellect between themselves and the Higher Power."[37] That is, they are not detached or critical. It is generally agreed that persons who remain entirely unmoved by the ceremonies do not experience cures.

The cured skeptics typically have a devout parent or spouse, suggesting either that their skepticism was a reaction-formation against an underlying desire to believe, or at least that the pilgrimage involved emotional conflict. In this connection, all cured skeptics have become ardent believers.

A point of considerable theoretical interest, to be discussed again, is that the emotions aroused by Lourdes or by the healing ritual described earlier, may be not only intense, but as unpleasant as those created by the illness itself. The sufferings of a debilitated invalid in a prolonged healing ritual or on the long trip to Lourdes must often be severe; yet their effect is usually beneficial. This suggests that the effects of strong emotions on one's well-being depend on their meaning or context—that is, on how the person interprets them. Intense emotional arousal, for example, if it occurs in a setting of hopelessness and progressive isolation of the patient from his usual sources of support, may contribute to his death. If he experiences the same arousal in a setting of massive human and supernatural encouragement so that it carries a context of hope, it can be healing.[38]

In short, the healing ceremonials at Lourdes, like those of primitive tribes, involve a climactic union of the patient, his family, the larger group, and the supernatural world by means of a dramatic, emotionally charged, aesthetically rich ritual that expresses and reinforces a shared ideology.

OTHER FORMS
OF NONMEDICAL HEALING

Lourdes may serve as one example of institutionalized religious healing in the West. An adequate survey of Western forms of nonmedical healing would have to include other institutionalized

[37] Cranston (1955), p. 125.
[38] See Schachter (1965).

religious healing such as Christian Science, and secular therapies ranging from homeopathy, which considers itself a form of medicine, through medicine-related methods such as osteopathy and chiropractic, to healers who function as individuals with idiosyncratic theories. Together these practitioners probably treat many more persons than do physicians,[39] but they do not warrant extended attention for our purposes because of the lack of dispassionate, objective information about most of them. In general, they do not seem to involve any healing principles beyond those already considered.

One feature they all share that is worth emphasizing because, as we shall see, it is highly relevant to psychotherapy, is the ability to evoke the patient's expectancy of help, a factor also involved in religious healing. Two sources of this expectancy are discernible. The first is the personal magnetism of the healer, often strengthened by his own faith in what he does. As an investigator who interviewed many such healers writes: "The vast majority of the sectarians sincerely believe in the efficacy of their practices . . . the writer has talked to [chiropractors] whose faith was . . . nothing short of evangelistic, whose sincerity could no more be questioned than that of Persia's 'whirling dervishes.' "[40] However, the success of peddlers of obviously worthless nostrums and gadgets attests to the fact that the healer need not necessarily believe in the efficacy of his methods to be able to convince his patients of their power.

Another source of the patient's faith is the ideology of the healer or sect, which offers him a rationale, however absurd, for making sense of his illness and the treatment procedure, and places the healer in the position of transmitter or controller of impressive healing forces. In this he is analogous to the shaman.

[39] Healing cults are astonishingly popular. A survey (Reed, 1932) found some 36,000 sectarian medical practitioners, exclusive of esoteric and local cults, which equaled almost one-fourth of the total number of medical practitioners at that time, to whom people paid at least $125,000,000 annually. One physician found that 43 percent of his private patients and 26 percent of his clinic patients had patronized a cult during the three months preceding their visits to him. Inglis (1965) cites an estimate of 35 million patients of chiropractors in the United States. See also Steiner (1945).

[40] Reed (1932), pp. 109–10.

Often these forces are called supernatural, but the healer[41] may pose as a scientist who has discovered new and potent scientific principles of healing, thus surrounding himself with the aura that anything labeled scientific inspires in members of modern Western societies. These healers characteristically back up their pretensions with an elaborate scientific-sounding patter and often add an imposing array of equipment complete with dials, flashing lights, and sound effects.

The apparent success of healing methods based on various ideologies and methods compels the conclusion that the healing power of faith resides in the patient's state of mind, not in the validity of its object. At the risk of laboring this point, an experimental demonstration of it with three severely ill, bedridden women may be reported.[42] One had chronic inflammation of the gall bladder with stones, the second had failed to recuperate from a major abdominal operation and was practically a skeleton, and the third was dying of widespread cancer. The physician first permitted a prominent local faith healer to try to cure them by absent treatment without the patients' knowledge. Nothing happened. Then he told the patients about the faith healer, built up their expectations over several days, and finally assured them that he would be treating them from a distance at a certain time the next day. This was a time in which he was sure that the healer did *not* work. At the suggested time all three patients improved quickly and dramatically. The second was permanently cured. The other two were not, but showed striking temporary responses. The cancer patient, who was severely anemic and whose tissues had become waterlogged, promptly excreted all the accumulated fluid, recovered from her anemia, and regained sufficient strength to go home and resume her household duties. She remained virtually symptom-free until her death. The gall bladder patient lost her symptoms, went home, and had no recurrence for several years. These three patients were greatly helped by a belief that was false—that the faith healer was treat-

---

[41] Oursler (1957) provides readable, anecdotal surveys of faith healing groups and individuals in the United States.
[42] Rehder (1955).

ing them from a distance—suggesting that "expectant trust"[43] in itself can be a powerful healing force.

If, as pointed out earlier, depression and certain other emotional states seem to retard healing, it seems reasonable to assume that hope could enhance it, and this is strongly suggested by miracle cures and the example just cited. A final bit of evidence is worth reporting because scientifically it is virtually impeccable. Patients about to undergo an operation for detached retina were interviewed before the operation and rated on a scale of "acceptance," including such items as trust in the surgeon, optimism about the result, and confidence in ability to cope. Scores on this scale correlated very highly with speed of healing after the operation, rated independently by the surgeon.[44]

One cannot conclude this review of nonmedical healing without mentioning the possibility that some individuals, like Quasalid, may have a gift of healing that defies scientific explanation. In this it resembles the charisma of certain political leaders. Nor can one rule out the possibility—indeed the evidence for it is quite persuasive—that some healers serve as a kind of conduit for a healing force in the universe, often called the life force, that, for want of a better term, must be called supernatural.[45] That is, it cannot be conceptually incorporated into the secular cosmology that dominates Western scientific thinking. Many will reject the notion out-of-hand on this account. Others, of whom I am one, are ever mindful of Hamlet's admonition to Horatio and prefer to keep an open mind.

A fitting conclusion for this chapter is supplied by two quotations which highlight the striking similarity between religious healing in primitive groups and in the Christian world, with respect to the interaction of patient, healer, group, and supernatural forces. The first sums up primitive healing, the second Christian spiritual healing:

The medicine man is a soul doctor. . . . He gives peace by confessing his patient. His rigid system, which ignores doubt, dispels fear, restores

---

43 The phrase is from Weatherhead (1951), p. 26, and is his characterization of religious faith as it refers to healing.
44 Mason *et al.* (1969).
45 See Oursler (1957), Inglis (1965).

confidence, and inspires hope . . . the primitive psychotherapist works not only with the strength of his own personality. His rite is part of the common faith of the whole community which not seldom assists *in corpore* at his healing act. . . . The whole weight of the tribe's religion, myths, and community spirit enters into the treatment.[46]

The intercession of people united in love for Christ . . . and the laying on of hands . . . by a priest or minister or other person who is the *contact-point . . . of a beloved, believing and united community standing behind him and supporting his ministration to a patient who has been taught to understand the true nature of Christian faith . . .* is the true ministry of the Church.[47]

SUMMARY

This review of nonmedical healing of bodily illness highlights the profound influence of emotions on health and suggests that anxiety and despair can be lethal; confidence and hope, life-giving. The current assumptive world of Western society, which includes mind-body dualism, incorporates this obvious fact with difficulty and, therefore, tends to underestimate its importance.

The core of the techniques of healing reviewed in this chapter seems to lie in their ability to arouse the patient's hope, bolster his self-esteem, stir him emotionally, and strengthen his ties with a supportive group, through several features that most methods share. All involve a healer on whom the patient depends for help and who holds out hope of relief. The patient's expectations are aroused by the healer's personal attributes, by his culturally determined healing role, or, typically, by both. The role of the healer may be diffused, as at Lourdes, where it resides in participating priests.

All forms of healing are based on a conceptual scheme consistent with the patient's assumptive world that prescribes a set of activities. The scheme helps him to make sense out of his inchoate feelings, thereby heightening his sense of mastery over

46 Ackerknecht (1942), p. 514.
47 Weatherhead (1951), p. 486. Author's italics.

them. Nonmedical healing rituals are believed to mobilize natural or supernatural healing forces on the patient's behalf. Often they include detailed confessions followed by atonement and reacceptance into the group. Many rituals also stress mutual service, which counteracts the patient's morbid self-preoccupation, strengthens his self-esteem by demonstrating that he can do something for others, and, like confession, cements the bonds between patient and group. Confession and mutual service contribute to the feeling that performance of the healing ritual confers merit in itself. If the patient is not cured, he nevertheless often feels more virtuous. If he is cured, this may be taken as a mark of divine favor, permanently enhancing his value in his own and the group's eyes. This may also help maintain the cure, for if he relapses he is letting the group down. Finally, in religious healing, relief of suffering is accompanied not only by a profound change in the patient's feelings about himself and others, but by a strengthening of previous assumptive systems or, sometimes, conversion to new ones.

BIBLIOGRAPHY

Ackerknecht, E. H. "Problems of Primitive Medicine." *Bulletin of the History of Medicine* 11 (1942):503–21.

Adland, M. L. "Review, Case Studies, Therapy and Interpretation of the Acute Exhaustive Psychoses." *Psychiatric Quarterly* 21 (1947):38–69.

Barber, T. X. "Death by Suggestion: A Critical Note." *Psychosomatic Medicine* 23 (1961):153–55.

Cannon, W. B. "Voodoo Death." *Psychosomatic Medicine* 19 (1957):182–90.

Cranston, Ruth. *The Miracle of Lourdes.* New York: McGraw-Hill, 1955.

Deren, Maya. *Divine Horsemen: The Living Gods of Haiti.* London: Thames & Hudson, 1953.

Everson, T. C., and Cole, W. H. *Spontaneous Regression of Cancer.* Philadelphia: W. B. Saunders, 1966.

Field, M. J. "Witchcraft as a Primitive Interpretation of Mental Disorder." *Journal of Mental Science* 101 (1955):826–33.

Fox, J. R. "Witchcraft and Clanship in Cochiti Therapy." In *Magic, Faith and Healing*, edited by A. Kiev, pp. 174–200. New York: Macmillan, 1964.

Frank, J. D. "Emotional Reactions of American Soldiers to an Unfamiliar Disease." *American Journal of Psychiatry* 102 (1946):631–40.

Gillin, J. "Magical Fright." *Psychiatry* 11 (1948):387–400.

Henry, W. E. "Some Observations on the Lives of Healers." *Human Development* 9 (1966):47–56.

Huxley, Elspeth. "Science, Psychiatry—or Witchery? *New York Times Magazine* (May 31, 1959):17–19.

Imboden, J. B.; Canter, A.; and Cluff, L. E. "Convalescence from Influenza." *Archives of Internal Medicine* 103 (1961):393–99.

Imboden, J. B.; Canter, A.; Cluff, L. E.; and Trevor, R. W. "Brucellosis, Ill: Psychological Aspects of Delayed Convalescence." *Archives of Internal Medicine* 103 (1959):406–14.

Inglis, B. *The Case for Unorthodox Medicine*. New York: G. P. Putnam's Sons, 1965.

Jahoda, G. "Traditional Healers and Other Institutions Concerned with Mental Illness in Ghana." *International Journal of Social Psychiatry* 7 (1961):245–68.

Janet, P. "Miraculous Healing," *Psychological Healing*, vol. 1, chap. 1. New York: Macmillan, 1925.

Kiev, A., ed. *Magic, Faith and Healing*. New York: Macmillan, 1964.

Kinkead, E. *In Every War but One*. New York: W. W. Norton, 1959.

LaBarre, W. "Confession as Cathartic Therapy in American Indian Tribes." In *Magic, Faith and Healing*, edited by A. Kiev, pp. 36–49. New York: Macmillan, 1964.

Lederer, W. "Primitive Psychotherapy." *Psychiatry* 22 (1959):255–63.

Leighton, A. H. "Contribution to the Therapeutic Process in Cross-cultural Perspective—A Symposium." *American Journal of Psychiatry* 124 (1968):1176–78.

Lesse, S. "Psychodynamic Relationships Between the Degree of Anxiety and Other Clinical Symptoms." *Journal of Nervous and Mental Diseases* 127 (1958):125–30.

Lévi-Strauss, C. *Anthropologie Structurale*. Paris: Librairie Plon, 1958.

Mason, R. C.; Clark, G.; Reeves, R. B.; and Wagner, B. "Acceptance and Healing." *Journal of Religion and Health* 8 (1969):123–30.

Nardini, J. E. "Survival Factors in American Prisoners of War of the Japanese." *American Journal of Psychiatry* 109 (1952):241–47.

Opler, M. E. "Some Points of Comparison and Contrast Between the Treatment of Functional Disorders by Apache Shamans and Modern Psychiatric Practice." *American Journal of Psychiatry* 92 (1936): 1371–87.

Oursler, W. *The Healing Power of Faith.* New York: Hawthorn Books, 1957.

Prince, R. "Contribution to the Therapeutic Process in Cross-cultural Perspective—A Symposium. *American Journal of Psychiatry* 124 (1968):1171–76.

Rasmussen, K. "An Eskimo Shaman Purifies a Sick Person." In *Report of the Fifth Thule Expedition (1921–24): Intellectual Culture of the Igluik Eskimos,* 7 (1929):133–41. Copenhagen: Gyldendalske Boghandel, Nordisk Forlag.

Reed, L. S. *The Healing Cults: A Study of Sectarian Medical Practice —Its Extent, Causes and Control.* Chicago: University of Chicago Press, 1932.

Rehder, H. "Wunderheilungen, ein Experiment." *Hippokrates* 26 (1955):577–80.

Richter, C. P. "On the Phenomenon of Sudden Death in Animals and Man." *Psychosomatic Medicine* 19 (1957):191–98.

Rosen, J. N. "A Method of Resolving Acute Catatonic Excitement." *Psychiatric Quarterly* 20 (1946):183–98.

Sachs, W. *Black Anger.* New York: Grove Press, 1947.

Schachter, S. "The Interaction of Cognitive and Physiological Determinants of Emotional State." In *Psychobiological Approaches to Social Behavior,* edited by P. H. Leiderman and D. Shapiro, pp. 138–73. London: Tavistock Publications, 1965.

Schmale, A. H. "Relationship of Separation and Depression to Disease." *Psychosomatic Medicine* 20 (1958):259–77.

Speck, R. V., and Rueveni, U. "Network Therapy—A Developing Concept." *Family Process* 8 (1969):182.

Spiro, M. G. *Burmese Supernaturalism: A Study in the Explanation and Reduction of Suffering.* Englewood Cliffs, N.J.: Prentice-Hall, 1967.

Steiner, L.: *Where Do People Take Their Troubles?* New York: International Universities Press, 1945.

Strassman, H. D.; Thaler, M. B.; and Schein, E. H. "A Prisoner of War Syndrome: Apathy as a Reaction to Severe Stress." *American Journal of Psychiatry* 112 (1956):998–1003.

Torrey, E. F. *The Mind Game: Witchdoctors and Psychiatrists.* New York: Emerson Hall, 1972.

Warner, W. L. *A Black Civilization: A Social Study of an Australian Tribe.* New York: Harper, 1941.

Weatherhead, L. D. *Psychology, Religion and Healing.* New York: Abingdon-Cokesbury Press, 1951.

Webster, H. *Taboo, a Sociological Study.* Stanford, Calif.; Stanford University Press, 1942.

Will, O. A. "Human Relatedness and the Schizophrenic Reaction." *Psychiatry* 22 (1959):205–23.

By Bernard Grad

Healing by the Laying On of Hands: A Review of Experiments

Healing by the laying on of hands is a very ancient practice, Aristophanes reporting the practice in Athens four centuries before the beginning of the Christian era. Indeed, evidence for the much earlier existence of laying on of hands is provided by the Ebers Papyrus, which includes it as a form of medical treatment used in Egypt prior to 1552 B.C. The Bible has numerous references to the laying on of hands and its spiritual as well as physical qualities. In the early centuries after the founding of the Christian Church, healing, along with preaching and administering the sacraments was considered the core of Christian work, and the laying on of hands was an important part of Christian healing. Later, when it was abandoned by the Church, the laying on of hands was taken up by several kings of Europe and became known as the Royal Touch. During all of this time healing by the laying on of hands was taken on faith, the scientific attitude being all but nonexistent. In 1784 a commission, which included Lavoisier and Benjamin Franklin, was appointed by the King of France to investigate the existence of a "magnetic fluid" which Mesmer claimed was at the core of the laying on of hands. The commission concluded that the magnetic fluid did not exist and that its medical effects were due to "sensitive excitement, imagination and imitation." However, a committee of the Medical Section of the Academie des Sciences examined animal magnetism again in 1831 and accepted Mesmer's viewpoint. Nevertheless, this had little impact, for the mechanistic materialistic direction of physics, chemistry, and biology was well underway by this time, a direction which grew ever stronger with the decades to our own time. In that interval, the methods of biological investigation became more sophisticated, but so strong was the reductionist materialistic bias in the scientific community that no one attempted to test the efficacy of the laying on of hands in carefully controlled experiments involving animals and plants where the possibility of the results being due to "sensitive excitement, imagination and imitation" was unlikely. In any case, in 1957 a series of such experiments was undertaken to test the effect of the laying on of hands as practiced by a man (OE) who claimed some success in healing by this means in humans and domestic animals in the decade that preceded these experiments.

REVIEW OF EXPERIMENTS

Because of the limited space available for housing animals and the limited funds of their maintenance, it was necessary to select small, inexpensive animals as the test object. Mice fulfilled these requirements as well as the statistical one that sufficient numbers of animals be tested in each group of each experiment. The mice were treated by the laying on of hands in groups. This was done by placing them in an "ice-cube tray" type of container made of galvanized iron and divided into compartments, each one large enough to hold a mouse comfortably. The size of the tray was constructed so that all the mice were covered when held between the palms of OE's hands. A wire mesh covered the tray to prevent them from escaping. The laying on of hands was given for fifteen minutes, morning and evening, for a minimum of five days per week.

Experience showed that it was necessary that the mice be calm during the treatment. To eliminate their nervousness about being confined in the trays, they were placed in the trays twice daily, five days a week for two weeks before starting the experiment, during which time they were also gently stroked for one to two minutes by a laboratory assistant to accustom them to the handling required during the experiment apart from the laying-on-of-hands treatment itself. Mice not calmed by this procedure were eliminated from the experiment. All mice were subjected to this quieting procedure before they were separated into control and treated groups, and the procedure was stopped when the treatment period of the experiment began.

The laying on of hands was carried out by placing the mice in the metal container, which, in turn, was placed on the palm of one hand while the other palm rested lightly on top of the wire mesh covering the box. Thus, the hands did not touch the mice underneath the wire mesh, nor were the hands moved during treatment.

Control mice were also placed in the trays—in some experiments they were given no treatment at all while in others they were treated by a lab assistant who made no special claim to healing. Still other controls were given a "heat" treatment produced by heating tapes adjusted to produce the same temperature in the trays as produced by laying on of hands by OE.

THE EFFECT ON GOITER

OE claimed considerable success in treating patients with thyroid disease in the decade before the animal experiments were begun. Therefore, the first animal studies were designed to test the efficacy of the laying on of hands in animals exposed to experimental conditions which would make them goitrous. These conditions included feeding the mice a diet deficient in iodine and dissolving the goitrogen, thiouracil, in their drinking water. Under these conditions, the thyroid increases to several times its usual size, and the aim of the studies in these experiments was to see whether the rate of growth of the thyroid of mice exposed to the laying on of hands would differ significantly from those not so treated.

In the first experiment there were two control and one treated group comprising seventy mice in all. All the groups were placed in the metal trays at the same time, but only the treated group received the laying on of hands, while one of the control groups was exposed to heat as described earlier, the remaining control did not receive heat or any other treatment. For the first twenty days of the experiment, the mice in the treated group were "handled" by OE as described earlier, while for the next twenty days a lab assistant, JB, handled them in the same way. (Subsequent experimentation showed that JB could also produce significant changes in animals and plants by the laying on of hands.)

The weights of the thyroid glands of all three groups increased in size during the forty days on the goitrogenic regimen, but the mice that received the laying on of hands increased in size more slowly and significantly so. By itself, heat did not reliably influence the goitrogenic process and therefore the effect of the laying on of hands could not be ascribed to the warmth which developed in the metal trays during the treatment.

In another experiment, the influence of the laying on of hands was tested indirectly, that is by having OE hold wool and cotton cuttings in his hands for fifteen minutes on the day the experiment was started and several times again until the fourth week of the forty-two-day experiment. The thirty-seven mice in this experiment were housed four or five per cage and exposed to ten grams of the cuttings, one hour per day, six days per week throughout the experiment. The cuttings were dropped into the cage and an hour later the mice were found getting on top of the cuttings. The treated mice were given cuttings held between OE's hands, while the control mice received identical but untreated cuttings. As in the previous experiment, the rate of development of a goiter in the treated mice was significantly slower than that of the controls. Obviously, heat emanating from the hands was not a factor in this experiment. Additional details of these studies have been provided elsewhere [1].

Other studies showed that not only did the laying on of hands slow down the rate of the development of a goiter in mice fed a goitrogenic diet, but it also accelerated the return of such goiters to normal when a normal iodine diet was substituted for the goitrogenic one. In this case also, the effect was apparent both when the laying on of hands was done directly on the animals or indirectly via cloth cuttings.

THE EFFECT ON WOUND HEALING

The effect of the laying on of hands on wound healing in mice was investigated in two experiments as follows: pieces of full skin about the size of a twenty-five-cent piece were removed from the backs of anesthetized mice and weighed as were paper outlines of the wound area obtained as described in an earlier publication [2]. The paper projections of the wound areas were also weighed one, eleven, and fourteen days after wounding to assess the size of the wounded speed of healing. In each experiment, there were three groups as in the first goiter experiment described earlier, that is, two control groups, one treated by heat and the other left untreated after being transferred to the metal trays. The third group received the laying on of hands as just described and the wounds healed significantly faster in this group than in the other two, between which there were no statistically significant differences. The same results were obtained in both experiments [2].

A subsequent more complex double-blind study was conducted at the University of Manitoba with Drs. R. J. Cadoret and G. I. Paul [3]. It involved one hundred mice in each of three groups: untreated controls, and two groups receiving the "laying on of hands" treatment, one group by OE and the other by medical students. All the individuals concerned with the care and feeding of the animals and the measurement of their wounds were unaware of which mice had been assigned to each of the three experimental groups. As a further precaution against identification of a particular treatment group by those concerned with treatment, the cages were placed inside paper bags during the treatment sessions. In half of each group, the bags were stapled shut during the treatment; in the other half, they were left open. In the open-bag series, OE and the students placed their hands inside the bags, one hand on top of the treatment cage, the other supporting the cage from below. In the closed-bag series, they held the cage in the same manner but on top of the paper bags. In neither case were the mice touched directly during the treatments.

In this double-blind investigation as in the earlier less elaborate studies on wound healing, those treated by OE healed at a more rapid rate than did the remaining two groups in both the open- and closed-bag series, but the differences were statistically significant only in the case of the open-bag series. A further finding was that the mice treated by the students (who were quite skeptical about the laying on of hands) healed more slowly than the mice that received no laying on of hands treatment at all, but these results were not statistically significant. Analysis also showed that there was no significant difference between the closed-bag and the open-bag series.

One of the reasons for placing the cages in paper bags during the treatment was to introduce another variable into the experiment, that is, to see whether the treatment influence could pass through paper. The results were inconclusive in this regard because the stapling of the bags had the unforeseen and unfavorable effect of agitating the mice. Apparently, holding the hands over the closed bag had the effect of adding heat to the mice under conditions of little or no air exchange and the mice responded by biting through the bag to gain access to the air. The mice in the open-bag series did not demonstrate this agitated behavior. Therefore, the disturbance of the mice, rather than the physical barrier of the paper bags, could account for the differences between the open-bag and closed-bag series. The basic finding, however, remains that OE was able to increase the rate of healing of skin wounds of mice relative to the controls in this double-blind experiment.

THE EFFECT ON PLANT GROWTH

In subsequent investigations on the effect of the laying on of hands on biological systems, the test object was barley seeds. The reason for this was twofold: to see whether the laying on of hands was effective in the plant as well as animal realm and to try to find a simple and less time-consuming assay.

Pilot studies revealed that the germination of control and treated barley seeds on blotting paper did not result in significant differences, at least under our conditions. Therefore further experiments were conducted with the seeds buried in soil. The earlier studies also showed that it was necessary that the plant experiment be conducted under conditions which would involve somewhat less than optimal growth. To this end, the seeds were first watered with a 1 percent solution of sodium chloride, then dried for several days after which the watering with tap water was applied so that the plants would grow but not flourish. This procedure was so devised so as to create a lack in the plants which would be responsive to the laying-on-of-hands treatment paralleling the responsiveness observed in the iodine-deficient and wound-healing investigations. However, most useful, at least from the point of view of simplifying the procedures, was the finding in preliminary experiments that when the solutions poured on the plants were treated by the laying on of hands, significant stimulations of plant growth occurred over the controls. Therefore, in subsequent experiments it became unnecessary to lay hands directly on the plants themselves. Furthermore, only the initial saline solution poured over the seeds need be treated; all subsequent waterings for both control and treated plants involved untreated water. The preliminary experiments have been described in a previous publication [4].

In the first series of plant experiments in which these preliminary findings were tested, OE treated the 1 percent sodium chloride solution in an open beaker, supporting it in one hand, while holding the other over the solution's surface for fifteen minutes. The seeds watered with the treated saline yielded significantly more plant material than did untreated saline. To test whether such significant differences in growth between two groups of pots could occur when each group was treated by the same untreated saline solutions, the first experiment was repeated in every detail except that the treatment of the saline by the laying on of the hands was not done. The resulting growth in the two groups of plants was almost identical and, therefore, the differences observed in the first experiment was indeed due to some change in the saline solution which had received the laying-on-of-hands treatment [4].

In the second series involving four plant experiments, the 1 percent saline solution in glass bottles fitted with ground glass stoppers was treated by holding the bottles between the hands for thirty minutes. The seeds watered with the saline treated in this way grew significantly taller than the seeds watered with control saline in two out of four experiments and produced significantly more seedlings and more plant material in the third experiment. Subsequent determinations of the sodium concentration and pH in both control and laying on of hands–treated solutions failed to reveal any differences, and therefore the observed significant differences in growth between these two different types of saline must have been due to other causes [5].

In the last of the plant experiments, three subjects other than OE were investigated. These included a fifty-two-year-old man (JB) who was psychiatrically normal and who apparently had a special facility for promoting plant growth. The other two subjects were patients in a psychiatric hospital and included a twenty-six-year-old woman (RH) with a depressive neurotic reaction, and a man (HR), thirty-seven years old and suffering from a psychotic depression. The aim of the experiment was to see whether a 1 percent saline solution held between the hands of a person with a "green thumb" would promote plant growth above that obtained with an untreated control solution and above that treated by depressed patients. A secondary purpose of this study was to test whether the saline treated by the depressives would inhibit plant growth vis-à-vis those watered by the untreated saline.

The four sterile normal saline solutions utilized in this study were in sealed bottles, each of the three subjects holding one such bottle between the hands for thirty minutes, the remaining bottle being left untreated. The saline of each bottle was poured on a group of eighteen pots, each containing twenty seeds, all seventy-two pots being randomized on a table. Subsequent waterings were with untreated tap water. This was a multiblind study; further details of the experimental procedure have been described elsewhere [6].

The barley seedlings watered by the saline treated by JB while in a confident mood grew significantly faster than those watered by the saline solutions of the remaining three groups, thus confirming the main hypothesis of this study. However, the secondary aim of the experiment, namely, that persons in low spirits would depress plant growth if watered by solutions held by them, was only partially achieved in that HR's plants grew less rapidly than those of the controls, but those of RH did not.

The different effect of the saline solutions of the two depressed persons can perhaps be understood as follows: when asked to hold the saline bottle between his hands for thirty minutes, HR was in a depressed, agitated state. He never requested to know why he was being asked to hold the bottle, but instead assumed that he was being prepared for a treatment which he did not wish to receive. Assurances to the contrary were of no avail. In this case, it is assumed that something associated with his depressed state altered the saline solution inside the bottle, inhibiting growth of the plants over which it was subsequently poured.

When RH was first approached with the bottle, she was somewhat forlorn. Upon querying why she was asked to hold the bottle, she was told that the saline would then be poured over the plants to test its effect on their growth. She found this idea interesting, brightened up considerably, and held the bottle much as a mother might cradle a baby. Her mood during the period when she held the bottle was not low as might have been expected from a person in hospital ill with depression, but positive as was apparent from her interest in the experiment. Continuing the same reasoning applied to HR, something associated with her positive attitude altered the saline solution so that its effect on plant growth was greater than that of HR's solution and that of the control. This same phenomenon was even more marked in the case of JB [7].

Inasmuch as the saline solutions in this experiment and in the previous series were altered while in glass-stoppered and even sealed bottles, whatever was causing the change in them must have penetrated the glass, and it is hypothesized that this something is an energy with characteristics which vary at least with the emotional state of the person doing the laying-on-of-hands treatment. It should be noted, however, that evidence supporting an individual's ability to influence solutions in such a way as to stimulate plant growth is still not proof of a gift of healing. It remains to be shown that a positive effect on plant growth is significantly correlated with any therapeutic effects. Further careful investigation is obviously indicated here.

The implications of the latter experiment are numerous: if a man's mood can influence a saline solution which he is holding, then it would appear natural to assume that the housewife's mood could influence the quality of the food she is preparing for a meal. Indeed, in some countries menstruating milkmaids were not permitted in that part of the dairy where cheese was prepared, presumably because of the unfavorable effect on the bacterial cultures. Similar prohibitions exist in the silkworm industry. Furthermore, folklore has it that the canning of perishables, the stiffening of beaten eggwhite, and the survival of cut flowers are all negatively influenced when in contact with a menstruating woman. Such attitudes find some explanation in the experiment just described in that many women, though by no means all, become depressed just prior to and during the early days of menstruation, and it is the depression, not the menstruation, which might account for a negative effect. Thus it is predicted that a depressed man would have a similar influence on the processes cited above. On the positive side, persons who love plants are generally said to be very successful in growing them. The same applies to the rearing of animals or children.

LAYING ON OF HANDS AND THE PLACEBO EFFECT

The findings of the experiments on plants reported here have relevance also for the placebo effect, which has been defined as "any response attributable to a pill or potion other than that due to its pharmacodynamic or specific properties." Some would widen this definition to include not only pills but other procedures, such as psychotherapy [8]. That such responses are common is shown by the comprehensive review of Haas, Fink and Hartfelder, who reported that 40.6 percent of 14,177 patients, with illnesses ranging from simple headache to multiple sclerosis, obtained relief from placebo pills [9]. Other surveys also reported high placebo relief figures for certain symptoms [10, 11].

The placebo effect can be quite powerful, even to the extent of reversing the normal pharmacological action of drugs. For example, prostigmine induced abdominal cramps, diarrhea, hyperemia, hypersecretion, and hypermotility of the stomach in a subject who later responded similarly to placebo injection and atropine sulfate [12]. However, atropine sulfate is known normally to inhibit gastric activity. The tendency of medicine has been to look upon the use of the placebo as a kind of deception permissible under certain circumstances. This is understandable inasmuch as the placebo effect is too often unpredictable to place any real reliance on it; it is preferable to search for drugs with specific pharmacological actions. However, the experiments described in this paper suggest an explanation which may be involved in the phenomena of the placebo effect and indicate a process which may be at the core of healing and of development generally.

The tendency in the past was to explain the effect of the placebo in terms of the expectations of the patient. That is, the prescribing of the placebo was seen as a kind of positive suggestion to the patient, but the experiments described in this paper suggest that the feelings and expectation of the physician may be at least as important. If these are positive and hopeful, they may communicate themselves directly to the patient in the form of an appropriate facial expression or glance or handshake or some other gesture or expression of assurance. Moreover, the positive emotions of the physician may also produce some effect similar to the laying on of hands either on the remedy or directly on the patient. This is parallel to the situation in the experiments when OE and JB's positive feelings may have caused the transmission of "something" to the saline solution they were holding, which, when poured on the plants, accelerated their growth.

Other studies show that the investigator himself can have a definite, measurable effect on the subject being tested, and this quite separate from any bias regarding the drug under investigation. For example, two investigators measured gastric secretion in healthy humans in response to an oral placebo. In one group of subjects, a 12 percent increase in gastric acidity was observed and in another group an 18 percent decrease was observed following the administration of the placebo [13]. These differing results were consistent when each of the experimenters was used. This is similar to the situation where two types of psychotherapists were found by Truax and Carkhuff [14] and the two types of effects produced by different subjects on plant growth in the present study.

It is a well-known fact that enthusiastic reports describing the therapeutic action of many drugs when first appearing on the market are often followed by a subsequent marked decrease in such effects. This is another example of the placebo effect and has prompted the old saying that physicians should be sure to use those drugs while they still have the power to heal. The importance of the beliefs of the physician regarding the therapeutic efficacy of any remedy he administers is interestingly revealed by the following case report:

A patient who suffered from asthma for many years, during which time he had become refractory to epinephrine, presented himself to a physician who then gave him a new medication recently received from a pharmaceutical company. The results were favorable: when given the pill, he was free of asthma; when it was stopped, the asthma returned. Later, when the physician substituted a placebo for the medication without the patient's knowledge, the physician was not surprised that the asthma was not relieved. Shifts from the agent to placebo and back again were carried out with consistent results in favor of the agent. In due course, the physician approached the company for additional supplies of the therapeutic agent, but to his astonishment was told that *he* had been receiving placebo all along, in order to check out the possible role of the placebo effect in the many enthusiastic reports the company had received regarding the therapeutic agent itself [13].

Two explanations are possible: the physician's belief transmitted itself either directly to the patient via some verbal or nonverbal communication, or indirectly via the pill, in the same way that the feelings of JB affected the growth of the plants via the saline solution poured over them. The effect of the pill on the patient was positive because the physician hoped (perhaps unconsciously) that the pill would cure the patient. On the other hand, when he believed that he was dealing with the placebo, there was no generation of positive emotion and therefore the effect was nil.

THE LAYING ON OF HANDS
AND PSYCHOTHERAPY

In our experiments it was observed that agitated and nervous mice that did not sit quietly in the cages during the laying-on-of-hands treatment did not respond favorably to such treatment. That is, attitudes of agitation appeared to prevent them from receiving from the healer whatever was necessary for acceleration of wound healing. This was the reason for training them to sit quietly in the holder and getting them used to the treatment boxes for several weeks before the experiment began.

Those who claim success in healing by the laying on of hands or related procedures also state that patients should not be in a state of active opposition to the treatment if they hope to be healed. Some have even stated that while it is desirable for the patient to have faith in the healer, it is not necessary, but that it is enough if the person wishing to be healed is neutral in his feelings and has an open mind in regard to the laying on of hands.

An analogous situation exists in psychotherapy, where it is well known that the prognosis of patients who do not come to treatment voluntarily is poor. That is, an attitude of acceptance is expected before therapy can begin. Again, once therapy has begun, as Freud pointed out, patients must have faith in their physicians to help them "fight out the normal conflict with the resistances which we have discovered in them by analysis" [15].

In general medical practice, the faith a patient has in his doctor has long been recognized as an important factor in his restoration to health. Furthermore, a physician whose bedside manner is such as to encourage such feelings will also make it easier for any therapeutic mechanism to function more effectively [16].

In addition to the receptivity of the patient, the mood and personal qualities of the therapist or healer are also significant in determining tthe efficacy of the therapeutic relationship. Persons who claim to have the gift of healing have often stated that the work of healing is not done by themselves but by a Higher Power with whom they claim to be in contact. This they do through evoking some positive emotion in themselves, such as submission to the will of God or the affirmation that "Jesus saves," or some prayer.

Interestingly enough, the question as to whether prayer itself is effective in helping sick people recover more rapidly than otherwise was first raised in the scientific community and tested by Galton [17]. That was in 1883 and since that time few further studies in this field have been published [18, 19], and their findings were not conclusive. Of course, the healings at Lourdes have received a great deal of attention.

Although the laying on of hands is usually associated in the public mind with prayer, both OE and JB did not pray while practicing the laying on of hands in the plant and animal studies reported in this paper, nor did they seek to influence the outcome of the results by prayer, although both men were not atheists or agnostics. However, care was taken to see that both were in a positive frame of mind during the laying-on-of-hands treatment.

In this connection, Sister Justa Smith tested OE's ability to stimulate by the laying on of hands the activity of the enzyme trypsin as measured by its action on a known substrate *in vitro* [20]. During a three-week period during the summer of 1967, consistent and statistically significant stimulations of enzyme activity were obtained by OE by means of the laying on of hands. However, in the autumn of the same year, the same procedure by him had no influence on the enzyme at all. She attributes the positive results to the fact that he was in a positive frame of mind during the first series of tests and in a negative frame of mind during the second series.

In line with these findings is the well-known importance of a physician's bedside manner: a confident, cheerful manner may do much to hasten healing. The importance of the therapist's emotions in the healing process is especially recognized by psychotherapists, some of whom are required to undergo a prolonged investigation of their inner emotional life so as to ensure a certain minimum of emotional health.

However, even among trained and practicing therapists, Truax and Carkhuff showed that there were "good" and "bad" ones, in that the former who bring to bear high levels of accurate empathy, unconditional positive regard, and therapist genuineness tend to produce positive changes in personality functioning beyond that usually seen in matched control groups [14]. By marked contrast, patients receiving relatively low levels of the three above-mentioned conditions show negative changes in personality functioning. That is, while good therapists tended to produce better psychological functioning, bad ones tended to produce further regressive behavior. The situation here may be similar to the positive effects produced by OE and JB on the plants and the negative effects observed with HR. Qualities such as unconditional positive regard, accurate empathy, and genuineness are attitudes which are either present in certain situations or not. That is, they cannot be "put on," and yet are apparently decisive in therapy [21]. That these qualities may in fact be at least as important as specific training is suggested by the high consistency of improvement rates found with various therapies conducted by physicians without psychiatric training and those with intensive psychoanalytic experience [22], and by the similar improvement rates for various types of neurotics treated by different forms of psychotherapy [23]. Indeed, Poser showed that undergraduate students with no training or experience as psychotherapists but enthusiastic at the time of the experiment achieved slightly better results than trained psychotherapists during group therapy with 295 psychotic patients, the criterion of therapeutic behavioral change being the psychological test performance before and after five months of therapy [24]. These findings support a trend toward a greater use of trained nonprofessional personnel as aides in the treatment of ever-increasing numbers of mentally ill patients [25, 26].

CONCLUSIONS

Due to the preliminary nature of these experiments great caution must be exercised in drawing any conclusions regarding the nature of the laying on of hands. A few tentative remarks, however, can be made.

First, we observed in our experiments that the laying-on-of-hands procedure significantly inhibited the development of goiters in mice, accelerated wound healing in mice, and stimulated growth (or more precisely, lessened the inhibition of growth) of "injured" barley seeds. Further evidence for the wide-ranging biological effects of this procedure comes from our preliminary studies with yeast cultures, as well as Sister Justa Smith's experiments in which the laying on of hands stimulated the activity of the enzyme trypsin *in vitro*. These latter experiments by Smith are of particular interest since they demonstrated changes at a molecular level in a substance treated outside of a living system. Krieger has also reported a statistically significant change *in vivo* in hemoglobin levels in patients treated with the laying on of hands and meditation [27].

Our experiments demonstrated that the laying on of hands effect is not restricted to one individual (OE) but could also be observed in other people (JB) who may not even conceive of themselves as "healers." Experiments have also been conducted with other healers. Miller demonstrated that two well-known healers (AW and OW) were able to cause an 830 percent increase in the growth rate of rye grass from a distance of six hundred miles [28]. In another experiment, one of these healers (OW) was reported to produce a striated dark-wave motion in a diffusion cloud chamber six hundred miles away. This motion occurred one and a half minutes after the command to cause this motion was given and continued for seven minutes, two minutes after OW stopped concentrating on producing this. After a rest period, the experiment was repeated with the same result. Normally, the type of perturbations which appear in the diffusion cloud chamber are vapor trails due to cosmic rays, not wave motions of the type produced by OW. Prior to the long distance experiment, when OW placed her hands on either side of the cloud chamber, a wave motion appeared parallel to the position of her hands. When she positioned her hands at right angles to the first position, the direction of the wave motion also changed accordingly so that it continued to be parallel to the position of her hands [29]. Other relevant studies include those reporting the hastening of the resuscitation of anaesthetised mice [30, 31], the inhibition of tumor growth in mice [32] and the inhibition of fungal growth in petridish culture [33, 34] by having human subjects concentrate with those aims in mind.

Much more research is required to establish the nature of such observed effects and little can be said at this point about the actual mechanism or mode of action of the laying on of hands. Still it is reasonably clear that the observed phenomena cannot be accounted for *solely* in terms of suggestion or any known physical or chemical forces. The stimulation of cell growth produced in wound-healing and plant-growth studies by the laying on of hands could not have been produced by suggestion inasmuch as the effects were produced on mice and barley seeds which by all normal criteria are not suggestible. Moreover, the fact that the stimulation of growth could occur upon watering with saline solutions which were treated in closed glass bottles indicates that the effect is not due to some chemical substance that might have passed from sweat or breath into the water. The effect must, therefore, be due to some agent which can penetrate the barrier of glass. The evidence against the possibility that the growth-promoting effect was caused by heat emanating from the hands of the person holding the bottle was presented earlier [1].

As mentioned earlier, in the experiments with sealed bottles, there were no significant differences between the control and treated saline solutions in the concentration of a variety of elements or in the pH of the solutions. However, when the transmission spectra of these solutions were determined by infrared spectrophotometry, differences were detected between the control and treated solutions in the 2,800 to 3,000 millimicron range, the treated solutions showing lower transmission spectra than the controls[4]. Subsequent double-blind experiments involving two independent laboratories confirmed the divergence in the transmission spectra between treated solutions and controls. The decreased transmission of the treated solutions suggests that either the ionic properties or the dipole movement of a significant number of water molecules in the sealed bottles was changed as a result of the laying on of hands treatment. The significance of these findings must await further investigation.

One way of conceptualizing the observed results is to assume the existence of some sort of "energy." This hypothetical "energy" may lie somewhere in the electromagnetic spectrum although we have no direct evidence to suggest this. It is proposed that this "energy" is involved in the phenomena observed in the laying on of hands, as well as in psychotherapy and the placebo effect. This "energy" may be generated in the patient by feelings of trust in the physician or remedy, or generated in the physician or healer and then transferred to the patient. Some anecdotal support for this hypothesis is provided by the majority of so-called healers who frequently claim to experience a "flow of energy" during the laying-on-of-hands treatment. Also, inasmuch as we noted both favorable and unfavorable responses in our experiments, there may be a dual aspect to this "energy," with one promoting normal growth and development and the other inhibiting this growth.

As to the nature of the "energy" itself, little can be said from the present studies. However, the idea that there is a force associated with life is an ancient one, and in more recent centuries Galvani, Mesmer, and Reichenbach promoted this idea. Galvani's work in the early discovery of electricity is well known, but less known is that he made a distinction between animal electricity and ordinary electricity because of their different characteristics. Later, he proposed that animal electricity was a life energy specific to the organic kingdom. Mesmer also put forward such ideas, and some of his work entered the "body scientific" in the form of hypnosis and suggestion, though the core of his ideas was either dismissed or misunderstood. Reichenbach, a German chemist and industrialist, and discoverer of creosote, spent decades developing the idea of "odic force," but his work was not accepted by most scientists of his time.

Even in our own time when the rejection of a life force had become entrenched among most scientists, people like the philosopher Henri Bergson, the embryologist Driesch, the biologist Gurwitsch, and others proposed the ideas of a life force. At least as original and sweeping in his outlook in this regard was Wilhelm Reich, who called the life force "orgone," which according to him was not only present in living organisms but was present in the atmosphere as well [35].

For many, the "life energy" paradigm is difficult to accept, but what then are the alternatives? We may be using the term "energy" because we do not yet possess a more refined way of describing and conceptualizing the nature of the phenomena. In any case, the "energy" paradigm provides a useful conceptual framework from which to design further experiments, and at this stage, further investigation is what is needed.

In the past, research in the area of healing evoked such strong skepticism that investigation was discouraged. At the present time, the skepticism persists, and rightly so, but a new attitude of openness is beginning to emerge, which should lead to ever better experiments so badly needed in a field so old and yet so new.

REFERENCES

1. B. R. Grad, "The Biological Effects of the 'Laying On of Hands': Implications for Biology." A.S.P.R. Symposium. (Metuchen, N.J.: Scarecrow Press, 1976).

2. B. Grad, "Some Biological Effects of the 'Laying On of Hands': A Review of Experiments with Animals and Plants." *Journal of the American Society for Psychical Research* 59 (April 1965):94–127.

3. B. Grad, R. J. Cadoret, and G. I. Paul, "The Influence of an Unorthodox Method of Treatment on Wound Healing in Mice," *International Journal of Parapsychology* 3 (Spring 1961):5–24.

4. B. Grad, "A Telekinetic Effect on Plant Growth," *International Journal of Parapsychology* 5 (Spring 1963):117–33.

5. B. Grad, "A Telekinetic Effect on Plant Growth, II: Experiments Involving Treatment of Saline in Stoppered Bottles," *International Journal of Parapsychology* 6 (Autumn 1964):473–98.

6. B. Grad, "The 'Laying On of Hands': Implications for Psychotherapy, Gentling and the Placebo Effect," *Journal of the American Society for Psychical Research* 61 (1967):286–305.

7. B. Grad, "The 'Laying On of Hands': Implications for Psychotherapy and the Placebo Effect," *Corrective Psychiatry and Journal of Social Therapy* 12, no. 2 (1966):192–202 and no. 6 (1966): 472–75.

8. D. Rosenthal and J. D. Frank, "Psychotherapy and the Placebo Effect," *Psychological Bulletin* 53 (1956):294.

9. H. Haas, H. Fink, and G. Hartfelder, "The Placebo Problem," *Psychopharmacology Service Center Bulletin* 2 (July 1963):1–65.

10. H. K. Beecher, "The Powerful Placebo," *Journal of the American Medical Association* 159 (1955):1602–06.

11. H. K. Beecher, *Measurement of Subjective Responses* (New York: Oxford University Press, 1959).

12. S. Wolf, "Effects of Suggestion and Conditioning on the Action of Chemical Agents in Human Subjects—The Pharmacology of Placeboes," *Journal of Clinical Investigation* 29 (1950):100–09.

13. Cited in J. S. Bell, "The Placebo Effect in Drug Evaluation," *Applied Therapeutics* 6 (1964):933–34.

14. C. B. Truax and R. R. Carkhuff, "For Better or for Worse or the Process of Psychotherapeutic Personality Change," In *Recent Advances in the Study of Behaviour Change in Proceedings of the Academic Assembly on Clinical Psychology*, pp. 118–57, sponsored by the Department of Psychology and the Department of Psychiatry, McGill University, Montreal, 1963.

15. S. Freud, *Introduction to Psychoanalysis.* (Garden City, N.Y.: Garden City Publishing Company, 1943).

16. A. Meares, *The Management of the Anxious Patient* (Philadelphia: W. B. Saunders, 1963), p. 151.

17. F. Galton, *Inquiries into Human Faculty and Its Development* (London: Macmillan, 1883), pp. 277–94.

18. C. R. B. Joyce and R. M. C. Welldon, "The Objective Efficacy of Prayer: A Double-Blind Clinical Trial," *Journal of Chronic Diseases* 18 (1965):367–77

19. P. J. Collipp, "The Efficacy of Prayer: A Triple Blind Study," *Medical Times* 97 (1969):201–204.

20. J. W. Smith, "The Influence of Enzyme Growth by the 'Laying-On of Hands,' in the Dimensions of Healing: A Symposium," The Academy of Parapsychology and Medicine (Los Altos, California, 1972).

21. R. D. Chessick, "Empathy and Love in Psychotherapy," *American Journal of Psychotherapy* 19 (1965):205–19.

22. H. J. Eysenck, "The Effects of Psychotherapy," *International Journal of Psychiatry* 1 (1965):99–144.

23. K. E. Appel, W. T. Lhamon, J. M. Myers, and W. A. Harvey, *Long-Term Psychotherapy in Psychiatric Treatment* (Baltimore: Williams and Wilkins, 1953).

24. E. C. Poser, "Effect of Therapists' Training on Group Therapeutic Outcome," *Journal of Consulting Psychology* 13 (1966):283–89.

25. E. C. Poser, "Training Behaviour Therapists," *Behavior Research and Therapy* 5 (1967):37–41.

26. I. M. Marks, J. Connolly, and R. S. Hallam, "Psychiatric Nurse as Therapist," *British Medical Journal* 3 (1973):156–60.

27. D. Krieger, "The Response of *In-Vivo* Human Hemoglobin to an Active Healing Therapy by Direct Laying-On-of-Hands. *Human Dimensions* 1, no. 3 (1972):12–15.

28. R. Miller, "The Effect of Thought upon the Growth of Remotely Located Plants," *Journal of Pastoral Counseling* 6 (1971–1972): 61–63.

29. R. N. Miller, P. B. Reinhart, and A. Kern, "Scientists Register Thought Energy," *Science of Mind* (July 1974):12–16.

30. G. Watkins and A. M. Watkins, "Possible PK Influence on the Resuscitation of Anaesthetised Mice," *Journal of Parapsychology* 35 (1971):257–72.

31. R. Wells and J. Klein, "A Replication of a 'Psychic Healing' Paradigm," *Journal of Parapsychology* 36 (1972):144–49.

32. G. H. Elguin, "Psychokinesis in Experimental Tumorigenesis" (abstract), *Journal of Parapsychology* 30 (1966):220.

33. J. Barry, "Essais relatif à l'influence de la pensée sur la croissance des champignons," *Revue Métapsch* 2 (1966):43–66.

34. J. Barry, "General and Comparative Study of the Psychokinetic Effect on a Fungus Culture," *Journal of Parapsychology* 13 (1968): 166–76.

35. Wilhelm Reich, *Selected Writings: An Introduction to Orgonomy.* (New York: Noonday Press, 1973).

By Harris L. Coulter

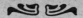

Homoeopathic Medicine

ASSUMPTIONS ABOUT HEALTH AND DISEASE

Any system of medical practice takes its origin in a set of assumptions about health and disease. Sometimes these assumptions are conscious and explicit. More often they are unconscious; the practitioner is unaware of them. The homoeopathic and allopathic approaches to therapeutics are based on sets of assumptions about disease, health, and the curative process. Furthermore, these two sets of assumptions are opposed to one another in many important respects. The different therapeutic procedures employed by homoeopathy and allopathy originate in different interpretations of observed physiological and pathological processes.

From Hahnemann* onwards, the homoeopathic physicians have characterized the processes of health and disease in vitalistic terms. They have talked of a "vital force," "power of recovery," or "natural force" in the body—a force which reacts to external stimuli. This reactive power is manifested in the symptoms of disease, just as it also makes its presence felt in the rhythmic al-

From *Homoeopathic Medicine* (Falls Church, Va.: American Foundation for Homoeopathy, 1972). Reprinted by permission.
* Samuel Hahnemann (1755–1843), the founder of the homoeopathic system of medicine.

terations of the body's functions in health; the alternation of sleep and wakefulness, the menstrual function in women, etc. Disease symptoms represent the form taken by this power when reacting to a morbific stimulus in the internal or external environment.

The vitalistic assumption is of primordial importance for homoeopathic therapeutics, since it imposes a particular interpretation of the symptom. Regardless of how disagreeable or even painful it may be, the symptom is still the visible manifestation of the organism's reactive power. And since this reactive power always strives for cure, for harmony in the functioning of the organism, and always strives to adjust the balance between the body and its environment, the symptoms are not the signs of a morbific, but of a curative, process. They point out to the physician the route taken by the body in coping with some particular stress; hence they are the best guides to treatment. Since the body's reactive force endeavors to cope with a given stress by producing *a particular set of symptoms,* the physician's duty is to promote the development of this very set of symptoms. The curative medicine is the one which supports and stimulates the organism's incipient and inchoate healing effort.

Homoeopathy stresses the importance of the body's natural discharges—urine, stool, menses, and especially skin eruptions. The organism's natural tendency in health is to rid itself of waste substances through these natural outlets, and a similar process is at work in disease. The suppression of natural secretions and eruptions can give rise to serious systemic disorders. Skin eruptions are the manifestation of nature's effort to throw off some internal toxin or waste matter. The suppression of eczema by local applications has been known to produce colitis, asthma, and bronchitis. The suppression of syphilitic and gonnorrhoeal skin symptoms can give rise to a myriad of chronic manifestations. Medicines must strengthen and intensify the processes adopted by the organism to cope with morbific stimuli and must never counteract these processes.

If we now attempt to elucidate the assumptions about health and disease current in orthodox practice, we find ourselves in a quandary, because modern allopathic medicine does not admit to any explicit set of assumptions in this area. A writer has observed that modern medicine shies away from any general theory of the organism, of health, and of disease.[1] A little thought, however, will disclose two important tenets of modern allopathic medicine. One relates to the symptom—allopathic medicine does not generally regard the symptom as a sign of the body's reaction to morbific environmental stimuli, but rather as a wound inflicted upon the body by morbific stimuli. Far from considering that the body reacts dynamically to external stimuli, allopathic medicine tends to view the body as the passive recipient of blows delivered from the outside.

The other major tenet of allopathic medicine is the "disease entity" or "clinical entity." Knud Faber has written that the physician "cannot live, cannot speak, cannot act, without [it]."[2] What is the meaning of the disease entity? It means that the symptoms —the "wounds which the environment inflicts upon the body"— can be grouped into typical patterns and viewed as discrete diseases. Thus allopathic medicine operates with a relatively static group of discrete "diseases." This is to be contrasted with the dynamic doctrine of disease categories employed in homoeopathy.

While, in allopathic medicine, the persons within each disease category will differ from one another in certain respects, for purposes of diagnosis and treatment the common elements are considered to be of greater significance than the points of difference. The physician bases his treatment upon the elements which the patients within each category possess in common.

These common elements may be bacterial, symptomatic, morphological, or other. What interests us is the logical idea that these common elements are the phenomena of primary interest to the physician.

There is a psychological connection between the disease-entity concept and the view that the symptom is a lesion inflicted by a morbific stimulus. The entity is built up from the prominent or striking symptoms; attention is directed to these symptoms, and it is thus natural to regard them as harmful manifestations. Fever is a good example. While the homoeopathic physician will regard fever as a benign symptom, reflecting the body's effort to overcome the morbific influence at work on the body, the orthodox physician will take the contrary view and administer medicines which lower the fever. (It is fair to note that the contrary interpretation of fever is also occasionally given in the allopathic medical writings, but then how is the physician to distinguish the benign fever from the one which is harmful?) Many of the medicines used in allopathic practice aim to oppose or counteract one or several prominent disease symptoms.

We may carry the analysis a step further and note that the allopathic physician's attitude toward the symptom determines his attitude toward the "vital force." He cannot admit the existence of such a force in the body and at the same time administer medicines which counteract or suppress the symptoms which are the very manifestations of this force. Hence he instinctively rejects the vital-force doctrine.

Thus the homoeopath and the regular physician start off with divergent interpretations of the symptom. The concept of the vital force is of considerable moment for the day-to-day practice of medicine in the homoeopathic school, and its rejection by medical orthodoxy has a similarly pronounced effect on the practice of allopathic medicine.

This concept is significant in yet another way. Its acceptance by homoeopathy symbolizes the deeply held conviction of this school that the internal processes of the organism are (1) extremely complex and not to be wholly comprehended by the physician—so that therapy may not be based upon this assumed knowledge, and (2) linked to one another in such a way as to make all parts of the organism interdependent—so that any attempt at treatment must be treatment of the whole patient, treatment which is proportioned to all parts and systems of the body and not merely treatment of one organ or part of the body.

Thus the reader should not be misled by the homoeopathic use of the expression, "vital force." It in no way implies a "mystical," "eighteenth-century," or "unscientific" approach to medicine. It does not imply any particular view of the essential nature of the organism but has a practical meaning in compelling the physician: (1) to take a humble view of his own ability to penetrate intellectually into the human body, and (2) to bear in mind at all times that any treatment must be treatment of the whole body, the whole man.

In thus stressing the ultimate unknowability of the body's physiological and psychological processes, homoeopathy is in agreement with the most recent standpoint of theoretical physics and of Jungian analytical psychology, both of which accept the ultimate indeterminacy of the phenomena investigated and call for a symbolic, "as if," approach to their understanding.

That the holism of the homoeopathic view of the organism is not without relevance for modern medicine is clear to anyone who has followed the discussion—during the last twenty years or so—of the typical defect of modern orthodox medical practice, which is precisely that the physician fails to pay sufficient attention to the wholeness of the patient, fails to adjust his treatment to the whole man. There is even a "crisis in medical education"—meaning that the medical student fails to acquire a feeling for the wholeness of the patient—and programs are elaborated for adjusting the medical school curriculum in such a way as to impart this feeling to the student.

Such efforts cannot be successful, however, in the absence of an integrated theory of the whole man. The mere reorganization of the curriculum, exhortations to the medical student to pay more attention to the psychological, sociological, or epidemiological background of his patients, can have no effect unless integrated into a therapeutic theory whose point of departure is a theory of the whole organism.

Allopathic medicine, however, does not possess such a theory and manifests no interest in acquiring one. The closest it comes to a basic theoretical tenet is its concept of the disease entity.

In contrast, homoeopathy does possess a precise theory of the organism—one which enables its practitioners to comprehend the significance of individual symptoms as well as the dynamic interaction among symptoms in health and disease. When asked how he can be sure that this theory is valid, the homoeopathic physician will respond that it has served for 150 years as the basis for the successful homoeopathic treatment of disease and the preservation of health. And if the homoeopathic physician *can* cure his patients consistently and methodically on the basis of this theory, this set of assumptions, who is to say that it is wrong? Practice is the only test. No one is justified in attacking the assumption of the vital force, and its theoretical and practical corollaries, unless he can produce a better theory—one which yields better practical results.

The Physician's Knowledge of the Organism and the Effects of Medicines

The physician's first task is to know what his patient is suffering from. His second task is to cure this patient. Thus he first needs a key to understanding the organism and, secondly, a key to the effects of medicines.

Let us first take up the problem of ascertaining what ails the patient. The physician has two sources of knowledge. The first is sense-perception, defined as including (1) that which is perceivable by the physician and (2) that which is perceivable by the patient and which can be elicited from him by careful questioning. The second source of knowledge—defined, in allopathic medicine, as "objective"—includes the various tests which have been devised for measuring the chemical composition of the blood and the other bodily fluids, for examining and analyzing the structure of the tissues, for measuring blood pressure, for recording brain waves, and the like. Generally speaking, these data are not directly sense-perceptible, and this knowledge is not symptomatic knowledge. It is knowledge of the physiological and pathological changes occurring in the body during disease.

The homoeopathic and orthodox physicians take opposed views of the nature and importance of these two kinds of knowledge. The former attribute prime importance to sensory knowledge of the patient's symptoms and secondary importance to the so-called "objective" disease parameters. With the latter, this emphasis is reversed. Allopathic physicians attribute greater importance to the "objective" information and less to the "subjective" symptoms.

The difference stems from homoeopathy's orientation toward the dynamic and changeable vital force, as opposed to allopathic medicine's concentration on the static disease entity. This initial difference in approach leads to different views of the relative importance of the symptoms and the "objective" pathological or physiological data.

Homoeopathy holds that the disease process first affects the vital force, where its presence is manifested by a change in the patient's general well-being—before any "objective" changes can be noted in the patient's fluids or tissues. These pathological changes are the *result* of the alteration in the vital principle and not its *cause*. The initial morbid changes in the state of the vital force are, therefore, expressed only as symptoms. Symptoms are chronologically prior to pathology. For this reason they are also prior in importance. The ongoing pathological changes are, at all stages, preceded by symptomatic changes. Attention to these symptomatic changes will enable the physician to forestall the pathological deterioration.

The homoeopathic physician of today will conduct the same chemical, microscopic, and other tests of the patient's tissues and fluids as are done by the allopathic physician, but he is always aware that they yield knowledge of the *consequences* of pathological alterations in the vital force. Tissue and fluid changes are chronologically posterior to the alterations in the vital force itself, and knowledge of these changes must therefore be of secondary importance for treatment.

The alterations in the vital force are to be perceived only by a most careful and exhaustive analysis of symptoms. Hahnemann exhorted the physician to observe with extreme care everything that was to be seen with the eyes or perceived in any way by the other senses. Above all, the physician was to question the patient minutely about his perceptions and sensations. If the physician's interrogation and observation of the patient were sufficiently thorough, as Hahnemann thought, he would have all the information needed to effect a cure in those cases where cure is possible.

"The internal essential nature of every malady, of every individual case of disease, as far as it is necessary for us to know it, for the purpose of curing it, expresses itself by the *symptoms,* as they present themselves to the investigations of the true observer in their whole extent, connection, and succession.

When the physician has discovered all the observable symptoms of the disease that exist, he has discovered the disease itself, he has attained the complete conception of it requisite to enable him to effect a cure."[3]

Hahnemann had strong objections to the cursory and superficial way in which most physicians examined their patients and proposed a far more comprehensive technique for observing and registering these all-important indicators of disease.

"For example, what is the character of his stools? How does he pass his water? How is it with his day and night sleep? What is the state of his disposition, his humor, his memory? How about the thirst? What sort of taste has he in his mouth? What kinds of food and drink are most relished? What are most repugnant to him? Has each its full natural taste, or some other unusual taste? How does he feel after eating or drinking? Has he anything to tell about the head, the limbs, or the abdomen? . . . What did the patient vomit? Is the bad taste in his mouth putrid or bitter or sour, or what? Before or after eating or during the repast? At what period of the day was it worst? What is the taste of what is eructated? Does the urine only become turbid on standing, or is it turbid when first discharged? . . . Does he start during sleep? Does he lie only on his back, or on which side? Does he cover himself well up, or can he not bear the clothes on him? Does he easily awake, or does he sleep too soundly? How does he feel immediately after waking from sleep? How often does this or that symptom occur? What is the cause that produces it each time it occurs? Does it come on whilst sitting, lying, standing, or when in motion? Only when fasting? . . . how the patient behaved during the visit—whether he was morose, quarrelsome, hasty, lachrymose, anxious, despairing, or sad, or hopeful, calm, etc. Whether he was in a drowsy state or in any way dull of comprehension; whether he spoke hoarsely or in a low tone or incoherently, or how otherwise did he talk? What was the color of his face and eyes, and of his skin generally? What degree of liveliness and power was there in his expression and eyes? What was the state of his tongue, his breathing, the smell from his mouth, and his hearing? Were his pupils dilated or contracted? How rapidly and to what extent did they alter in the dark and in the light? What was the character of the pulse? What the condition of the abdomen? How moist or hot, how cold or dry to the touch, was the skin of this or that part, or generally? Whether he lay with head thrown back with mouth half or fully open, with the arms placed above the head, on his back, or in what other position? What effort did he make to raise himself? And anything else in him that may strike the physician as being remarkable."[4]

Thus the homoeopath must record a long list of symptoms, including many which would be ignored by the orthodox physician. He must pay special attention to the "modalities": Is the particular symptom aggravated or relieved by heat, cold, motion, rest, noise, quiet, wetness, dryness, and changes in the weather? In the homoeopathic view all these symptoms are important in giving the detailed knowledge of the patient's state, which the physician must have if he is to effect a cure. These changes in the symptoms produced by different environmental conditions are often the key to the correct medicine.

The allopathic physician takes a contrary view, feeling that the measurement of physiological and pathological parameters are more reliable guides to treatment precisely because they are "objective," while the "subjective" symptoms are too ephemeral and unstable to be reliable. While he does note the symptoms generally, he does not go into them in the exhaustive way urged by Hahnemann, and the diagnosis will always rely more heavily upon the "objective" parameters than upon the "unstable" or "evanescent" symptoms.

The attempt to balance symptoms and "objective" findings places this physician in a dilemma. Symptoms are very numerous, as homoeopathic experience indicates. But the orthodox physician is not interested in *all* the patient's symptoms, only in the "important" ones, the ones which characterize unambiguously the presence of some typical disease process. But the "importance" of a given symptom is, of course, related to the diagnosis which is ultimately accepted. The physician may simply discard all the symptoms which do not fit the diagnosis, ascribing them to the patient's tendency to neurosis or hypochondria. Or he may retain some of them on the ground that the case is "atypical." What is important is that he does not base the diagnosis on all possible observable symptoms but arbitrarily accepts some of them and discards others. Hahnemann remarked in this connection:

" 'What do we care,' say the medical teachers and their books, 'what do we care about the presence of many other diverse symptoms that are observable in the case of disease before us, or the absence of those that are wanting? The physician should pay no attention to such empirical trifles; his practical tact, the penetrating glance of his mental eye into the hidden nature of the malady, enables him to determine at the very first sight of the patient what is the matter with him, what pathological form of the disease he has to do with, and what name he has to give it . . .' "[5]

Hahnemann felt that therapy should not be based upon a conclusion about the internal state of the organism, because this knowledge is unstable and arbitrary—reflecting an arbitrary selection among the symptoms. The allopathic physician cannot take into account all the symptoms presented by the patient because he would not know what to do with them anyway. Many cannot be referred to some accepted pathological process. But these may be the very ones which best define the illness from which the patient is suffering. Who is to say that they are unimportant?

Here it may only be suggested that an important reason for allopathic medicine's insistence upon "objective" data as the basic for diagnosis is that reliance upon sense-perception alone —upon the symptoms—leads to a tremendous proliferation of possible disease states. Any physician knows that the variety among patients is inexhaustible. If symptoms alone are to be the guide, where is the physician to find a principle for grouping the individual cases into recognizable categories?

Homoeopathy was confronted with the same problem. Hahnemann refused to group patients according to their pathological indications. In his view this blurred the small but significant differences among patients. He maintained that each case is unique and that the physician's task is not to ignore this uniqueness but to find some *methodical* way of adapting treatment to the specific needs of each patient.

The solution was found through a complete reorientation of medical thought. Hahnemann decided that diseased states must be classified—not in terms of their prominent symptoms—but in terms of the *medicines which cure them*.

This introduces our discussion of the physician's second task, as defined above—how to find a reliable guide to the operations of medicines.

Here the same contrast between the homoeopathic and allopathic approaches may be noted as held for their differing approaches to diagnosis. Homoeopathy maintains that, for evaluating the mode of action of a medicinal drug, sensory perception of the symptoms is a more reliable guide than the "objective" measurement of physiological parameters.

The methods for evaluating the effectiveness of drugs in allopathic medicine are numerous, but their underlying principle is the same: given the existence of such-and-such a disease entity, find a medicine whose mode of action will oppose or counteract the fundamental processes at work in the disease.

Hahnemann worked to develop an alternative procedure for ascertaining the curative powers of medicines, one which would meet all the criteria which he had set himself:

1) The procedure must avoid recourse to the disease entity:

2) The procedure must be based primarily upon sensory data; just as physiological processes are best described by their sense-perceptible manifestations, the alterations in these processes caused by medicines are also best described in sensory terms.

Hahnemann's solution to this problem was his adoption of the Law of Similars as the foundation-stone of homoeopathic therapeutics. The Law of Similars has figured in medical history since the time of Hippocrates. While it has had different meanings at different times, in Hahnemann's formulation it meant that each medicinal substance will cure the patient whose total set of symptoms corresponds precisely to the set of symptoms produced by the same substance when administered to a healthy person.

Hence the name, homoeopathy, from the Greek: *homoion pathos,* meaning "similar disease."

If a healthy person takes any drug or medicinal substance on a regular basis for several days or weeks, he will come to manifest a set of symptoms which are peculiar to the particular drug or substance.* In homoeopathic philosophy, this procedure is known as "proving" the medicine (from the German: *Pruefung,* meaning "test" or "trial"). Calomel by its physiological action produces diarrhoea, frequent bloody and mucous stools, increased secretion of bile, and salivation. When a case of disease is characterized by these symptoms, very small doses of calomel (*Mercurius dulcis*) will be curative. *Belladonna* is indicated homoeopathically when the patient presents dilated pupils, violent congestion of blood to the head with throbbing headache, high fever

---

* Persons who are particularly sensitive to a given drug will manifest the drug's symptomatology to a more marked degree. Those who are less sensitive will yield a less striking symptom picture.

with hot red skin, cerebral excitement, dryness of mouth and throat, muscular twitchings (the symptoms frequently encountered in scarlet fever). Any physician will recognize these symptoms as the well-known toxic effects of *Belladonna*.

Thus, when the homoeopathic physician has a complete and exhaustive listing of the patient's symptoms, he compares this with the listings of symptoms in the homoeopathic books of provings. When there is precise correspondence between the patient's symptoms and the symptoms of some particular medicine, as listed in the books of provings, this medicine will act curatively.

It will be seen that Hahnemann's assumption that the symptom is a benign manifestation is perfectly adapted to therapy based upon the Law of Similars. If the symptom is recognized as the expression of the organism's effort to counteract morbific stimuli and to rid itself of disease, the medicine which stimulates the organism in precisely this direction is the one which will act curatively. Thus in homoeopathy the symptoms, which are the sense-perceptible evidence of the disease process, are at the same time sufficient to characterize the effects of medicines upon the organism. The disease process and the operations of medicines are described by sensory phenomena.

THE HOMOEOPATHIC THERAPEUTIC METHOD

Hahnemann aimed to elaborate a therapeutic method which would enable the physician to account for the minute distinctions among patients and among remedies. The thrust of this system was to be contrary to that of orthodox medicine—which often classifies patients under the same diagnosis despite quite significant symptomatic differences and which also fails to distinguish among medicines with approximately similar modes of action.

Hahnemann presented his system in the form of the three rules: 1) prescription of the drug according to the Law of Similars, 2) the minimum dose, and 3) the single remedy.

1.) *The Law of Similars*. The homoeopathic physician must

select his remedy on the basis of the *totality* of the patient's symptoms. This leads to a further distinction between the homoeopathic and the allopathic views of the relative importance of symptoms. While orthodox medicine stresses the obvious and striking symptoms, those which cause the patient the greatest unease, homoeopathy views these as of lesser importance than the symptoms peculiar to the given patient—the ones which he manifests and which another patient would not manifest under the same circumstances. As Hahnemann wrote, "the more common and undefined symptoms: loss of appetite, headache, debility, restless sleep, discomfort, and so forth, demand but little attention when of that vague and undefined character, if they cannot be more accurately described, as symptoms of such a common nature are observed in almost every disease and from almost every drug."[6] "The most singular, most uncommon signs furnish the characteristic, distinctive, and peculiar features."[7] "The more striking, singular, uncommon, and peculiar (characteristic) signs and symptoms of the case of disease are chiefly and most solely to be kept in view."[8]

The medicine which resembles the patient's syndrome in only its more common features will have little or no curative effect. The highly similar remedy, the *similimum,* derives its curative power from its close resemblance to the fleeting but strongly characteristic symptoms of the patient. The key to the remedy is furnished by the small differences which distinguish one patient from another, one case of "pneumonia" or "scarlet fever" from another. These are the details which "individualize" the case, which reveal the peculiar features, the wholeness, of the disease and of the remedy. To ensure that these details were preserved in all their freshness and purity, Hahnemann urged the physician to take down the patient's symptoms in the *patient's own words* whenever possible. Homoeopathic experience has shown that the patient's own novel way of expressing his sensations is often paralleled precisely in the records of the provings, and these rare and peculiar symptoms are often of the greatest value to the physician.

Homoeopathic physicians since Hahnemann's time have made further study of the different grades of symptoms and of their relative importance. They have found that mental symptoms, when well defined, are usually the most useful. Then come the general symptoms: the patient's overall reaction to heat, cold, movement, foods, wet or dry weather, etc. Finally come the particular symptoms: those relating to a part of the body. In all three of these categories the symptoms which are absolutely dominant are the "strange, rare, and peculiar" symptoms which qualify the given patient and distinguish him from all others with similar mental, general, or particular symptoms.

The homoeopathic analysis of symptoms provides a sound method for "treating the patient and not the disease." This is an oft-mentioned desideratum in orthodox medicine but one which is difficult, if not impossible, to attain with a method based upon the concept of the disease entity. The disease entity, of necessity, directs the physician's attention away from the rare and peculiar symptoms (since they cannot usually be associated with any pathology) and toward the common symptoms of the various cases subsumed under a single disease name.

This attention to the common symptoms of disease is what makes orthodox medicine "scientific" in its own estimation. These physicians endeavor to treat the fever, the inflammation, the severe headache, the thirst, the restlessness, etc. which are striking features of very many different diseases. The homoeopath, on the contrary, denies the utility of these common symptoms precisely because they are common to so many diseases and so many cases of the same disease: he maintains that the scientific method is the one which enables the physician to take into account the minute but significant differences between one patient and another.

If patients are to be distinguished minutely from one another, it must also be possible to distinguish remedies in the same way. And just as the unusual symptoms are the key to the uniqueness of the particular patient, so these same symptoms in the provings are the key to the uniqueness of the particular remedy. Hahnemann's comments about the relative valuelessness of such common symptoms as headache, nausea, diarrhoea, and the like—when manifested by the sick patient—are equally applicable to these symptoms when manifested in the provings of remedies. Nearly every proving will yield a group of these common symptoms, and for that reason they are of little value for treatment. What is significant are the "modalities": which conditions relieve the headache or the nausea, which aggravate them, etc. It is found that remedies can be distinguished from one another on the basis of the modalities and that these are often the key to correct prescribing.

The remedy prescribed according to the Law of Similars is "specific" to a particular disease syndrome, a particular conglomeration of symptoms, and homoeopathy thus provides an answer to the time-honored dispute in medical history over the meaning of the "specific medicine." In the orthodox tradition the "specific" has meant the medicine which was of use in a particular disease even though no explanation of its action was forthcoming, the best examples being quinine (*Cinchona*) in malaria (intermittent fever) and mercurial compounds in syphilis. Hahnemann's provings of these two substances revealed them to be homoeopathic to certain instances of their respective "diseases," and he rightly observed that their popularity over the centuries stemmed from the fact that they were truly curative in these cases because homoeopathic to their symptoms. In the light of the homoeopathic experience, therefore, "specific" means homoeopathic to a particular set of symptoms. Every medicine or substance used as a medicine is the specific remedy for the group of symptoms which it develops when proved on healthy persons. Quinine is specific to certain cases of malaria, and mercury is specific to certain syphilis syndromes. Neither is specific to all cases of disease lumped by some physicians under the headings, "malaria," or "syphilis." The specificity is not to the disease name but to certain symptom-syndromes which, in the case of malaria and syphilis, happen to be syndromes often encountered in persons suffering from these diseases.

In the orthodox tradition, on the other hand, where medicines are grouped together in terms of their general effect on some organ or system of the body, there is no method for making precise distinctions among them. The homoeopathic physician is trained to spot the one medicine, or the group of complementary medicines, out of the 2,000-odd substances in the homoeopathic pharmacopoeia, which the patient before him needs. He will make regular use of perhaps 800 different medicines in his day-to-day practice.

This ability to make small distinctions among patients and among superficially similar disease processes is the natural corollary of the concern for the whole man which is central to homoeopathy. The homoeopathic physiological assumptions imply the conviction that the organism must be viewed as an integrated whole, and the Law of Similars gives the physician a technique for distinguishing the whole state of one patient from the whole state of another. Thus homoeopathy is holistic (i.e., synthesizing), as contrasted with the analytical approach of orthodox medicine. The latter bases treatment on what appear to be the common elements in a series of slightly different cases. Homoeopathy largely ignores these common elements, the prominent symptoms, and bases treatment on the small differences between one patient and another. The holism of homoeopathy applies to the medicine as well as to the patient. The provings, in principle, yield *all* the symptoms of the remedy, and the indicated remedy is the one whose symptoms match *all* the symptoms of the patient.

Another important difference between the homoeopathic and the allopathic approaches to therapeutics stems from the homoeopathic awareness of the existence of "primary" and "secondary" symptoms of drugs. Hahnemann discovered in 1796 that any drug administered to a healthy person gives rise to two consecutive sets of symptoms, the second set being in a sense the "opposite" of the first. Hahnemann wrote, with respect to the primary and secondary symptoms of *Opium:* "A fearless elevation of spirit, a sensation of strength and high courage, an imaginative gaiety, are part of the direct primary action of a moderate dose on the system: But after the lapse of eight or twelve hours an opposite state sets in, the indirect secondary action; there ensue relaxation, dejection, diffidence, peevishness, loss of memory, discomfort, fear ..."[9] Initially he felt that both sets of symptoms were symptoms of the drug, but he later concluded that the *"secondary" symptoms expressed the reaction of the organism to the drug.* Thus it seems that the primary symptoms represent the actual effect of the drug on the organism, and the "secondary" symptoms represent the vital reaction of the organism to the drug.

The "secondary" symptoms are merely another manifestation of the reactive power of the vital force and of its ability to overcome morbific stimuli impinging upon the body from the external environment.

Hahnemann and his followers have held that the primary symptoms are the ones to be recorded in the provings. When the medicine is given whose primary symptoms are identical with the symptoms of the disease, the organism's reaction to the drug (expressed in the form of the secondary symptoms) will be the "opposite" of the disease symptoms and will thus neutralize or annihilate the "disorder of the vital force" which is the disease.

Hence the frequently observed "aggravation" of the disease after administration of the indicated remedy. Since the primary symptoms of the remedy are identical with the symptoms of the disease, these latter are at first intensified; this, in turn, stimulates the reactive power of the organism (the "secondary symptoms" of the provings) which overcomes and nullifies the primary symptoms (the "disease" symptoms), thus removing the disease.

2.) *The Minimum Dose.* Hahnemann's second rule was the result of his experience with the phenomenon of disease aggravation. Finding that the administration of medicines in substantial doses according to the Law of Similars led to aggravation of the patient's symptoms, he reduced his doses drastically. In the process he found that the strength of the "primary" symptoms was lessened while that of the "secondary" symptoms remained unimpaired. Since the curative effect of the remedy is a function of the "secondary" symptoms, this discovery permitted a continuing reduction in dose size.

As early as 1800 Hahnemann referred in a writing to a dose of arsenic "one ten-millionth the usual size," and after this time he made general (although not exclusive) use of the so-called ultramolecular dose.

Since this ultra-molecular dose has become the hallmark of homoeopathy, some explanation of it must be made. Medicines are prepared for homoeopathic use by diluting one part of the original substance (if a solid) or tincture (if a liquid) in nine parts of milk sugar or of an 87% solution of alcohol and distilled water. The mixture is triturated in a mortar or succussed in a bottle for some time until the medicinal substance is uniformly distributed throughout the diluent, and it is then known as the 1 X dilution. The mixture can also be made in the proportion 1 to 99 and is then known as the 1 C dilution.

The process can be repeated as many times as is desired, and the remedies are prepared and used in all dilutions from 1 X or 1 C up to 30 X, 200 X, and beyond, the former being known as "low" and the latter as "high" dilutions.

According to the Avogadro Law, however, the number of molecules in one gram/mole of any substance is approximately 1×10^{24}. Therefore, when medicines are diluted beyond the 12 C or 24 X levels, it is statistically improbable that a single molecule of the original medicinal substance will remain in the milk-sugar or alcohol used as the diluent (assuming that a homogeneous solution has been achieved at each stage). And since homoeopathy makes frequent use of medicines diluted well beyond the Avogadro limit, these physicians are often accused of employing pure placebos.

A more controversial aspect of the dilution of remedies is the belief that the succussion and trituration of these remedies at the various stages of their preparation actually increase the power of the remedy, so that the "high dilutions" provoke a more powerful response, by the organism, than the "low dilutions."

A corollary is that some substances which are quite inert in their natural state—such as certain metals, silica, charcoal, and others—develop medicinal powers when prepared according to the above procedures. Hahnemann, for example, recommends dilutions of metallic gold as the antidote for suicidal tendencies.[10] It is felt that most mineral remedies, and those derived from the animal kingdom, act more powerfully in the higher dilutions.

Several comments may be made on the homoeopathic dilutions. In the first place, their value has been proven by much clinical experience. Thousands of homoeopaths have used them and are using them today. These dilutions have been found highly effective when used according to the correct indications. In the second place, a series of biological, chemical, and physical experiments have uniformly demonstrated the existence of some physico-chemical, or other, force in the ultra-molecular dilutions. In

1928, H. Junker added various substances, in dilutions up to 10^{-27}, to bacterial cultures and found that they affected the growth of the bacteria. J. Patterson and W. Boyd in Scotland found that the Shick test for diphtheria was changed from positive to negative by oral administration of alum-precipitated toxoid in a dilution of 10^{-60} or of *Diphtherinum* (a homoeopathic preparation of throat swabs from diphtheria patients) in a dilution of 10^{-402}. W. Persson in Leningrad investigated the effects of dilutions up to 10^{-120} on the rate of fermentation of starch by ptyalin and on the lysis of fibrin by pepsin and trypsin; in 1954 W. Boyd announced positive results from a retest of Persson's findings with respect to the effect of dilutions of mercuric chloride up to 10^{-61} on the rate of hydrolysis of starch by diastase.[11] These findings appear to be strong evidence against any suggestion that the homoeopathic infinitesimal doses are mere placebos.[12]

Furthermore, it is worth noting that orthodox medicine has never made an effort to test this aspect of homoeopathy under controlled conditions. Criticism of the ultra-molecular dose has been strictly *a priori*—with vague references to common sense which is a notoriously unreliable guide in medical matters.

Use of the ultra-molecular dose, in any case, is not an essential principle of homoeopathy. Hahnemann insisted on the "minimum dose," which is an ambiguous concept in view of the associated doctrine that increased dilution of the substance actually enhances its power. Homoeopathic physicians, like Hahnemann himself, make use of the whole range of dilutions, from the lowest to the highest.

3.) *The Single Remedy*. Hahnemann's third rule requires the physician to administer one remedy at a time. Here again his rule contrasts with orthodox practice which permits the use of several drugs at once or in combination.

The homoeopathic principle is not arbitrary but stems logically from the other elements of the homoeopathic system. The physician may give only one drug at a time because the provings are only of a single substance. The physician may not give two remedies at once (i.e., on the ground that their combined symptoms match all of the symptoms of the patient) because, when two remedies are administered at the same time, they yield additional symptoms which are neither those of substance A nor of substance B, but of A and B combined. Administration of two remedies at the same time introduces an unknown into the picture, and the purpose of Hahnemann's new method was to eliminate just such speculative and unreliable procedures from medicine.

Homoeopathy is in no way averse to the use of chemical compounds *provided they have been proved as such*. Thus, *Ferrum metallicum* yields one set of symptoms, and *Phosphorus* yields another set. Phosphate of iron (*Ferrum phosphoricum*) yields symptoms of both *Ferrum metallicum* and *Phosphorus*, but, in addition, has a distinctive action not found in either of its components. The characteristic symptoms produced by *Ferrum phosphoricum* mark it as a distinctive single remedy, and it must be prescribed on the basis of the symptoms from its own proving, not on the basis of a mixture of *Ferrum metallicum* and *Phosphorus* symptoms.

The homoeopathic materia medica contains provings of numerous such chemical compounds: potassium sulphate, protoiodide of mercury, sodium carbonate, to mention only a few.

In orthodox practice, the use of medicinal mixtures is justified on the ground that each medicine has a specific function inside the body and is directed "against" some specific aspect of the disease in question. Homoeopaths disapprove of this practice not only because the medicines are not given in accordance with the Law of Similars, but also because such mixtures yield new and unpredictable combined effects which may be harmful to the patient. Here, as elsewhere, the homoeopathic approach is consistently holistic—demanding the matching of the whole symptomatology of the patient with the symptomatology of a single remedy.

In conclusion, it should be stressed that the rationale for prescribing the remedy in homoeopathic practice is very different from its rationale in orthodox practice. The homoeopath views disease as a derangement or disturbance of the body's economy, of the vital force. Since this disturbance cannot be known directly by the physician, because of the complexity of the internal processes involved, it must be cognized indirectly by means of the patient's symptoms. The symptoms reveal the course taken by the vital force in counteracting the morbific environmental stimulus. The remedy is administered with the aim of helping the organism to react along these lines. The only remedy which can produce this effect is the *single substance,* administered in the *minimum dose,* and in *strict conformity with the Law of Similars.*

Thus, the homoeopathic refusal to base remedy selection on bacteriological factors has a logical basis. While no homoeopath denies the indisputable fact that germs, bacteria, viruses, etc., can cause or aggravate diseases in various ways,* this does not mean that the most appropriate mode of therapy is one which attempts to "kill" the germ or bacterium or virus within the organism. Germs are merely another type of morbific external force. Once inside the body, they promote a reaction just like any other such stimulus. In bacterial diseases, as in all others, the homoeopath attempts to further the reaction of the organism, and experience shows well that this procedure is as successful in this class of diseases as in others.

Thus, the homoeopath disapproves of the use of bactericidal medicines, feeling that killing the assumed bacterial or viral disease "cause" within the body does not lead to a true or permanent cure, since it in no way strengthens the organism. In fact, this type of medication may well weaken the organism and affect adversely its inherent recuperative powers, leaving the patient prone to a relapse or to infection with another disease. It is well known that antibiotics can at times upset the balance of microorganisms within the body and thus permit the ingress of pathogenic varieties.

Similarly, in the homoeopathic view, the other typical medicines used in orthodox practice—substances which stimulate or depress some physiological function, deal only with particular manifestations of the disease process and fail to reach the root.

Killing the germ inside the body does not eliminate the disease cause. The "cause" is not the germ but the preexisting state of the

---

* In 1832, Hahnemann suggested that the cause of the Asiatic cholera epidemic of that year was probably "an enormous...brood of excessively minute, invisible, living creatures" (*Lesser Writings,* p. 758). He still called for remedies prescribed on a symptomatic basis. Many of these remedies were taken over by allopathic medicine.

organism which permits the germ to exist and multiply there. Enhancing or blocking some physiological function does not remove the disease cause but only diverts the vital force into different channels. The "cause" is the preexisting state of the organism which in time gives rise to an observable pathological process. It is non-material and cannot be cognized directly. Knowledge of it is obtained only through the minute homoeopathic analysis of the patient's symptoms. This cause can be removed only through administration of the similar remedy.

REFERENCES

1 Ian Stevenson, "Why Medicine Is Not a Science," *Harpers* (April 1949):36–39.

2 Knud Faber, "Nosography in Modern Medicine," *Annals of Medical History*, Vol. IV, 1922, p. 63.

3 Samuel Hahnemann, *Lesser Writings* (New York: William Radde, 1852), p. 443.

4 Samuel Hahnemann, *The Organon of Medicine*. 6th ed., translated and a preface by William Boericke, M.D. Indian edition (Calcutta: Roysingh and Co., 1962), notes to Sections 88–90.

5 Hahnemann, *Lesser Writings*, p. 714.

6 Hahnemann, *Organon*, Section 153.

7 Hahnemann, *Lesser Writings*, pp. 181, 444.

8 Hahnemann, *Organon*, Section 153.

9 Hahnemann, *Lesser Writings*, pp. 266–67.

10 Hahnemann, *Lesser Writings*, p. 695.

11 See James Stephenson, M.D., "A Review of Investigations into the Action of Substances in Dilutions Greater than 1×10^{-24} (Microdilutions)," *Journal of the American Institute of Homoeopathy* 48 (1955):327–55.

12 Some results of research on the physical basis of the action of microdilutions are reported in James Stephenson, M.D. and G. P. Barnard, "Fresh Evidence for a Biophysical Field," *Journal of the American Institute of Homoeopathy* 62 (1969):73–85.

PART FOUR

TECHNIQUES OF SELF-REGULATION

Introduction

For a man who wears the shoe, the whole earth would indeed seem as if covered with soft leather.

Yoga Vasistha

The principal strategy of Western scientific medicine has been to identify specific causes or manifestations of disease and then to proceed with physical and chemical therapeutic interventions. There is, however, a complementary approach that aims at decreasing the susceptibility to disease by strengthening the inherent capacities of the organism. This basic strategy appears in most of the ancient systems of healing. For example, in traditional Chinese medicine the *i liao* aspect (active intervention) is contrasted with the *yang sheng* (strengthening the natural power of the body); the latter forms the basis of the traditional therapeutic methods of acupuncture, herbalism, diet, and exercise. In Hippocratic medicine, the emphasis is on supporting the *vis medicatrix naturae* (healing force of nature).

Recently there has been increasing lay and professional interest in ancient meditation, relaxation, and yogic self-control techniques as well as in the newly developed biofeedback technology. These techniques are diverse, yet they all seem to share certain basic features of training the ability of a person to mentally control physiological processes. A consideration of these techniques draws attention to a neglected implication of psychosomatic medicine, namely, if certain states of mind can produce *psychosomatic disease*, then other psychological states may lead to *psy-*

chosomatic health. The self-regulatory techniques are providing the means to enhance human capacities for psychosomatic self-regulation and are already contributing to a reformulation of our scientific conception of mind/body relationships.

For example, for many years reports have reached the West of Hindu yogic feats of physiological self-mastery such as stopping the heart, controlling bleeding, lowering body metabolism, and modifying pain. Until recently such claims were dismissed as impossible. They were impossible because the prevailing assumptions of Western psychology and medicine did not allow for voluntary control of internal states. Internal physiological processes were regulated by the "autonomic," or "involuntary," nervous system, which, by definition, operated outside of voluntary control. However, new evidence derived from animal and human research has changed the current thinking about the human nervous system and opened the door to serious investigation of some of the ancient techniques of psychosomatic self-regulation.

A new science of psychosomatic self-regulation is taking shape, drawing together the techniques and insights of the ancient meditative practices, the principles of learning theory and behavior modification and the sophisticated physiological monitoring technology of Western science. The early findings suggest that we have radically underestimated human capacities for voluntary control of internal states. Indeed, in light of the new research many of the ancient healing practices such as those described in earlier chapters do not seem as far-fetched, and concepts like the *vis medicatrix naturae* may soon be extended and reinterpreted in modern terms.

The implications for health care are profound. Self-regulatory techniques promise to provide a new range of therapeutic options. In some cases it may be possible to prescribe a course of relaxation or biofeedback training instead of a drug. Or self-regulatory therapies may serve as an adjunct to medical therapy (for example, by helping to overcome side effects of drugs or speeding recovery from surgery or physical illness). But perhaps most important, the self-regulatory techniques promise to place the locus of control with the patient and enable patients to take a more active role in assuming responsibility for their therapy. Self-regulatory techniques, however, are not limited to therapy. In fact, their most extensive use may be as educational tools. Individuals may soon be able to learn, as part of their general education, how deliberately to control their own physiological and psychological states much as they learn other basic skills.

This section begins with a chapter on yogic therapy taken from a document prepared for the Ministry of Health of the Government of India. This selection provides a brief introduction to the philosophical principles and therapeutic strategies underlying yogic therapy. The basic approach, which derives from a belief in the unity of mind and body, utilizes a wide range of techniques aimed at strengthening the inherent psychophysiological mechanisms of adaptation rather than combating the specific agents of disease. For a full discussion of the specific postural (*Asanas*), breathing (*Pranayamas*), meditational, nutritional, and hygienic practices, the reader is referred to the original monograph. The authors, Swami Kuvalyananda and Dr. S. L. Vinekar served as directors of research at one of the institutes established in India to investigate the scientific basis of indigenous medical practices, which include yoga and the traditional Hindu system of medicine called *Ayurveda*. In this chapter the perspectives of a traditional teacher of yoga and a medical doctor are combined to present an early, and admittedly oversimplified, integration of ancient yogic practices and Western physiology. It should be remembered, however, that yogic therapy—that is, the application of yogic techniques in the treatment of disease—is a relatively recent phenomenon. At its inception, yoga was concerned with psychological and spiritual development, not medical therapy. Nevertheless, many yogic techniques, particularly those of the more physical branch called Hatha Yoga, are now being used in a wide range of therapeutic and health-promotive applications.

In the chapter that follows, Herbert Benson, a cardiologist, examines the commonalities underlying various meditation and relaxation techniques. Benson, one of the first researchers in the United States to investigate meditation, identifies a basic psychophysiological pattern that he calls the *relaxation response*. This innate, integrated pattern consisting of decreases in sympathetic nervous system activity, heart rate, blood pressure, respiratory rate, metabolism, and muscular activity is the physiological counterpart of the flight-or-fight response. The flight-or-fight response, frequently and often inappropriately elicited in modern society, has been implicated in a variety of stress-related diseases, including hypertension. Benson presents some early clinical evidence that the regular elicitation of the relaxation response may serve to counteract the deleterious effects of stress. The relaxation response may be elicited in a variety of ways, many of which have been described in religious terms. Benson has separated the essential relaxation features common to these techniques from their cultural, and sometimes cultish, trappings and reintroduced them as a simple relaxation practice. However, it is useful to keep in mind that meditation was originally employed to effect a shift in consciousness and awareness of the individual, not necessarily to lower blood pressure, decrease muscle activity, or effect any of the other physiological parameters of relaxation. To investigate the utility of these meditation techniques as therapeutic or preventive health practices is productive, but does not exhaust the full psychological significance of these techniques.

In the last chapter of this section, Gary E. Schwartz introduces biofeedback and a new conceptual model of psychosomatic regulation and *dis*regulation. In terms of this model, many of the therapeutic interventions of contemporary medicine are seen to run counter to the inherent homeostatic mechanisms of the organism. Biofeedback, in contrast, is intended to enhance these self-regulatory capacities by providing the brain with new information about internal processes. This additional feedback, which augments the inherent homeostatic mechanisms, facilitates the learning of new options in physiological self-regulation. In biofeedback training subtle physiological processes are monitored, amplified, and presented to the person in the form of external feedback (for example, lights, sounds, or tactile stimuli). By contrast, in many forms of meditation, self-regulation is learned by turning off awareness of external stimuli and attending to very subtle internal signals. Both techniques can extend human capabilities for psychosomatic self-regulation. In his critical review of the current research, Schwartz illustrates the clinical applications of biofeedback that may prove useful in the treatment or prevention of many disorders. He is quick to point out, however, that biofeedback is neither a panacea nor a passing fad. Rather, it is likely to be most effective when combined with other learning strategies including the adjustment of excessive environmental demands and maladaptive lifestyles.

By *Swami Kuvalayananda and S. L. Vinekar*

Principles
of Yogic Therapy

Yoga is generally supposed to deal with only the mind and spirit. But a diligent reading of the Yoga Sutras (aphorisms) of Patanjali will convince anyone that they treat the body and mind as a whole. Hence they include certain "physical" exercises like Asanas (postures) and Pranayamas (breathing exercises), as a prelude to the higher psychological practices. All these, as claimed by the Sutras themselves, aim at bringing about an integration in the psychophysiological processes as a first step towards the attainment, according to Patanjali, of *samadhi*.[1] These practices are intended to stabilize the psychophysiological mechanism so that there is less tendency towards an imbalance in the face of external and internal stimuli. Yoga thus does not divide the body and mind into water-tight compartments but recognizes the close interrelationship between the two.

The yogic concept of the working of body and mind is that there is a homeostatic mechanism in both, which contributes to a balanced, integrated functioning (*samadhi*) even in the face of normal, external and internal stimuli (*klesa's*), i.e., that every person has an inherent power of adaptation. At the same time, though the tendency of body and mind is to obtain a functional balance, every irritation or stimulus, from without or within (be

From *Yogic Therapy: Its Basic Principles and Methods* (New Delhi: Ministry of Health, Government of India, 1963).

it mechanical, chemical, electrical, biological or psychological), does bring about a certain amount of psychophysiological disturbance (*viksepa*). How long this *viksepa* will last will depend upon the relative strength of the stimuli, on the one hand, and the homeostatic ability of the body and mind, on the other. It is the aim of Yoga to devise ways and means to help the body and mind maintain their state of balance, or regain it quickly if lost, in the face of such disturbing factors.

The word "Yoga" is used to indicate both the "end" as well as the "means" and signifies "integration" or *samadhi* (from *sm+a +dha*—to put together as one whole). *Vyadhi* (from *vi+a+dha* —to put out, to disconcert) is opposite of this, i.e., dis-integration; it contributes to a feeling of being "ill" at ease and hence it is a "disease"-producing process.[2]

An acute disease, though it indicates a failure on the part of the body to meet the offending factor adequately, still indicates that the body is putting up a successful "fight" to eradicate or neutralize the disturbing element. It is thus only a temporary disturbance, and, as such, in the view of Yoga, it is better to leave the body alone. The body in most cases can take care of itself. It is best to help the body in its fight by not taxing it with further work. Thus, to an extent, Yoga would seem to agree with modern "naturopathy." However, it should not be said that yogic therapy is against resorting to any specific method of eradication of the offending factors, providing that one knows how to do so, without harming the body or mind. A thorn, for example, that pricks and disturbs the "equilibrium," is better out than left to Nature to deal with. So too, if one knows the exact agent or agents that are responsible for a disturbance, and also how to eradicate the same, without disturbing, for long, the normal functioning of the body itself, only then would one be justified in resorting to such methods. Yoga is not opposed to such a proper and judicious treatment of acute diseases, as is generally supposed. In fact, most of the Yogins have been found to use herbal and Ayurvedic remedies for such purposes and are found to keep a good stock of them to help themselves and others in certain cases.

It is a different story, however, with subacute and chronic disorders. These fall in a different category and indicate that the body is failing in its fight and is inadequately equipped. A chronic disease process is a sign of some maladjustments or faults in our forces of adaptation. According to Yoga, these mostly consist of: (1) a faulty circulation of blood and lymph, leading to chronic congestions and stagnation of waste products in certain regions, which have a toxic effect on the body as a whole; and (2) a faulty system of neuromuscular and neuroglandular reactions.

These two, that is, chronic congestions and faulty neuro-musculo-glandular reactions are interdependent. Thus, a disturbance in the vasomotor control disrupts the rhythm of vaso-dilatation and vasoconstriction and gives rise to general or local circulatory disturbances. When the nerves, muscles, and glands are deprived of a good blood supply, they fail to react adequately and thus a vicious circle ensues, each disturbance contributing to the other. So, if one is to set the process right, one has to find out the causes that lead to these two disruptions. They may be due to one or more of the following: bad postural and other habits, deficiencies or lack of proper control in diet, or certain psychological disturbances, that is, conflicts within. It is best to attend to all of these and see that they are all set right. According to Yoga, which looks upon man as "a whole," a mere exercise treatment, or just a change in diet or psychological attitude, though it may afford some relief, does not constitute a complete rational treatment for a person.

Acute diseases, too, generally leave some effect on the body and mind, though there may not be any apparent sign of the mischief done. They leave behind some imbalances, which may take the body long to overcome, and at times, may even make it nearly impossible for the body to recover completely. It is the duty of the attending physician not to leave the patient to his fate the moment he is "on his feet," but to advise him of some adequate methods of rehabilitation to be practiced for a length of time, depending upon the nature of the disease process and the damage suffered. A person can be said to be "cured" only when he is entirely free from the vestiges of the disease process. It is a pity that, in the busy routine work-a-day-world of today, these rehabilitative procedures are rarely adopted, with the result that the person, though apparently healthy and moving about, is not at all capable of meeting adequately the many stresses of life. This renders him easily prone to either other acute attacks or to some chronic disorder. Since very few people can claim to be completely safe from attacks of acute diseases, Yoga, therefore, recommends the practice of at least some of its procedures to keep oneself "positively" healthy and "buoyant."

In the treatment of diseases, there are two ways of looking at things: one is to investigate the offending factor, help in its eradication, and leave the body to recoup itself once freed from the hands of the "marauders." The other way is to help the body itself to put up a brave and successful fight against the offenders and come out victorious by dint of its own efforts. The body has its own inherent powers of developing specific immunity and also has a general capacity of resisting the onslaughts of offending factors successfully.

Since the discovery of "microbes" and the part they play in the causation of disease, orthodox medicine has concentrated mostly on the first approach. It is not that modern doctors are ignorant of the second, but, in practice, much less attention is generally given to this strategy. After the treatment of an acute disease, patients are generally left to their own fate. At the most, some vitamin tablets or a general "tonic" is recommended. The net result is that the body is left weakened and inefficient while still exposed to the ravages of the disease. Of course, this new idea of taking care of every patient even after he is rendered free from acute attacks is slowly gaining ground and is being accepted more and more in the medical world, especially in the field of physical medicine. Still, as matters stand at present, physical medicine is more occupied with the problem of rehabilitation of the physically disabled, especially with locomotor disabilities, than with rehabilitation of those that suffer from functional disorders, as a result of either repeated acute attacks or other maladjustments.

The attitude of Yoga towards the problem of disease, as towards everything else, is that one has to fortify one's own self rather than waste time in eradicating this or that particular offending factor. The simile that is given is that of a forest full of thorns. If one were to go through such a forest, it would be foolish to remove the thorns one by one, and then move forward. It would be wiser and easier to wear a pair of good shoes to protect one's feet, "For a man who wears the shoe, the whole earth would indeed seem as if covered with soft leather."[3] One of the meanings of the word "Yoga" is *sannahana*—to be armoured or well-prepared. Thus, Yoga lays great stress on strengthening the inherent defensive mechanisms of the body and mind rather than attacking and eradicating individual offending factors. In the treatment of diseases, too, the emphasis is on the development of the inner natural powers of the body and mind to help gain homeostatic balance. In doing so, yogic therapy gives special attention to the various eliminative processes and the processes of reconditioning that are inherent in the body, that is, developing one's powers of adaptation and adjustment.

One of the aims of Yoga is to encourage positive hygiene and health. Positive health does not mean merely freedom from disease, but a jubilant and energetic feeling of well-being with high levels of general resistance and the capacity to cultivate successfully an immunity against specific offending agents. It does not mean merely an ability to work *somehow* but a capacity which does not allow a person to be slothful or lazy. *Styana* and *alasya*—sloth and laziness—are considered psychophysiological disturbances in Yoga. They are a sign of ill health, an imbalance whether on the physical or psychological level, and must be dealt with seriously. Unfortunately such a strict view about positive health is rarely held in modern orthodox systems of medicine. Hygiene and its methods, today, are mostly concerned with problems of sanitation, prevention of disease by eradication of disease agents through various insecticides, etc., prevention of pollution of air and water, care of food, general cleanliness, development of specific immunity through vaccine and sera, etc. These are all highly necessary from the point of public health measures, but, with all due deference to the good intentions of modern medicine, it may be pointed out that they are all "negative measures." While they do prevent the spread of certain diseases, they also render the individual more and more delicate and incapable of "standing on his own legs" and actively fighting a disease process while depending upon his own inherent powers and capacities. As it is, it seems the modern man is being gradually deprived of his internal capacity to fight his own battles, and is being made to lean increasingly on external measures to save him from such disturbing factors. The net result is that the body does not at all "learn" to meet the "offenders" and, if caught unawares, finds itself incapable of fighting them. It is a law of Nature that whatever is thrown into disuse slowly atrophies and ultimately disappears. Man in his attempts to get more and more "comforts" has been gradually depriving himself of the natural rugged resistance and health of his forefathers.

In the "Great War" that is being waged between man and microbes today, it seems that while man has been winning battles, he is losing the war. It is known that microbes have been evolving strains that are stronger and more highly resistant to the new chemicals and drugs invented or discovered by man, so much so that man has to change his method of attack every few years. It is perhaps too early to say who will win this war. So far, man is having apparently an upper hand by bringing in new weapons. While all this is going on, man himself is losing his power of inner resistance for the reasons mentioned above. In addition, the growing industrialization of today, and the rapid changes in social structure, etc., force him to meet much more complex situations than his forefathers had to, and he seems to be rather unprepared for them.

Even though infectious diseases are on a decrease, due principally to better public health measures, there has been a rise in metabolic and psychosomatic disorders. All these are chronic disorders of adaptation. Science seems to be groping about for some external help in the form of substitution therapies, tranquillizers, etc., but it is increasingly being appreciated that the approach should be from the other side, that is, the internal systems of man have to be trained to cope with the new situations and circumstances. In other words, man has to be trained to cultivate his own powers of adaptation and adjustment.

The foregoing paragraphs have been written not with the intention of deprecating the value of public health measures but only to show another aspect of their results. Along with the eradication of deleterious agents from the external environment of man, it is high time that hygiene also gave more attention to methods of cultivation, and widening the range, of the inherent powers of adaptation and adjustment in man's internal environment so as to help him enjoy positive health and not just freedom from disease. Yoga, it must be pointed out, lays great stress on this aspect. It does so through three integral steps:

(1) cultivation of correct psychological attitudes,

(2) reconditioning of the neuro-muscular and neuro-glandular systems—in fact, the whole body—to enable the individual to withstand greater stress and strain, and at the same time,

(3) emphasizing a health-giving diet, and encouraging the natural processes of elimination, whenever it is necessary, by resorting to special lavages and baths.

These constitute the three general measures of yogic therapy.

Cultivation of correct psychological attitudes is of high significance in yogic therapy. One's attitude towards things in general, and towards one's circumstances of life in particular, according to Yoga, have an important bearing, direct or indirect, on the genesis of not only psychosomatic, chronic, metabolic, and other disorders, but also of infectious ones.

It has already been pointed out that the approach of Yoga towards the problem of disease is an integral one. It does not view man as consisting of so many unrelated parts but takes him as a whole, or to be more correct, as an integral part of a larger whole—the cosmos. It is not that modern medicine is blind to this, but in treatment and practice, there seems to be a preoccupation with specificity in diseases. Thus, pneumonia, for example, is considered mostly to be a disease of the lungs proper, and not a disease of the body as a whole, and therefore attention and efforts are concentrated on and directed to that organ in the main. It is assumed that the reactions of the body which constitute the disease process are due to an attack by certain organisms on the lung—and that once that part is rendered free from the attack, the general reactive processes will stop automatically and the patient will be "cured." It is contended that this "curative process" is inherent in every living being; medicine has only to help the person repulse the particular attack and destroy or neutralize the offending factors. There is nothing irrational in this. In fact, medicine has succeeded in making an immense progress in affording "relief" to humanity through this approach. But, as is well known to every doctor, no ideal drug or method has so far been discovered which destroys or neutralizes the offending factors alone but does not disrupt normal tissues to some degree. No wonder then that, after the so-called cure, a person may be left debilitated and handicapped and with much less of his own inherent powers of resistance and immunity.

To use a metaphor, it is like a big house whose inhabitants are capable of fighting and warding off external attacks but when attacked by some marauders the police are called in. The police, being unable to distinguish between the "friends" and the "foes" resort to indiscriminate firing and end up killing some members of the household as well as the enemy. The result is that when the police leave all is "quiet," but the house is left without a good portion of its own defense force. It is true that modern medicine attempts to make this "firing" as discriminate and controlled as possible, and some measure of success has been achieved in this. But still it has not yet been able to find such "ideal" drugs.

Many times the body is thrown into disorder because of some internal mismanagement, due to certain deficiencies and inefficiency in, or lack of proper coordination between, the various internal organs. Functional disorders belong mostly to this group. Deficiencies are filled by modern medicine by what is known as "substitution therapy," supplying the want by giving an extra amount of substances required by the body (nowadays these "substitution" items mostly consist of synthetic products). Also at times, a special and well-regulated diet may be prescribed. But, the efficiency of organs, and cooperation between them, cannot be brought about by mere ingestion of anything. They are set right by training the organs once again, directly or indirectly, and re-establishing a proper coordination and harmony between the various parts. This is now being recognized as the special field of physical medicine; but, unfortunately, as stated before, physical medicine seems to be thoroughly preoccupied with orthopedic problems, that is, disabilities of locomotion.

Apart from the metabolic disorders, referred to above, there is another large group of diseases, not so well defined, which is included under "psychosomatic" disorders. With these disorders there is an element of somatic dysfunction as well as a significant psychological component with each one contributing to the other. Thus, modern medicine has come to accept that mind plays a significant role in at least a number of diseases.

Yoga seems to go a step further than this. The mind has a very significant role to play not only in psychosomatic diseases, but also in every other form of disease, including the *acute* ones. The mind, when it is disturbed, may make the body prone to attacks by external organisms by lowering general resistance and also bring about an incoordination between various organs, thus lowering the efficiency of the body (and of itself). Thus according to the principles of Yoga, every psychophysiological disturbance (*viksepa*), every emotion, especially a negative and destructive one, apart from causing distress and depression, also interferes with the tonic rhythm of muscles and vessels (*angamejayatva*) and to a disturbance of respiration (*svasa-prasvasa*).[4] The disturbance of the tonic rhythm of muscles and vessels, according to Yoga, acts as a trigger to start a chain of reactions; even the disturbance of respiratory rhythm is, in part, due to this *angame-jayatva*. The rationality of this concept can be gauged when we visualize the physiological effects of this process. Any sudden increase in the tone of muscles makes a higher demand on circulation, respiration, sugar metabolism, and other metabolisms, to feed the muscles *better* in order to maintain the required tone. If, along with this increased demand, there is also a general constriction of blood vessels due to a state of emotion, the heart and lungs will be taxed all the more, as they will have to work against the resistance offered by the narrowed vessels. To meet these demands, the autonomic nervous system as well as the endrocrine system will be placed in a different state of activation with higher adreno-sympathetic activity. If the process is continued long enough, the thyroid will also be stimulated to further action.

The chain of disturbances does not end here. The process affects not only the skeletal musculature but the body as a whole; thus, the contractile tissue of the various internal organs—intestines, heart, lungs, bronchioles, blood vessels, etc.—is also affected by it, and this gives rise to a disturbance in the behavior of internal organs as well, and changes the entire "postural substrate" of the person. If the process goes on for a long time, that is, chronically, it may either give rise to congestion and stagnation, in the case of decreased tone or to abnormal wear and tear, if the tone is increased. This, along with disturbances in glandular secretions affecting all the body fluids, makes the body more prone to attacks by foreign organisms, that is, to various infective diseases, or give rise to various chronic, functional, and metabolic disorders.

Thus, *angamejayatva,* or "the disturbance of the tonic rhythm of muscles and vessels," seems to be rightly treated by Yoga as a general precursor of *vyadhi,* or "disease." In trying to go to the very root of the trouble, Yoga concentrates on efforts to prevent, as well as set right, this basic and primary factor.

There was a time when modern medicine looked upon a disease process in terms of individual organs, tissues and cells. Thus, as Drs. Weiss and English put it, "the view point of disease bequeathed to us from the nineteenth century could be indicated in the following formula: Cellular disease → structural alterations → physiological (or functional) disturbance.

In the twentieth century, this formula underwent alteration in some situations. For example, in essential hypertension and vascular disease, the formula was altered to read: Functional disturbance → cellular disease → structural alteration.[5]

The authors further remark, "We are still in the dark as to what may precede the functional disturbance, as in the example just cited, of essential hypertension and resulting vascular disease. It seems probable that future investigations will permit us to say that it is possible for a psychological disturbance to antedate the functional alteration. Then the formula would read: Psychological disturbance→ functional impairment→ cellular disease→ structural alteration."

It is interesting to note that, ages ago, Yoga not only presented the same concept of disease but offered a psychophysiological mechanism for the whole process and also suggested ways and means to re-establish equilibrium.

In this sense modern medicine seems inclined to agree with this ancient concept of Yoga. Its latest trends have been towards the recognition of a "pathodynamics" of disease *in the whole body* rather than viewing disease in terms of the pathology of individual organs, tissues or cells. These latter are nowadays being regarded as mere "nodal points" in an incessant flux of biochemical and biophysical processes involving of necessity all the body fluids. The part played by the mind in the deviations of such a flux is also receiving more and more attention these days. On the other side, the advent of physical medicine has not only brought to light the special value of controlled and guided exercise in therapy, but recent work in that field has established the importance of the role played by tonic impulses in maintaining functional efficiency of not only the neuro-muscular mechanism but of practically the whole body. It is interesting to note that the ways and means suggested by Yoga are in line with these most modern findings.

REFERENCES

1. *Patanjala Yoga Sutra,* II-2.
2. *Patanjala Yoga Sutra,* I-30.
3. *Yoga Vasistha* (Bombay: Nirnayasagar Press).
4. *Patanjala Yoga Sutra,* I-31.
5. Weiss, E. and English, O. S., *Psychosomatic Medicine* (Philadelphia: W. B. Saunders, 1957).

By Herbert Benson

❧ ❧

The Relaxation Response: Techniques and Clinical Applications

Emotional stress is a well-known aspect of the modern Western world. However, there is a simple way for the individual to alleviate stress and thus moderate or control many of its undesirable effects—effects which may range from simple anxiety to heart disease. The "relaxation response," an integrated physiologic response, appears to counteract the harmful physiologic effects of stress and can be elicited by a simple mental technique.

The essential elements of the technique have long been familiar to man, and although they have usually been framed in the vocabularies of religions and cults where the elicitation of the relaxation response has played an important role, the response and the technique can be described in ordinary language and beneficially applied.

THE CONCEPT OF STRESS

The concept of stress has been difficult to define and difficult to quantify. Stress can be usefully defined through its physiologic correlates, particularly elevations in blood pressure. Elevated

From *Harvard Business Review* 52, no. 4 (July–August 1974): 49–57. Copyright © 1974 by the President and Fellows of Harvard College. Reprinted by permission of Herbert Benson and Harvard Business Review.

blood pressure is consistently related to environmental situations that require behavioral adjustment by the individual and thus may be described as stressful. The behavioral adjustments associated with socioeconomic mobility, cultural change, urbanization, and migration are examples of such environmental situations [23].

Relevant findings were obtained in a comparison of high school and college graduates in managerial positions within the same corporation. The high school graduates experienced more general illness during the one-year period of observation and displayed more signs of cardiovascular disease and high blood pressure (hypertension). The investigators in this study postulated that the high school graduates perceived more threats and challenges in their life situations than the college graduates because of the greater discrepancy between their lives and their childhood experiences: the relative ill health of the high school graduates is regarded as part of the price they pay for "getting ahead in the world."

In other investigations, undertaken in several Pacific islands, higher blood pressure was found to be associated with the degree of Westernization. Migration from rural to urban areas in these same islands was also correlated with a rise in the prevalence of elevated blood pressure. Adrian M. Ostfeld and Richard B. Shekelle of the University of Illinois clearly summarized why these situations apparently require behavioral adjustment:

"There has been an appreciable increase in uncertainty of human relations as man has gone from the relatively primitive and more rural to the urban and industrial. Contemporary man in much of the world is faced every day with people and with situations about which there is uncertainty of outcome, wherein appropriate behavior is not prescribed and validated by tradition, where the possibility of bodily or psychological harm exists, where running or fighting is inappropriate, and where mental vigilance is called for" [32].

The Fight-or-Flight Response

Stressful situations that require behavioral adjustment appear to elevate blood pressure by means of a physiologic response popularly referred to as the "fight-or-flight response," first described by Dr. Walter B. Cannon of the Harvard Medical School. When an animal perceives a threatening situation, its reflexive response is an integrated physiologic response that prepares it for running or fighting. This response is characterized by coordinated increases in metabolism (oxygen consumption), blood pressure, heart rate, rate of breathing, amount of blood pumped by the heart, and amount of blood pumped to the skeletal muscles.

The existence of this integrated response in lower animals was substantiated by the Swiss Nobel laureate, Dr. Walter R. Hess. By stimulating the brain of the cat, he demonstrated that the controlling center for the fight-or-flight response is located within a specific area of the brain called the hypothalamus. When this area is electrically stimulated, the brain and other portions of the nervous system respond by controlled outpouring of epinephrine and norepinephrine (also called adrenalin and noradrenalin), which leads to the physiologic changes noted in the fight-or-flight response. These two compounds are the major chemical mediating substances of the sympathetic nervous system. Significantly, the over-activity of this functional division of the nervous system has been implicated in the development of many serious diseases. Thus the fight-or-flight response is an integrated physiologic mechanism leading to coordinated activation of the sympathetic nervous system.

A Czech scientist, Dr. Jan Brod, and his associates have demonstrated the physiologic characteristics of the fight-or-flight response in man in the laboratory setting. First, control measurements were made in a group of healthy young adults in a resting position. These subjects were then given a mental-arithmetic problem to solve: from a four-digit number like 1,194, subtract consecutive serial 17s. A metronome was set clicking in the background, and others around the subjects made statements such as: "I did better than that. You're not doing very well." Then new measurements were taken of blood pressure, blood pumped by the heart, and blood pumped to the skeletal muscles. All had increased.

Other situations requiring behavioral adjustment also lead to the fight-or-flight response. All humans use the same basic physiologic mechanisms to respond to individually meaningful, stressful events. Although the fight-or-flight response is still a necessary and useful physiologic feature for survival, the stresses of today's society have led to its excessive elicitation; at the same time, its behavioral features, such as running or fighting, are usually socially inappropriate or unacceptable. These circumstances may lead to persistent hypertension. Those who experience greater environmental stress and, therefore, more frequent elicitation of the fight-or-flight response have a greater chance of developing chronic hypertension.

The Importance of Hypertension

High blood pressure, or hypertension, is of far greater significance to man than as just an index of stressful circumstances. It is one of the important factors—if not the most important—predisposing man to heart attack and stroke. These diseases of the heart and brain account for more than 50 percent of the deaths each year within the United States. Therefore, it is not surprising that various degrees of hypertension are present in 15 percent to 33 percent of the adult population of the United States, affecting between 23 million and 44 million individuals.

Heart attacks and strokes have always been diseases leading to death, predominantly in the elderly. However, it is highly disturbing that these diseases are now affecting a younger population. The late American cardiologist Dr. Samuel Levine pointed out that in families he followed for decades in which both fathers and sons experienced heart attacks, the average age at the time of the first attack was 13 years earlier for the sons than for their fathers. Many cardiologists feel that we are in the midst of an epidemic of these diseases. If hypertension could be prevented, this epidemic might be alleviated. Consequently, situations requiring behavioral adjustment, which may lead to hypertension, are of considerable concern.

THE RELAXATION RESPONSE

What can be done about everyday situations that lead to stress and its consequences? It is unlikely that the rapid pace of Western life will slow down significantly; and as far as our present standard of living depends on that pace, it is unlikely that most executives would want it to slow down. The need for behavioral adjustment will probably continue, and therefore individuals should learn to counteract the harmful effects of the physiologic response to stress. One possibility is the regular elicitation of the relaxation response [7].

The relaxation response is an innate, integrated set of physiologic changes opposite to those of the fight-or-flight response. It can be elicited by psychologic means. Hess first described this response in the cat. He electrically stimulated another specific area of the hypothalamus and elicited what he called "a protective mechanism against overstress (which promotes) restorative processes" [24].

Like the fight-or-flight response, the relaxation response is also present in man. Until recently, the relaxation response has been elicited primarily by meditational techniques—the reader will find information about the effects of some of these techniques in the accompanying table.

"Fight-or-Flight" Response	Relaxation Response
Increased sympathetic nervous system activity	Decreased sympathetic nervous system activity
Increased body metabolism	Decreased body metabolism
Increased breath rate	Decreased breath rate
Increased heart rate and blood pressure	Decreased heart rate and blood pressure
Marked increase of blood flow to muscles	

The physiologic changes consist, in part, of decreased oxygen consumption, respiratory rate, heart rate, and muscle tension. Increases are noted in skin resistance and EEG alpha wave activity. These changes are distinctly different from the physiological changes noted during quiet sitting or sleep. These changes are hypothesized to result from an integrated, hypothalamic response leading to decreased sympathetic nervous system activity. The neurophysiologic and neuroanatomic pathways from the cortex to the diencephalon remain to be definitively established [21].

TECHNIQUES FOR ELICITING THE RELAXATION RESPONSE*

Autogenic training is a technique of medical therapy which is said to elicit the trophotropic response of Hess or the relaxation response. Autogenic therapy is defined as ". . . a self-induced modification of corticodiencephalic interrelationships" which enables the lower brain centers to activate "trophotropic activity" [28]. The method of autogenic training is based on six psychophysiologic exercises devised by a German neurologist, J. H. Shultz, which are practiced several times a day until the subject is able to voluntarily shift to a wakeful *low-arousal* (trophotropic) state. The "Standard Exercises" are practiced in a quiet environment, in a horizontal position, and with closed eyes [28]. Exercise 1 focuses on the feeling of heaviness in the limbs, and Exercise 2 on the cultivation of the sensation of warmth in the limbs. Exercise 3 deals with cardiac regulation, while Exercise 4 consists of passive concentration on breathing. In Exercise 5, the subject cultivates the sensation of warmth in his upper abdomen, and Exercise 6 is the cultivation of feelings of coolness in the forehead. Exercises 1 through 4 most effectively elicit the trophotropic response, while Exercises 5 and 6 are reported to have different effects [28]. The subject's attitude toward the exercise must not be intense and compulsive, but rather of a quiet, "let it happen," nature. This is referred to as *passive concentration* and is deemed absolutely essential [29].

Progressive relaxation is a technique which seeks to achieve increased discriminative control over skeletal muscle until a subject is able to induce very low levels of tonus in the major muscle groups. Jacobson, who devised the technique, states that anxiety and muscular relaxation produce opposite physiologic states, and therefore cannot exist together. Progressive relaxa-

---

* © 1974 The William Alanson White Psychiatric Foundation, Inc., from *Psychiatry* 37 (1974):41–44. Reprinted by special permission.

tion is practiced in a supine position in a quiet room; a passive attitude is essential because mental images induce slight, measurable tensions in muscles, especially those of the eyes and face. The subject is taught to recognize even slight contractions of his muscles so that he can avoid them and achieve the deepest degree of relaxation possible [26].

Hypnosis is an artificially induced state characterized by increased suggestibility [22]. A subject is judged to be in the hypnotic state if he manifests a high level of response to test suggestions such as muscle rigidity, amnesia, hallucination, anesthesia, and post-hypnotic suggestion, which are used in standard scales such as that of Weitzenhoffer and Hilgard [40]. The hypnotic induction procedure usually includes suggestion (autosuggestion for self-hypnosis) of relaxation and drowsiness, closed eyes, and a recumbent or semisupine position [5]. Following the induction procedure, an appropriate suggestion for the desired mental or physical behavior is given.

So far it has not been possible to find a unique physiologic index which defines the hypnotic state [5]. Physiologic states vary the same way during hypnosis as they do during waking behavior. Suggested states of arousal or relaxation are accompanied by *either* increased or decreased metabolic rate, heart rate, blood pressure, skin conductance, and respiratory rate, corresponding to the changes seen when these states are induced by nonhypnotic means [5]. If the control state is the same as the suggested state, then, of course, no change in physiologic parameters will be seen [4]. For example, the study by Whitehorn et al. reported that the control oxygen consumption value of 217 ml/min was not significantly changed by hypnosis. However, subjects in this experiment were trained to relax before control readings were taken. Therefore, hypnotic suggestion to relax produced no further change [41].

Sentic cycles is another psychophysiologic technique, devised by Manfred Clynes. A sentic "cycle" is composed of eight sentic states. A sentic "state" is a self-induced emotional experience, and the sequence of states used by Clynes is: no emotion, anger, hate, grief, love, sex, joy, reverence. A subject practices a cycle by thinking the state—for example, anger—and responding with finger pressure on a key (which transduces the pressure for

COMPARISON OF METHODS FOR

TECHNIQUE	PHYSIOLOGIC MEASUREMENT		
	Oxygen Consumption	Respiratory Rate	Heart Rate
Transcendental Meditation [39, 38]	Decreases [39, 37]	Decreases [1, 39]	Decreases [39, 37]
Zen and Yoga [25, 31]	Decreases [2, 36]	Decreases [3, 31, 36]	Decreases [3, 36]
Autogenic Training [28]	Not measured	Decreases [28]	Decreases [28]
Progressive Relaxation [26]	Not measured	Not measured	Not measured
Hypnosis with Suggested Deep Relaxation [5, 22, 4, 17]	Decreases [19]	Decreases [5]	Decreases [5]
Sentic Cycles [16]	Decreases [16]	Decreases [16]	Decreases [16]
Cotention [15]	Not measured	Decreases [35]	Not measured

recording) as he sits and listens to a tape recording. The recording states which sentic state is present and when the subject should press the key [16].

Burrow described two kinds of attention: *Cotention* and *ditention* [15, 35]. Cotention is the subject's "... focus on the object of its environment." It is concentration on one thing exclusively. Ditention is described as "ordinary" wakefulness, in which state the subject's interest shifts from object to object. The state of cotention is induced by relaxing the muscles, closing the eyes, and resting them on a point imagined to be the center of a curtain of darkness in front of the subject.

INDUCING THE RELAXATION RESPONSE

Alpha Waves	Blood Pressure	Muscle Tension	Skin Resistance
Increases [39, 37]	Decreases [13, 10, 12]	Not measured	Increases [39, 37]
Increases [25, 36]	No change [27, 36]	Not measured	Increases [3]
Increases [28]	Inconclusive results [28]	Decreases [28]	Increases [28]
Not measured	Inconclusive results	Decreases [26]	Not measured
Not measured	Inconclusive results [17]	Not measured	Increases [18, 20]
Not measured	Not measured	Not measured	Not measured
Present [34]	Not measured	Not measured	Not measured

Yoga has been an important part of Indian culture for thousands of years. It is claimed to be the culmination of the efforts of ancient Hindu thinkers to "give man the fullest possible control over his mind" [25]. Yoga consists of meditation practices and physical techniques usually performed in a quiet environment, and it has many variant forms. Yoga began as Raja Yoga, which sought "union with the absolute" by meditation. Later, there was an emphasis on physical methods in attempts to achieve an altered state of consciousness. This is termed Hatha Yoga. It has developed into a physical culture and is claimed to prevent and cure certain diseases. Essential to the practice of

Hatha Yoga are appropriate posture and control of respiration [33]. The most common posture is called Lotus (seated on the ground with legs crossed). This posture helps the spine stay erect without strain and is claimed to enhance concentration. The respiratory training promotes control of duration of inspiration and expiration, and the pause between breaths, so that one eventually achieves voluntary control of respiration. Bagchi and Wenger, in studies of Yoga practitioners, reported that Yoga could produce a 70 percent increase in skin resistance, decreased heart rate, and EEG alpha wave activity. These observations led them to suggest that Yoga is "deep relaxation of a certain aspect of the autonomic nervous system without drowsiness or sleep" [3].

Transcendental Meditation (TM) is currently a widely practiced form of Yoga. The technique, as taught by Maharishi Mahesh Yogi, comes from the Vedic tradition of India [30]. Instruction is given individually, and the technique is allegedly easily learned at the first instruction session. It is said to require no physical or mental control. The individual is taught a systematic method of repeating a word or sound, the mantra, without attempting to concentrate specifically on it. It involves little change in life style, other than the meditation period of 15 to 20 minutes twice a day when the practitioner sits in a comfortable position with closed eyes.

Zen is very like Yoga, from which it developed, and is associated with the Buddhist religion [31]. In Zen meditation, the subject is said to achieve a "controlled psychophysiologic decrease of the cerebral excitatory state" by a crossed-leg posture, closed eyes, regulation of respiration, and concentration on the Koan (an alogical problem—for example, What is the sound of one hand clapping?), or by prayer and chanting. Respiration is adjusted by taking several slow deep breaths, then inspiring briefly and forcelessly, and expiring long and forcefully, with subsequent natural breathing. Any sensory perceptions or mental images are allowed to appear and leave passively. A quiet, comfortable environment is essential. Experienced Zen meditators elicit the relaxation response more efficiently than novices [36].

The basic technique for the elicitation of the relaxation response is extremely simple. Its elements have been known and used for centuries in many cultures throughout the world. Historically, the relaxation response has usually been elicited in a religious context [7].

Four basic elements are common to all these practices: a quiet environment, a mental device, a passive attitude, and a comfortable position. A simple, mental, noncultic technique based on these four elements has recently been used in my laboratory. Subjects are given the following description of the four elements in the technique.

1. *A Quiet Environment.* One should choose a quiet, calm environment with as few distractions as possible. Sound, even background noise, may prevent the elicitation of the response. Choose a convenient, suitable place—for example, at an office desk in a quiet room.

2. *A Mental Device.* The meditator employs the constant stimulus of a single-syllable sound or word. The syllable is repeated silently or in a low, gentle tone. The purpose of the repetition is to free oneself from logical, externally oriented thought by focusing solely on the stimulus. Many different words and sounds have been used in traditional practices. Because of its simplicity and neutrality, the use of the syllable "one" is suggested.

3. *A Passive Attitude.* The purpose of the response is to help one rest and relax, and this requires a completely passive attitude. One should not scrutinize his performance or try to force the response, because this may well prevent the response from occurring. When distracting thoughts enter the mind, they should simply be disregarded

4. *A Comfortable Position.* The meditator should sit in a comfortable chair in as restful a position as possible. The purpose is to reduce muscular effort to a minimum. The head may be supported; the arms should be balanced or supported as well. The shoes may be removed and the feet propped up several inches, if desired. Loosen all tight-fitting clothing.

ELICITING THE RELAXATION RESPONSE

Using these four basic elements, one can evoke the response by following the simple, mental, noncultic procedure that subjects have used in my laboratory:

—In a quiet environment, sit in a comfortable position.

—Close your eyes.

—Deeply relax all your muscles, beginning at your feet and progressing up to your face—feet, calves, thighs, lower torso, chest, shoulders, neck, head. Allow them to remain deeply relaxed.

—Breathe through your nose. Become aware of your breathing. As you breathe out, say the word "one" silently to yourself. Thus: breathe in . . . breathe out, with "one." In . . . out, with "one" . . .

—Continue this practice for 20 minutes You may open your eyes to check the time, but do not use an alarm. When you finish, sit quietly for several minutes, at first with your eyes closed and later with your eyes open.

Remember not to worry about whether you are successful in achieving a deep level of relaxation—maintain a passive attitude and permit relaxation to occur at its own pace. When distracting thoughts occur, ignore them and continue to repeat "one" as you breathe. The technique should be practiced once or twice daily, and not within two hours after any meal, since the digestive processes seem to interfere with the elicitation of the expected changes.

With practice, the response should come with little effort. Investigations have shown that only a small percentage of people do not experience the expected physiologic changes [6, 39]. However, it has been noted that people who are undergoing psychoanalysis for at least two sessions a week experience difficulty in eliciting the response.

A person cannot be certain that the technique is eliciting these physiologic changes unless actual measurements are being made. However, the great majority of people report feelings of relaxation and freedom from anxiety during the elicitation of the relaxation response and during the rest of the day as well. These feelings of well-being are akin to those often noted after physical exercise, but without the attendant physical fatigue. The practice of this technique evokes some of the same physiologic changes noted during the practice of other techniques, such as those listed in the table. These physiologic changes are significant decreases in body metabolism—oxygen consumption and carbon dioxide elimination—and rate of breathing. Decreased oxygen consumption is the most sensitive index of the elicitation of the relaxation response [6].

Techniques that elicit the relaxation response should not be confused with biofeedback. Through biofeedback training, a subject can be made aware of an otherwise unconscious physiologic function, such as his heart rate, and learn to alter it voluntarily. He uses a device that measures the function—heart rate, for example—and "feeds back" to him information corresponding to each beat of his heart. He can then be rewarded (or reward himself) for increases or decreases in his heart rate and thus learn partial heart rate control. Other physiologic functions that have been shown partially controllable through biofeedback are blood pressure, skin temperature, muscle tension, and certain patterns of brain waves, such as alpha waves.

But, whereas biofeedback requires physiologic monitoring equipment and can usually be focused on only one physiologic function at a time, elicitation of the relaxation response requires no equipment and affects several physiologic functions simultaneously.

THERAPEUTIC POSSIBILITIES
FOR HYPERTENSION

I suggest that voluntary, regular elicitation of the relaxation response can counterbalance and alleviate the effects of the environmentally induced, but often inappropriate, fight-or-flight response.

For example, the regular elicitation of the relaxation response is useful in lowering the blood pressure of hypertensive subjects [10, 12]. Individuals attending an introductory transcendental meditation lecture were asked whether they would be willing to participate in a study of the effects of meditation on high blood pressure. Over 80 subjects with high blood pressure volunteered for the study. They agreed to postpone learning meditation for six weeks while their blood pressures were periodically measured and recorded to establish their premeditation blood pressures.

At the end of the six-week period, the subjects were trained to elicit the relaxation response through transcendental meditation. After at least two weeks of twice-daily meditation, the subjects' blood pressures were measured approximately every two weeks for at least nine weeks. Measurements were made at random times of the day but never during meditation. Throughout this entire period, the subjects were instructed to remain under the care of their physicians and to make only those changes in their medications that were prescribed by their physicians.

Of the original group, about 50 individuals altered the type or dosage of their antihypertensive medications during the course of the experiment. The data on these individuals were excluded from the study to avoid possible inaccurate interpretations caused by the altered regimens. There remained over 30 subjects who either did not alter their medications or took no antihypertensive medications. Comparisons were then made between these sub-blood pressures before and after learning meditation.

During the premeditation (control) period, the subjects' systolic blood pressures averaged 140 to 150 millimeters of mercury. (Systolic pressure is the measure of the highest component of blood pressure.) After nine weeks of regular elicitation of the relaxation response, this average dropped into the range of 130 to 140 millimeters. Their diastolic pressures (the lowest component of blood pressure) averaged 90 to 95 millimeters during the control period and dropped into the range of 85 to 90 millimeters by the ninth week of meditation. These decreases reflect a statistically significant change in blood pressure, from what is considered the borderline hypertensive range to the normal range of blood pressure [10, 12, 13].

An equally important result of the experiment was the change in blood pressure in the subjects who chose to stop meditation. Within four weeks both their systolic and their diastolic pressures had returned to their initial hypertensive levels.

Work remains to be done in this area, but these studies suggest that the regular elicitation of the relaxation response may be another means of lowering blood pressure. At the present time, standard medical therapy for hypertension involves the use of antihypertensive drugs. This pharmacologic method of lowering blood pressure is very effective, but it is sometimes accompanied by unpleasant side effects, and it is expensive. Indications are that the relaxation response affects the same mechanisms and lowers blood pressure by the same means as some antihypertensive drugs. Both act on the sympathetic nervous system.

Although it is unlikely that the regular elicitation of the relaxation response will be adequate therapy by itself for severe or moderate hypertension, it might act synergistically, along with antihypertensive drugs, to lower blood pressure, and may lead to the use of fewer drugs or decreased dosages. In borderline hypertension, the regular elicitation of the relaxation response may be of great value, since it has no pharmacologic side effects and might possibly supplant the use of drugs.

However, no matter how encouraging these initial results appear to be, no person should treat himself for high blood pressure by regularly eliciting the relaxation response. He should use the technique only under the supervision of his physician, who will routinely monitor his blood pressure to make sure it is adequately controlled.

OTHER THERAPEUTIC POSSIBILITIES

Individuals choose various means to alleviate their subjective feelings of stress, and heavy alcohol intake, drug abuse, and cigarette smoking are serious problems in our society. In a recent investigation, 1,862 individuals completed a questionnaire in which they reported a marked decrease in hard-liquor intake, drug abuse, and cigarette smoking after they had begun the elicitation of the relaxation response through the practice of transcendental meditation [14].

Details on decreased alcohol intake are as follows. Hard liquor was defined as any beverage of alcoholic content other than wine or beer, and its usage was divided into four categories:

1. Total nonusage of alcohol.
2. Light usage—up to three times per month.
3. Medium usage—one to six times per week.
4. Heavy usage—at least once per day.

Prior to the regular practice of meditation, 2.7 percent were heavy users of hard liquor. This percentage decreased to 0.4 percent after 21 months of the twice-daily practice of meditation. Medium users comprised 15.8 percent prior to meditation, after 21 months they were only 2.6 percent. Light usage of hard liquor decreased from 41.4 percent to 21.9 percent. Further, heavy and medium users tended to become light users or nonusers as they continued to meditate; and, whereas 40.1 percent were nonusers of alcohol prior to learning meditation, this percentage had increased to 75.1 percent after 21 or more months of meditation.

The questionnaire also surveyed the drug abuse patterns of the group—that is, the usage of marijuana, amphetamines, barbiturates, narcotics, LSD, and other hallucinogens. Following the start of the regular practice of meditation, there was a marked decrease in the number of drug abusers in all categories; and, as the practice was continued, there was a progressive decrease in drug abuse. After 21 months, most subjects were using no drugs at all.

For example, in the 6-month period before starting the practice of meditation, about 80 percent of this sample used marijuana, and of those about 28 percent were heavy users. After regularly eliciting the relaxation response for approximately 6 months, 37 percent used marijuana, and of those only 6 percent were heavy users. After 21 months of the practice, 12 percent continued to use marijuana, and of those almost all were light users; only one individual was a heavy user.

There was an even greater decrease in the abuse of LSD. Before starting the practice of meditation, 48 percent of the subjects had used LSD, and of these about 14 percent were heavy users (at least once per week). After 3 months of meditation, 12 percent of the subjects still took LSD, but after 21 months only 3 percent still took it.

For other drugs there were similar increases in numbers of nonusers after starting the practice of meditation. After 21 months, nonusers of the other hallucinogens rose from 61 percent to 96 percent; for the narcotics, from 83 percent to 99 percent; for the amphetamines, from 68 percent to 99 percent; and for the barbiturates, from 83 percent to 99 percent.

The smoking habits of the subjects also changed. Approximately 48 percent smoked cigarettes before starting meditation, and 27 percent of the sample were heavy users (at least one pack per day). After 21 months of meditation, only 16 percent still smoked cigarettes, and only 5.8 percent were heavy smokers.

This particular investigation was biased in several ways. The data were retrospective and subject to the limitation of personal recall. The group was not a random sample, nor was it chosen to be representative of the general population. Further there was no control population; there are no data concerning the patterns of alcohol intake, drug abuse, and cigarette smoking of a matched sample of nonmeditators. Only a prospective investigation can eliminate these biases. However, these data, as well as data from the other studies cited, suggested strongly that a beneficial effect may be derived from elicitation of the relaxation response.

I must emphasize again, however, that the relaxation response should not be viewed as a potential panacea for medical problems. An investigation of the response in the therapy of severe migraine and certain other kinds of headache, for example, has demonstrated the response to be of limited usefulness in these illnesses; it is recommended that this particular therapy be tried when other therapies of headache have proved unsuccessful [9]. Thus, the relaxation response should not be practiced for preventive or therapeutic medical benefits unless done so with the approval of a physician.

The side effects of the extensive practice of the relaxation response are worth brief discussion, although they have not been well documented.

When the response is elicited for two limited daily periods of 20 to 30 minutes, no adverse side effects have been observed. When the response is elicited more frequently—for example, for many hours daily over a period of several days—some individuals have experienced a withdrawal from life and have developed symptoms which range from insomnia to hallucinatory behavior. These side effects of the excessive elicitation of the relaxation response are difficult to evaluate on a retrospective basis, since many people with preexisting psychiatric problems might be drawn to any technique which evangelistically promises relief from tension and stress.

However, it is unlikely that the twice-daily elicitation of the response would do any more harm than would regular prayer.

As noted above, well over 50 percent of our present U.S. population will die of heart disease and related conditions, and these diseases appear to be attacking Americans at younger and younger ages. The frequent elicitation of the fight-or-flight response has been strongly implicated in the development of these diseases. The regular use of the relaxation response in our daily lives may counteract the harmful effects of the fight-or-flight response and thereby mitigate these extremely prevalent and dire diseases.

For centuries, people have used various techniques to elicit the relaxation response, but it is only now that we are recognizing its potential physiologic benefits. However, modern Western society has turned away from many of the traditional techniques that elicit the relaxation response, such as prayer. Our society has thus lost an important means of alleviating stress and maintaining equilibrium in a changing world. We can probably greatly bene-fit by the reintroduction of the relaxation response into our society.

BIBLIOGRAPHY

1. Allison, John. "Respiration Changes During Transcendental Meditation." *Lancet* 1 (1970):833–34.
2. Anand, B. K., et al. "Studies on Shri Ramananda Yogi During His Stay in an Air-tight Box." *Indian Journal of Medical Research* 49 (1961):82–89.
3. Bagchi, B. K., and Wenger, M. A. "Electrophysiological Correlations of Some Yoga Exercises." *Electroencephalography and Clinical Neurophysiology* 7, Supplement (1957):132–49.
4. Barber, Theodore X. "Physiological Effects of Hypnosis." *Psychology Bulletin* 58 (1961):390–419.
5. ———. "Physiological Effects of Hypnosis and Suggestions." In *Biofeedback and Self-Control 1970.* Chicago: Aldine-Atherton, 1971.
6. Beary, John F., and Benson, Herbert. "A Simple Psychophysiologic Technique Which Elicits the Hypometabolic Changes of the Relaxation Response." *Psychosomatic Medicine* 36 (1974):115–20.
7. Benson, Herbert; Beary, John F.; and Carol, Mark P. "The Relaxation Response." *Psychiatry* 37 (1974):37–46.

8. Benson, Herbert; Greenwood, Martha M.; and Klemchuk, Helen. "The Relaxation Response: Psychophysiological Aspects and Clinical Applications." *Psychiatry in Medicine* 6, no. 1 (1975).

9. Benson, Herbert; Klemchuk, Helen M.; and Graham, John R. "The Usefulness of the Relaxation Response in the Therapy of Headache," *Headache* 14 (1974):49–52.

10. Benson, Herbert; Marzetta, Barbara R.; and Rosner, Bernard A. "Decreased Blood Pressure Associated with the Regular Elicitation of the Relaxation Response: A Study of Hypertensive Subjects." In *Stress and the Heart,* edited by R. S. Eliot. Contemporary Problems in Cardiology, vol. 1. Mt. Kisco, N.Y.: Futura, 1974.

11. Benson, Herbert; Rosner, Bernard A.; and Marzetta, Barbara R. "Decreased Systolic Blood Pressure in Hypertensive Subjects Who Practiced Meditation," *Journal of Clinical Investigation* 52 (1973): 8a.

12. Benson, Herbert; Rosner, Bernard A., Marzetta, Barbara R.; and Klemchuk, Helen. "Decreased Blood Pressure in Pharmacologically Treated Hypertensive Patients Who Regularly Elicited the Relaxation Response," *The Lancet* 1 (1974):289–91.

13. ————. "Decreased Blood Pressure in Borderline Hypertensive Subjects Who Practiced Meditation," *Journal of Chronic Disease,* in press.

14. Benson, Herbert, and Wallace, Robert K. "Decreased Drug Abuse with Transcendental Meditation—A Study of 1,862 Subjects." In C. J. D. Zarafonetis ed., *Drug Abuse—Proceedings of the International Conference;* Lea and Febiger, 1972.

15. Burrow, Trigant. "Kymograph Studies of Physiological (Respiratory) Concomitants in Two Types of Attentional Adaptation." *Nature* 142 (1938):156.

16. Clynes, Manfred. "Toward a View of Man." In M. Clynes and J. Milsum, eds., *Biomedical Engineering Systems.* New York: McGraw-Hill, 1970.

17. Crasilneck, Harold B., and Hall, James A. "Physiological Changes Associated with Hypnosis: A Review of the Literature Since 1948." *International Journal of Clinical and Experimental Hypnosis* 7 (1959):9–50.

18. Davis, R. C., and Kantor, J. R. "Skin Resistance During Hypnotic States." *Journal of General Psychology* 13 (1935):62–81.

19. Dudley, Donald L., et al. "Changes in Respiration Associated with Hypnotically Induced Emotion, Pain, and Exercise." *Psychosomatic Medicine* 26 (1963):46–57.

20. Estabrooks, G. H. "The Psychogalvanic Reflex in Hypnosis." *Journal of General Psychology* 3 (1930):150–57.
21. Gellhorn, Ernst. *Principles of Autonomic-Somatic Interactions.* Minneapolis: University of Minnesota Press, 1967.
22. Gorton, Bernard E. "Physiology of Hypnosis." *Psychiatric Quarterly* 23 (1949):317–43 and 457–85.
23. Gutmann, Mary C., and Benson, Herbert. "Interaction of Environmental Factors and Systemic Arterial Blood Pressure: A Review." *Medicine* 50 (1971):543–53.
24. Hess, Walter R. *Functional Organization of the Diencephalon.* New York: Grune & Stratton, 1957.
25. Hoenig, J. "Medical Research on Yoga." *Confinia Psychiatrica* 11 (1968):69–89.
26. Jacobson, Edmund. *Progressive Relaxation.* Chicago: University of Chicago Press, 1938.
27. Karambelkar, P. V., et al. "Studies on Human Subjects Staying in an Air-tight Pit," *Indian Journal of Medical Res.* 56 (1968): 1282–88.
28. Luthe, Wolfgang, ed. *Autogenic Therapy,* vols. 1–5. New York: Grune & Stratton, 1969.
29. Luthe, Wolfgang. "Autogenic Therapy: Excerpts on Applications to Cardiovascular Disorders and Hypercholesterolemia." In *Biofeedback and Self-Control 1971.* Chicago: Aldine-Atherton, 1972.
30. Maharishi Mahesh Yogi. *The Science of Being and Art of Living.* London: International SRM Publications, 1966.
31. Onda, A. "Autogenic Training and Zen." In W. Luthe, ed. *Autogenic Training.* New York: Grune & Stratton, 1965.
32. Ostfeld, Adrian M., and Shekelle, Richard B. "Psychological Variables and Blood Pressure." In *The Epidemiology of Hypertension,* J. Stamler, R. Stamler, and T. N. Pullman, eds. New York: Grune & Stratton, 1967.
33. Ramamurthi, B. "Yoga: An Explanation and Probable Neurophysiology." *Journal of the Medical Association* 48 (1967):167–70.
34. Segal, Julius, ed. *Mental Health Program Reports—5.* Washington, D.C.: National Institute of Mental Health, 1971.
35. Shiomi, K. "Respiratory and EEG Changes by Cotention of Trigant Burrow." *Psychologia* 12 (1969):24–28.
36. Sugi, Yasusaburo, and Akutsu, Kunio. "Studies on Respiration and Energy-Metabolism During Sitting in Zazen." *Research Journal of Physical Education* 12 (1968): 190–206.
37. Wallace, Robert K. "Physiological Effects of Transcendental Meditation." *Science* 167 (1970):1751–54.

38. Wallace, Robert K., and Benson, Herbert. "The Physiology of Meditation." *Scientific American* 226 (1972):85–90.
39. Wallace, Robert K.; Benson, Herbert; and Wilson, Archie F. "A Wakeful Hypometabolic State." *American Journal of Physiology* 221 (1971):795–99.
40. Weitzenhoffer, Andre M., and Hilgard, E. *Stanford Hypnotic Suggestibility Scale*. Palo Alto: Consulting Psychologists Press, 1959.
41. Whitehorn, J. C., et al. "The Metabolic Rate in Hypnotic Sleep." *New England Journal of Medicine* 206 (1932):777–81.

By Gary E. Schwartz

Biofeedback and the Treatment of Disregulation Disorders

In one way or another, almost everything man does involves corrective information or feedback, both external and internal [1]. The concept of feedback in its simplest form is so obvious that it is often overlooked by health professionals and laymen alike. Everyone knows that it is essential to have external visual feedback and internal kinesthetic and proprioceptive feedback to learn to tie a knot or to serve a tennis ball. Placed in a more neurophysiological perspective, it becomes clear that the brain requires feedback of what it is doing and of its surroundings in order to appropriately regulate itself and its body [2].

The recent product of 20th-century biomedical technology, biofeedback is a special form of information. With the aid of modern electronics it is now possible to accurately monitor a variety of internal physiological processes and to convert these signals into novel forms of visual or auditory information that can be consciously perceived and processed by the brain, and consequently self-regulated by the brain. From an evolutionary perspective this is a unique event in human history, for man has provided the brain with a dynamic form of bioinformation not part of its original biological structure [3].

This capacity for new perception and regulation of the brain and body has stimulated extensive research on the voluntary control of neural, visceral and skeletal responses [4], and the application of biofeedback to the behavioral treatment of psychophysiological disorders [5]. Although I emphasize a neurophysiological interpretation of biofeedback and its application to the treatment of functional [6] or disregulation [2] disorders, this approach is recent in origin and does not reflect the historical development of biofeedback [7].

Much of the early research was derived from learning theory, emphasizing the application of instrumental [8] or operant [9] conditioning procedures. As noted by a number of authors [10–12], investigators taking a feedback approach emphasize the role of information in self-regulation, whereas researchers taking a learning approach tend to emphasize incentives or motivation in the development and maintenance of self-control. As we will see, information and incentives are *both* important to the clinical application of biofeedback procedures, and their integration is emphasized in current neurophysiological theory.

Yogis and meditators have long claimed unusual powers of voluntary control over physiology and consciousness, but until recently these claims were dismissed by the scientific community. The theories or paradigms of the researchers could not explain such claims, and therefore they were dismissed as being inaccurate or fraudulent [13]. Not only did paradigms in medicine disallow the voluntary control of visceral and glandular responses, but so did the prevailing conditioning paradigms in psychology. However, with the development of biofeedback, coupled with advances in neurophysiology, new paradigms have evolved which seek to explain and extend these observations. In the process, this information is revising our conceptualization of health and disease, and therefore the means by which we treat disease.

Unfortunately, the fervor for biofeedback was so strong that it has become almost fanatical. The popular press has at times been filled with uncritical enthusiasm for any speculated application of biofeedback techniques. The electronics industry has taken advantage of this interest and has exploited biofeedback in both the medical and lay markets. At one extreme there are those today who argue that biofeedback can enable us to control any aspect of our biology at will; at the other extreme, a growing number dismiss biofeedback as a useless gimmick. It is this writer's opinion that neither of these extremes is appropriate, and that current research on biofeedback from a neurophysiological perspective not only expands our understanding of human self-regulation and its applications to medicine, but helps us recognize its limitations [14].

In order to more fully appreciate the potential and limitations of biofeedback for the treatment of psychosomatic disorders, it is essential to view biofeedback within a broader psychobiological perspective. Towards this end a brief introduction to psychosomatic disorders from the perspective of feedback and disregulation is presented. The relevance of this model to the development of more holistic approaches in medicine becomes clear when we consider how the traditional medical model is inadvertently perpetuating physiological disregulation by ignoring the role of negative feedback in homeostasis [2].

DISREGULATION: A NEUROPHYSIOLOGICAL MODEL OF PSYCHOSOMATIC DISORDERS

The concept of feedback is central to our understanding of health and disease. As originally posited by the French physiologist Claude Bernard in the last century, and elaborated by Walter Cannon in his classic volume, *The Wisdom of the Body* [15], there is a biological necessity to maintain physiological variables within adaptive limits for the purpose of survival. This is accomplished by homeostasis, a process requiring an intact nervous system. Homeostasis, therefore, is an *internal* negative ✓ feedback mechanism, devoted to the maintenance of the internal organs. It is negative in the sense that the feedback acts to dampen overresponding in a corrective and stabilizing manner.

However, what happens if the protective negative feedback circuit or loop is altered or made ineffective? It follows logically that normal self-regulation will not occur, and the system will become unstable. I have called this instability disregulation [2] and it is similar to Miller and Dworkin's [16] concept of anti-homeostasis.

The basic model is as follows: when the environment places demands on a person, the brain performs the necessary regulations to meet the specific demands. Depending upon the nature of these stresses, certain bodily systems will be activated, while others may simultaneously be inhibited. However, if this process is sustained to the point where the organ becomes damaged, the negative feedback loop of the homeostatic mechanism will normally be accentuated, forcing the brain to change its course of action. Often this negative feedback loop results in the experience of pain.

For example, if a person is very active and eating on the run, the stomach may fail to function properly. Consequently, the stomach may generate sufficient negative feedback to the brain, which is experienced as a stomachache. This corrective signal should serve the important function of causing the brain to change its regulation in specific ways, such as leading the person to slow down and to allow digestion to occur more normally. The pain serves a second function in that it "teaches" the brain what it can and cannot do if the stomach is to work properly. The adaptive brain is one that can learn through its mistakes, and learn to anticipate the needs of its organs for the sake of their health.

However, the brain may fail to regulate itself effectively to meet the stomach's needs. The reasons for this can be quite varied. There are four major stages where disregulation can occur [2].

Stage 1: Environmental Demands. The stimuli from the external environment may be so demanding that the brain (stage 2) is *forced* to *ignore* the negative feedback (stage 4) generated by the stomach (stage 3). This is the classic case of the person placed in unavoidable stress who must continue to act in certain ways despite negative feedback to the contrary. Many previous theories of psychosomatic disorders have emphasized this factor.

Stage 2: CNS Information Processing. The brain may be so programmed, initially through genetics and/or subsequently modified through learning, to respond inappropriately to the stimuli in the external environment. This is what we typically refer to as personality or life style. Thus, although feedback from the abused organ may be present, the person's brain may fail to react to it appropriately.

Stage 3: Peripheral Organ. The organ in question may itself be hyper- or hypo-reactive to the neural or hormonal stimulation

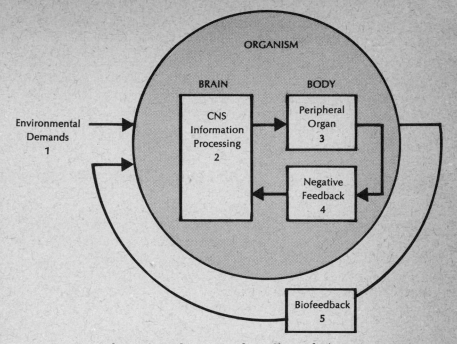

*Schematic of the stages where disregulation
can be produced*

This shows environmental demands (external, stage 1), entering via sensory inputs (not shown) the CNS information processing system (the brain, stage 2), which regulates a particular organ in the body (only one shown, stage 3), and is provided with information about the state of the organ via negative feedback (stage 4). Biofeedback (stage 5) represents an external feedback loop which augments the internal homeostatic mechanisms.

coming from the brain. This is the literal translation of what has sometimes been called the "weak organ" theory of psychosomatic disorders. It can explain why, in response to the same environmental stress, people differ in the organ that ultimately becomes dysfunctional. From this perspective, it is possible that the brain cannot regulate itself to compensate for the altered feedback it is receiving from the given organ, or in the case of a diseased organ, finds itself no longer capable of modifying the functioning of the organ.

Stage 4: Negative Feedback. Finally, the negative feedback derived from the organ in question may itself be inappropriate. In other words, it is possible for the protective negative feedback system to become less effective and, in extreme cases, be inactivated. An extreme example of this condition can be seen in persons born without the normal pain response system [17]. These individuals are constantly in danger of severely injuring themselves, for they lack the protective mechanism for detecting and coping with injury.

Although the etiology of disregulation can occur at any of these four stages, the general consequence of disregulation is the same in each case. By not responding appropriately to the negative feedback (stage 4) the brain (stage 2) fails to maintain stable regulation of the organ in question (stage 3) and disregulation (with its accompanying instability) emerges.

It is important to recognize that not only can disregulation occur at each of the four stages in the system, but also it is possible for problems to occur simultaneously at multiple stages. In the extreme case, if a person was (1) exposed to demanding stimulation in his environment, requiring continued adaptation (stage 1), *and* (2) his brain processed the sensory information and reacted inappropriately due to genetic and/or learning factors (stage 2), *and* (3) the peripheral organ itself reacted inappropriately due to genetic and/or maturational factors (stage 3), *and* (4) the feedback mechanism derived from this organ was also ineffective (stage 4), this *pattern* would combine so as to increase the likelihood that the person would develop a specific psychosomatic disorder. Since the brain and body are composed of multiple systems that must be coordinated in an integrated fashion, it becomes necessary to examine *each* of the components and then consider how they *combine* so as to produce the final outcome or disease.

This holistic perspective to psychosomatic disorders illustrates how the functioning of a *system as a whole* requires the adaptive coordination of all of its components in responding to a variety of environmental demands. By emphasizing the concept of feedback, the disregulation model provides a framework for understanding how biofeedback is viewed as the addition of a new corrective feedback loop (stage 5) to augment those inherent in man's natural biological structure (2). By taking a neurophysiological, multi-process perspective, the disregulation model also helps to delineate under what conditions biofeedback will be ineffective as a clinical tool. But before considering biofeedback's role in the treatment of disregulation, it is instructive to consider how the traditional medical model approaches these disorders.

MEDICINE AND THE
PERPETUATION OF DISREGULATION

One novel, and somewhat disturbing, implication of the disregulation model is that due to incomplete diagnosis and treatment of functional disorders, the traditional medical model inadvertently leads to the enhancement of disregulation, not only of bodily disease but of human behavior as well [2].

As we have seen, disregulation can be initiated and perpetuated at four stages. Often, the disregulation is initiated by stimulus demands from the outside environment (stage 1), coupled with the brain's reaction to them (stage 2). If the brain is exposed to (or exposes itself to) environmental conditions which ultimately cause an organ system (stage 3) to break down and develop a functional disorder, the appropriate internal negative feedback loops are activated (stage 4). This negative feedback serves a vital function, since it directs the brain (stage 2) to take corrective action if the organ is to survive. Even if the brain is busy attending to other stimuli in the outside environment, and thus fails to recognize the breakdown of a given organ, at some point the organ (if its negative feedback loop is intact) will generate sufficient negative feedback to redirect the brain's attention. The reader who has experienced a strong stomachache caused by overeating, eating under the wrong circumstances, or eating the wrong food, knows the power that negative feedback can have in commanding our attention and our subsequent behavior.

What *should* the brain's response be to this internal stimulation? From a neurophysiological perspective, it becomes clear that the brain should either change the external environmental demands (stage 1) or its behavior (stage 2) to maintain the health of the organ (stage 3). Consequently, the intrinsic pain of the disturbed stomach (stage 4) can help to keep our behavior in check by forcing us to stop eating, or to stop running while we are eating, or to not eat the dangerous food again.

However, for many sociological reasons, man is not content to follow his initial biological heritage. He either feels no longer competent to change his environment or behavior, or simply does not want to. However, due to his highly developed brain and the resulting development of culture, he is no longer constrained to deal with the negative feedback by responding to organ dysfunction in terms of the body's normal structure. Instead, the typical patient would rather change his body structure (stages 3 or 4) than change his life style (stage 2) or his environment (stage 1), the two factors which together augment or cause the bodily dysfunction in the first place. Simply stated, man may choose instead of modify stage 3 and/or 4 by *extrinsic biological intervention*. As would be predicted from the disregulation model, by artificially removing the negative feedback mechanisms, the brain is freed to continue behaving in *maladaptive* ways that could ultimately be deleterious to its survival. Lacking the stabilizing impact of the negative feedback regulation, the brain (and therefore its expression as behavior) thus goes more and more out of control [2].

Consider again the basic stomachache. At no time in human history has human culture so reinforced the practice of taking drugs to eliminate stomachaches caused by the brain's disregulation. The antacid commercials of the 1970s exemplify this value system. We see an obese man stuffing himself with apple pies or spaghetti. When he gets a functional stomachache, the conclusion is not "The stomach and the rest of the body was not meant to eat like that—your stomachache represents the necessary biological feedback mechanism that will help keep you from further abusing your body." Instead, what we hear is "Eat, eat—and if you get a stomachache, don't change your external environment or behavior—rather, eliminate the internal discomfort artificially by taking a pill instead." Or we see a family shopping at Christmas time, surrounded by crowds, struggling to hold the packages, rushing from counter to counter, continually inhibiting aggression caused by being bumped or offended in other ways. And in the process, one of the members of the family gets a stomachache. The conclusion to this scenario based on the disregulation model, "The stomach and the rest of the body was not meant to live like that—your stomachache represents the necessary biological feedback mechanism that will help you from further abusing your body," is not the message of the commercial. Rather, what we are told is "Shop, shop—and if you get a stomachache, don't change your external environment or behavior—rather, eliminate the discomfort artificially by taking a pill instead."

Simple antacids are mild drugs, and do not always work. When this happens, medicine comes to the rescue with stronger medication to quell the pain. When the organ becomes sufficiently abused so that an ulcer develops and internal bleeding occurs, does the person then listen to his stomach and radically change his external environment and behavior? Often not, what he does instead is to go to his surgeon and have the stomach repaired. Medicine, by dint of its continued ingenuity, is developing new and finer means of bypassing these normal adaptive feedback mechanisms. Thus, in extreme cases a patient can have a vagotomy, thereby eliminating the brain's capability to regulate the stomach directly. And if the trend in modern medicine continues, man in the future can look forward to the day when he can simply go to his local surgeon and be fitted with a new, artificial stomach.

Now we have a brain that is no longer constrained by the needs of its natural stomach. Consequently, according to the disregulation model, this brain is free to continue and even expand upon the inappropriate disregulation that was the initial cause of the problem. The stomach is only one organ, however, whereas modern medicine is using the same strategy for many of the systems of the body. Our culture is continually reinforcing the idea that if the brain and its body cannot cope with its external environment, then the body and brain will simply have to alter itself medically to adjust to the increasing maladaptive demands of the environment. According to the disregulation model, this prospect carried to its extreme would have serious consequences for the structure and survival of the human species as we now know it.

The reader should not be left with the conclusion that I am

against all medical intervention: On the contrary, a disregulation analysis helps delineate under what select conditions it is adaptive, not only in the short run but more importantly in the long run, for pharmacological and surgical intervention to be used. My point instead is that we should not come to the over-simplistic conclusion that the correction of stages 3 and 4 of disregulation using external medical intervention should be the *sole* approach to treatment. Rather, it may be necessary for us to accept and respect the wisdom and limitations of the body as it was originally designed [15] even though this may require more active self-regulation on the part of the brain to keep the health and behavior of the human organism intact. Biofeedback could play a role in helping to reinforce this conclusion by providing additional external feedback (stage 5 in Figure 1) to augment the inherent homeostatic mechanisms.

BIOFEEDBACK AND PHYSIOLOGICAL SELF-REGULATION: BASIC RESEARCH

There are now hundreds of studies demonstrating increased physiological control with feedback and reward. The list of responses brought under self-control includes systolic and diastolic blood pressure, heart rate, blood flow, sweat gland activity, skin temperature, body temperature, respiratory functions, genital responses, stomach motility, fine skeletal muscle control (including single motor units) and various changes in the electrical activity of the brain. Many of these studies are reprinted in a set of *Biofeedback and Self-Control* volumes [18–23] and are critically evaluated elsewhere [4].

A useful example of basic biofeedback research concerns blood pressure self-regulation in normotensive subjects. It is now well established that normal subjects can learn to regulate their systolic and diastolic blood pressure depending upon the nature of the feedback and instructions used. If subjects are given simple binary (yes-no) feedback for relative increases or decreases in systolic pressure at each beat of the heart, and are given minimal instructions about what they are to do (they are not told what specific response they are to control, nor are they told in what direction their physiology is to change), subjects learn in 25 one-minute trials to increase or decrease voluntarily their systolic pressure without producing similar changes in heart rate [24, 25]. Conversely, if the feedback is provided for increases or decreases in heart rate, and minimal instructions are again used, subjects rapidly learn to increase or decrease their heart rate without similarly changing their systolic pressure [26]. These data illustrate how biofeedback procedures can enable subjects to learn to control *specific* responses associated with the feedback. In more neurophysiological terms, if the brain is required to process the external feedback without any "preconceived notions," it readily learns to regulate those specific neural processes required to activate the periphery and thereby control the feedback.

Subjects can learn to regulate two or more responses simultaneously if feedback and reward is given for the desired *pattern* of responses. For example, if subjects are given feedback only when their systolic blood pressure and heart rate simultaneously increase ($BP^{up}HR^{up}$) or simultaneously decrease (BP_{down} HR_{down}), subjects now learn to regulate both responses [27]. Interestingly, teaching subjects to control patterns of responses uncovers biological linkages and constraints between systems not readily observed when controlling the individual functions alone [3, 11, 14]. For example, when subjects are taught to lower both their systolic pressure and heart rate simultaneously, they tend to show more rapid learning, produce somewhat larger changes, and experience more of the subjective concomitants of relaxation than when they are given feedback for either function alone [27]. When subjects are given pattern biofeedback for making these responses go in opposite directions ($BP^{up}HR_{down}$ or BP_{down} HR^{up}), regulation of the two responses is attenuated. These observations are important because they highlight the concept of physiological *patterning* in both basic research and clinical treatment [3, 11, 14] and emphasize natural physiological constraints that must limit the degree of neural control possible.

In all of the above-mentioned studies, subjects were given minimal instructions about the task. When subjects are specifically instructed to control their heart rate or blood pressure, however, the subject may demonstrate physiological control even in the absence of any feedback [28, 29]. However, it is a mistake to conclude that instructional control is identical to regulation gained through biofeedback. Whereas single system biofeedback leads to learned specificity, instructions often lead to more complex patterns of responses. Hence, the verbal instruction to control blood pressure leads to control of heart rate as well, whereas single system biofeedback for blood pressure with minimal instructions can lead to blood pressure control in the absence of heart rate control. It follows that the precise nature of the biofeedback *and* the specific instructions used *both* contribute to the final *pattern* of responses that the subject will learn to regulate. It should not be surprising for us to recognize that instructions differentially influence physiology, since the average adult brain can draw on a variety of neural strategies in its conscious repertoire to control the feedback, and depending upon the specific nature of the instructions, the strategies will vary.

This issue is of more than just academic importance. For example, in certain cases of hypertension the goal may be to lower peripheral resistance in the absence of heart rate changes, whereas for the treatment of angina pectoris the goal may be to lower the pattern of blood pressure and heart rate since the product of these two functions leads to reduced work of the heart and consequently reduced pain [30]. At the present time, however, we can only speculate as to what kinds of biofeedback procedures and instructions are best combined to produce these two different cardiovascular results, for there are as yet no controlled clinical studies on this issue.

CLINICAL APPLICATIONS OF BIOFEEDBACK: A CRITICAL OVERVIEW

At the present time there are over 50 published papers on clinical applications of biofeedback techniques. Most of these papers are based on collections of case studies, and it is difficult to interpret them. Several critical reviews have been written which cover a wide variety of clinical applications [5, 12, 16, 31, 32], including tension headache, asthma, bruxism, muscular rehabilitation, epilepsy, hypertension, cardiac arrhythmias, Raynaud's disease (a vasospastic disorder affecting the extremities), migraine, sexual responses, pain, and anxiety. Many of these reports represent only pilot studies, and while suggestive, all require carefully controlled clinical trials to evaluate them.

The clearest evidence for the efficacy of biofeedback therapy grows out of research on the regulation of skeletal muscle activity. This should not be surprising, since of all the bodily systems the skeletal muscles are under the most voluntary control, and feedback of their activity (both external and internal) is most extensive and available to the conscious brain. A clinical example is tension headaches, where the major symptom (pain) is often due to excessive and prolonged tension of the muscles in the forehead and neck. Budzynski and Stoyva et al. have demonstrated that biofeedback for changes in frontalis muscle activity can enhance a patient's ability to voluntarily decrease forehead tension, which in turn leads to reduced pain. In one experiment, they found that clinical improvement was significantly greater in the frontalis biofeedback treatment group compared to two control groups, one given false biofeedback, the other given no treatment at all [33].

There is little question that biofeedback can enhance the self-regulation of muscle activity. In fact, it has been demonstrated that subjects can gain control of individual motor units within a single muscle when provided with the appropriate biofeedback, even though these changes are well below the level of normal awareness [34]. However, Budzynski and Stoyva et al. are careful to point out that gaining control over frontalis tension with biofeedback in the laboratory is but a prerequisite for clinical improvement. Patients must also practice self-regulation in real-life situations outside of the laboratory in order for the biofeedback training to have any long-term clinical value. This observation is understandable within the disregulation model, since there is no reason to expect that enhancing self-regulation via the addition of external feedback will in and of itself compensate for headache disregulation, especially if the etiology and maintenance of the disorder involves excessive environmental stresses (stage 1) or maladaptive life styles (stage 2). Budzynski and Stoyva et al. are careful to tell their patients that they should use the enhanced awareness of muscle tension in their daily life as a signal for them to change their environment and/or their life style (including coping style) in order to maintain low tension levels. If they do not, disregulation will continue and their headaches will likely return.

There are numerous other applications of muscle tension biofeedback under investigation, including applications to various neuromuscular disorders such as hemiplegia due to stroke; reversible physiological blocks due to edema; and Bell's palsy [see 32]. The extent of muscle retraining depends in large measure on the precise nature of the etiology, including the extent of central (stage 2) and peripheral (stages 3 and 4) damage. It is likely that such work will continue to progress, and that feedback techniques may become a standard adjunctive treatment in physical rehabilitation.

There are other more general muscle biofeedback applications of relevance to psychosomatic medicine and psychiatry. Whatmore and Kohli [6] claim that the training of whole body muscle relaxation can be used as a treatment for such skeletal, autonomic, and affective disorders as functional backache and neck pain, hyperventilation syndrome, hypertension, ulcers, anxiety and depression. Like Jacobson [35] before them, they argue that chronic muscle tension in various parts of the body play an important role in the development and maintenance of disregulation disorders, and through muscle biofeedback these functional disorders can be eliminated. Their neurophysiological model of "dysponesis," including case studies involving prolonged muscle retraining collected over a 20-year period, is described in *The Physiopathology and Treatment of Functional Disorders* [6]. While this approach is promising, particularly in their consideration of possible neurophysiological mechanisms and emphasis on multi-process treatment programs, it must be recognized that their conclusions are based entirely on uncontrolled case reports. Carefully designed outcome studies have yet to be carried out demonstrating that the use of biofeedback training in the regulation of muscle tension has a central role in the treatment of these disorders.

A second major area of biofeedback therapy involves feedback for electroencephalographic (EEG) activity of the brain. The most well documented studies are those by Sterman and colleagues [36] in which biofeedback training for EEG activity recorded from the scalp over the sensory/motor cortex is used to reduce specific epileptic seizures. Sterman claims that one particular sensory/motor rhythm (SMR) between 12 and 14 hertz must be regulated by the patient in order for reduction of seizures to occur. However, this conclusion may be premature, since other rhythms in this same region such as sensory/motor alpha (8–13 hertz) may reflect similar brain processes. In any event, Sterman claims that when selected patients learn to exhibit sensory motor processes, reductions in seizures can occur. What is not known is whether training in general muscle relaxation (which by definition involves regulation of the sensory motor cortex) is sufficient for obtaining clinical improvement.

Like biofeedback for peripheral skeletal motor responses, it should not be surprising to learn that biofeedback for various EEG changes results in rapid self-control. This is because surface EEG typically reflects complex neural processes underlying normal voluntary control by the brain of its sensory, attentional, cognitive and skeletal processes [2]. However, the claim that training for EEG alpha (without regard for cerebral localization) will lead to general relaxation and altered states of consciousness [37] is now recognized as being simplistic [3, 14]. Furthermore, altered states of awareness can so readily be achieved through simple cognitive, attentional and somatic exercises already under a person's voluntary control [for example, 38, 39] that biofeedback for EEG may be irrelevant to this goal.

Stoyva and Budzynski [40] point out, however, that for certain patients, for example, those with insomnia, a multi-stage training procedure may be needed for inducing low arousal, drowsiness, and sleep: (1) training in forearm muscle relaxation (which is quite easy), followed by (2) training in frontalis muscle relaxation (which is more difficult), followed by (3) training in EEG theta (4–7 hertz) activity (which is quite difficult). What becomes clear is that blanket statements for or against the use of biofeedback techniques are premature and likely incorrect.

The last class of biofeedback applications involves feedback for visceral and glandular responses regulated by the autonomic nervous system. One major area of application under investigation involves the treatment of migraine headache. In an uncontrolled clinical trial Sargent and colleagues [41] have claimed that training migraine patients to simultaneously increase warmth in the fingers and decrease warmth in their forehead region using pattern temperature biofeedback leads to the reduction of migraine headaches. They combined biofeedback with instructions to imagine that one's hands were heavy and warm, based on a cognitive self-regulation therapy called autogenic training [42]. The rationale for using "autogenic-feedback" training was suggested to them by the experience of a research subject who, during the spontaneous recovery from a migraine attack, demonstrated considerable flushing in her hands with an accompanying 10° F rise in two minutes. In subsequent work with 19 patients with migraine headache, Sargent et al. reported improvement in 63 percent.

Despite these encouraging findings, it is not known whether these same results could have been obtained with autogenic phrases alone, or if comparable results might have been observed through spontaneous remission and/or a "placebo" effect. Again, the issue is not simply whether biofeedback can be used to regulate temperature. As recently reviewed by Taub [43], highly localized control of skin temperature can be trained with temperature biofeedback. What is not clear is whether temperature biofeedback training is necessary and/or sufficient for the treatment of migraine. Nor is it known whether biofeedback for other parameters such as blood flow in the inflicted area will be more beneficial. In this regard biofeedback for temperature and blood flow are currently considered as a potential adjunctive treatment for Raynaud's disease. Successful cases have been described [43–45], but the interpretation of these cases is unclear.

Biofeedback for disorders of cardiac rhythms such as tachycardias and preventricular contractions (PVCs) has been investigated by Engel and Bleecker [46]. There is little question that certain patients can reduce the frequency of PVCs by regulating heart rate. Interestingly, for some patients this is accomplished by decreasing sympathetic tone, in other cases it is achieved by decreasing parasympathetic tone. It appears that depending upon the specific etiology of the arrhythmia, different components of the neural innervation must be self-regulated to achieve clinical improvement.

A major application of autonomic biofeedback involves feedback for blood pressure in the regulation of essential hypertension. Based on our blood pressure findings obtained in normotensive subjects [24–27], we studied 7 patients with essential hypertension [47]. After between 5 and 16 control sessions, patients were given daily biofeedback sessions for lowering systolic pressure. Large decreases in pressure were obtained in 5 of the patients, ranging from 16 to 34 mm Hg after 12 to 34 training sessions. Using a more sophisticated subject design in which patients were taught to both decrease and increase pressure with systolic blood pressure biofeedback, Kristt and Engel [48] have replicated and extended these findings. In their study, daily blood pressure readings were obtained outside of the laboratory with a 3-month follow up. These data suggest that blood pressure biofeedback can be used to help hypertensive patients regulate their pressure. However, it is not known whether blood pressure biofeedback is either necessary or sufficient for achieving clinical improvement. For example, Jacobson [35] reported that large blood pressure decreases could be obtained through general muscle relaxation, and Whatmore and Kohli [6] have extended this observation using biofeedback for muscle tension.

The utility of biofeedback in visceral self-regulation appears to be especially well documented in the training of rectosphincteric responses for the treatment of fecal incontinence. Engel and colleagues [49] used pattern biofeedback for training external sphincter contraction in synchrony with internal-sphincter relaxation in six patients with severe fecal incontinence. During follow-up periods ranging from 6 months to 5 years, four of the patients remained completely continent and the other two were definitely improved. The technique was simple to apply and learning occurred within four sessions or less. Engel and colleagues emphasize that not only can sphincter activity be brought under voluntary control (a phenomenon long recognized) but that this control can be reintroduced in patients with chronic fecal incontinence, even when the incontinence is secondary to organic lesions. Clearly, the capacity for neural control must have been present in these patients for the biofeedback to have been effective.

A final example concerns the possible use of intestinal biofeedback in the treatment of functional diarrhea. Furman [50] reports that subjects can rapidly learn to reduce stomach and colon activity when given auditory biofeedback using a simple, electronic stethoscope. Furman applied this procedure to five patients with functional disorders of the lower gastrointestinal tract who manifested no organic findings. Response to treatment was uniformly positive. Furman claims that even patients who had experienced a lifetime of functional diarrhea and who had been virtually toilet bound are now enjoying normal bowel function. Although controlled studies have yet to be carried out using this technique, Furman's study illustrates how simple modes of feedback may be utilized by the patient and therapist as a team to aid in regaining control over a functional disorder.

THE PLACE OF BIOFEEDBACK IN THE TREATMENT OF DISREGULATION DISORDERS

It is clear that there are many potential applications of biofeedback in the treatment of physiological disorders. It is also clear that the exacting work of conducting controlled clinical studies to determine the validity and limitations of biofeedback for specific disorders with particular patients is just beginning. It will be years before definite conclusions can be drawn. Issues of expectancy, placebo responses, spontaneous remission and others, must be considered [2, 16, 31] since they apply to any behavioral or biological treatment in psychiatry and medicine.

However, biofeedback research is providing more than just a potential clinical technique. It is providing a new research tool for understanding functional disorders, and as I have illustrated, it is stimulating new neurophysiological analyses of normal and abnormal physiological self-regulation [2]. These analyses, in turn, serve to illuminate both the potential and limitations of biofeedback as a self-regulation therapy. They emphasize how biofeedback must be viewed as only one component of a multi-process approach to treatment if long-term clinical gains are to be obtained.

For example, one issue of historical relevance to the development of biofeedback therapy concerns the so-called direct versus indirect approach [45, 51]. The simple, direct approach is to provide the patient with feedback for a specific symptom for the purpose of self-regulating the symptom. Once self-regulation is acquired, the hope is that the symptom will remain under control and disappear. The indirect approach is broader in scope; it argues that patients should learn to regulate as many of the underlying components or processes contributing to the disorder as possible, including environmental and behavioral factors.

The indirect approach argues that biofeedback can be used to signal both the therapist and the patient that the patient is currently thinking, feeling or doing specific things that are detrimental to his physical or emotional health. A well-known example of this approach is the use of feedback in the treatment of obesity. In the same way that a scale helps direct the therapist and his obese patient in learning how to reduce food consumption and/or to increase exercise in order to reduce weight (rather than the patient spending hours on the scale attempting to lower his weight by thought processes alone), biofeedback for physiological disorders can be similarly employed. By means of the immediate, augmented feedback of stage 5 (with its associated increased bodily awareness) the patient can learn new ways of coping cognitively and behaviorally with his environment (stage 2 CNS information processing) and/or he can learn to alter his environment (stage 1) in such a way as to keep his physiological processes (stage 3) within safer limits. In this respect biofeedback is similar to current psychotherapies, for they all provide corrective feedback [45] in the cybernetic sense [1].

By recognizing that disregulation disorders can have multiple etiologies requiring a multi-process treatment program, it becomes possible to determine more precisely what combination of factors are contributing to the disorder in the individual patient, and what combination or pattern of treatment approaches should be used in each individual case [2]. For example, if it were found in a given hypertensive patient that the high pressure tended to occur in anger-arousing situations, the therapist could employ a variety of cognitive and behavioral approaches, including, for instance, role playing, as a means of teaching the person better ways of handling his aggression. Or, if the patient had difficulty relaxing in situations of moderate stress, the therapist could employ a variety of cognitive and behavior relaxation procedures, including muscle relaxation and meditation procedures, as a means of teaching the person better ways of reducing excessive tension. As part of the treatment, however, both the therapist and patient would profit from intermittent biofeedback (stage 5) of blood pressure to ensure that the treatment regime was effective. This use of feedback is similar to what the physician normally does when he monitors the patient's pressure as a means of titrating drug effects. The difference here, however, is the emphasis on the patient via the feedback (stages 4 and 5) taking a more active role in monitoring his physiological processes (stage 3) and in self-regulating his behavior (stage 2) and environment (stage 1).

There are numerous issues that need to be resolved, not the least of which is economy. Is biofeedback too expensive to be considered on a large-scale basis, especially if nonelectronic relaxation procedures in and of themselves prove sufficient to produce clinically significant long term changes [39]? It seems probable that certain patients with certain disorders will not require augmented biomedical instrumentation to achieve improvement, but at this point it is premature to conclude (and unlikely to happen) that this will be the case for all patients. The disregulation model helps us to appreciate the multiplicity of factors contributing to functional disorders, and helps us place factors such as secondary gain and suggestion (stage 1) and peripheral organpathology (stages 3 and/or 4) into a total treatment approach [2]. To the extent that severe pathology reduces the brain's ability to regulate the diseased organ via normal and humoral factors, the limitations of biofeedback and other behavioral approaches can be estimated. The theme of self-regulation (broadly defined) and biofeedback (in particular) provides the impetus for developing a field of "behavioral medicine" [5]. It places more responsibility for both sickness and health in the hands of the patient, and suggests new directions for preventive medicine by manipulating stages 1 and 2 before organic pathology in stages 3 and 4 has a chance to develop.

However, when we view functional disorders in terms of four stages of disregulation, and we recognize that a *combination* of stages can contribute to the final disorder in the individual patient, it becomes clear why increasing external feedback in and of itself may not be sufficient for long-term clinical gains, even with the use of home trainers and ambulatory feedback devices. As mentioned earlier, the corrective internal negative feedback loop (stage 4) in normal homeostasis not only provides information, but with few exceptions it also provides a strong incentive (that is, pain), for the brain (stage 2) to regulate itself for the sake of the organ's health (stage 3) and therefore ultimately its own. For this reason it is necessary for the therapist to consider both the information value and incentive value of biofeedback in the total treatment program. If the latter is lacking, the former will be short-lived at best.

In cases of extreme pain or embarrassment (such as in fecal incontinence), this adaptive mechanism provides a strong incentive for the patient to seek treatment and follow the regime. In these instances biofeedback may be particularly effective in aiding the patient to gain self-control. Unfortunately, in other disorders such as essential hypertension, this adaptive mechanism is minimal or lacking. As a result, not only does the patient lack the feedback that something is wrong, but when he receives this feedback from his physician, he still lacks the built-in internal negative feedback which would motivate him to recover.

A good illustration of this point comes from one of our hypertensive patients who, during the feedback sessions, was successful in lowering his pressure [45]. Over the five daily sessions of a typical week, he would lower his pressure by 20 mm Hg and thus earn a total of over $35.00 for participating in the research. However, we consistently noticed that after the weekend, he would enter the laboratory on Monday with elevated pressures again. In interviews with the patient, the problem became clear.

After earning a sizable amount of money, the patient would go to the race track on the weekend, gamble, and invariably lose. The likelihood of teaching this patient to "relax" while losing at the race track through simple laboratory blood pressure feedback would seem slim, indicating that there is a need to change other aspects of the patient's total life style, including developing some enduring incentive system for sustaining his health.

The motivation issue helps clarify the distinction between *learning* a self-regulation skill versus *using* that skill for the continued maintenance of one's health. The long-term effectiveness of biofeedback, or for that matter, any behavioral or biological treatment program involving self-control (for example, taking drugs), ultimately depends on the patient's motivation and ability to continue using the self-regulation skill. This distinction is an important one, for it helps us recognize the difference between developing behavioral procedures for helping patients to help themselves, as opposed to developing educational and social programs for leading patients to make effective, long-term use of the new behavioral technology. This writer is of the strong opinion that we are closer to solving the former than the latter. The ultimate clinical value of biofeedback and other self-regulation procedures for the treatment of disregulation disorders will hinge on our success in solving both of them.

REFERENCES

1. N. Wiener, *Cybernetics or Control and Communication in the Animal and Machine* (Cambridge: M.I.T. University Press, 1948).
2. G. E. Schwartz, "Psychosomatic Disorders and Biofeedback: A Psychobiological Model of Disregulation." In *Psychopathology: Experimental Models,* ed., J. D. Maser and M. E. P. Seligman (San Francisco: W. H. Freeman, 1976).
3. G. E. Schwartz, "Self-Regulation of Response Patterning: Implications for Psychophysiological Research and Therapy," *Biofeedback and Self-Regulation* (1976).
4. G. E. Schwartz and J. Beatty, eds., *Biofeedback: Theory and Research* (New York: Academic Press, 1976).

5. L. Birk, ed. *Biofeedback: Behavioral Medicine* (New York: Grune & Stratton, 1973).
6. G. E. Whatmore and D. R. Kohli, *The Physiopathology and Treatment of Functional Disorders* (New York: Grune & Stratton, 1974).
7. H. D. Kimmel, "Instrumental Conditioning of Autonomically Mediated Responses in Human Beings," *American Psychologist* 29 (1974):325–35.
8. N. E. Miller, "Learning of Visceral and Glandular Responses," *Science* 163 (1969):434–45.
9. D. Shapiro, A. B. Crider, and B. Tursky, "Differentiation of an Autonomic Response Through Operant Reinforcement," *Psychonomic Science* 1 (1964):147–48.
10. P. J. Lang, "Learned Control of Human Heart Rate in a Computer Directed Environment," in *Cardiovascular Psychophysiology,* ed. P. A. Obrist, A. H. Black, J. Brener and L. V. Dicara (Chicago: Aldine, 1974).
11. G. E. Schwartz, "Toward a Theory of Voluntary Control of Response Patterns in the Cardiovascular System," in *Cardiovascular Psychophysiology,* ed. P. A. Obrist, A. H. Black, J. Brener and L. V. DiCara (Chicago: Aldine, 1974).
12. D. Shapiro and R. S. Surwit, "Learned Control of Physiological Function and Disease," in *Handbook of Behavior Modification and Behavior Therapy,* ed. H. Leitenherg (New York: Prentice-Hall, 1976).
13. T. Kuhn, *The Structure of Scientific Revolutions* (Chicago: University of Chicago Press, 1967).
14. G. E. Schwartz, "Biofeedback, Self-Regulation, and the Patterning of Physiological Processes," *American Scientist* 63 (1975):314–24.
15. W. B. Cannon, *The Wisdom of the Body* (New York: W. W. Norton, 1939).
16. N. E. Miller and B. R. Dworkin, "Critical Issues in Therapeutic Applications of Biofeedback," in *Biofeedback: Theory and Research,* ed. G. E. Schwartz and J. Beatty (New York: Academic Press, 1976).
17. R. Melzack, *The Puzzle of Pain* (New York: Basic Books, 1973).
18. T. X. Barber, L. V. DiCara, J. Kamiya, N. E. Miller, D. Shapiro, and J. Stoyva, eds. *Biofeedback and Self-Control 1970: An Aldine Annual on the Regulation of Bodily Processes and Consciousness* (Chicago: Aldine-Atherton, 1971).

19. J. Kamiya, L. V. DiCara, T. X. Barber, N. E. Miller, D. Shapiro, and J. Stoyva, eds., *Biofeedback and Self-Control: An Aldine Reader on the Regulation of Bodily Processes and Consciousness* (Chicago: Aldine-Atherton, 1971).

20. J. Stoyva, T. X. Barber, L. V. DiCara, J. Kamiya, N. E. Miller, and D. Shapiro, eds., *Biofeedback and Self-Control 1971: An Aldine Annual on the Regulation of Bodily Processes and Consciousness* (Chicago: Aldine-Atherton, 1972)

21. D. Shapiro, T. X. Barber, L. V. DiCara, J. Kamiya, N. E. Miller, and J Stoyva, eds., *Biofeedback and Self-Control 1972: An Aldine Annual on the Regulation of Bodily Processes and Consciousness* (Chicago: Aldine, 1973).

22. N. E. Miller, T. X. Barber, L. V. DiCara, J. Kamiya, D. Shapiro, and J. Stoyva, eds., *Biofeedback and Self-Control 1973: An Aldine Annual on the Regulation of Bodily Processes and Consciousness* (Chicago: Aldine, 1974).

23. L. V. DiCara, T. X. Barber, J. Kamiya, N. E. Miller, D. Shapiro, and J. Stoyva, eds., *Biofeedback and Self-Control 1974: An Aldine Annual on the Regulation of Bodily Processes and Consciousness* (Chicago: Aldine, 1975).

24. D. Shapiro, B. Tursky, E. Gershon, and M. Stern, "Effects of Feedback and Reinforcement on the Control of Human Systolic Blood Pressure," *Science* 163 (1969):588–90.

25. D. Shapiro, B. Tursky, G. E. Schwartz, "Control of Blood Pressure in Man by Operant Conditioning," *Circulation Research* Supplement I (1970): 26–27, 27–32(a).

26. D. Shapiro, B. Tursky, and G. E. Schwartz, "Differentiation of Heart Rate and Systolic Blood Pressure in Man by Operant Conditioning," *Psychosomatic Medicine* 32 (1970):417–23(b).

27. G. E. Schwartz, "Voluntary Control of Human Cardiovascular Integration and Differentiation Through Feedback and Reward," *Science* 175 (1972):90–93.

28. I. R. Bell and G. E. Schwartz, "Voluntary Control and Reactivity of Human Heart Rate," *Psychophysiology* 12 (1975):339–48.

29. J. Brener, "A General Model of Voluntary Control Applied to the Phenomena of Learned Cardiovascular Change," in *Cardiovascular Psychophysiology*, ed. P. A. Obrist, A. H. Black, J. Brener and L. V. DiCara (Chicago: Aldine, 1974).

30. E. Braunwald, S. E. Epstein, G. Glick, A. S. Wechsler, and N. S. Braunwald, "Relief of Angina Pectoris by Electrical Stimulation

of the Carotid-Sinus Nerves," *New England Journal of Medicine* 227 (1967):1278–83.

31. D. Shapiro and G. E. Schwartz, "Biofeedback and Visceral Learning: Clinical Applications," *Seminars in Psychiatry* 4 (1972):171–84.

32. E. B. Blanchard and L. C. Young, "Clinical Applications of Biofeedback Training: A Review of Evidence," *Archives of General Psychiatry* 30 (1974):573–89.

33. T. H. Budzynski, J. M. Stoyva, C. S. Adler, and D. J. Mullaney, "EMG Biofeedback and Tension Headache: A Controlled Outcome Study," *Psychosomatic Medicine* 35 (1973):484–96.

34. J. V. Basmajian, "Electromyography Comes of Age," *Science* 176 (1972):603–09.

35. E. Jacobson, *Progressive Relaxation,* 2nd ed. (Chicago: University of Chicago Press, 1938).

36. M. B. Sterman, "Clinical Implications of EEG Biofeedback Training: A Critical Appraisal," in *Biofeedback: Theory and Research,* ed. G. E. Schwartz and J. Beatty (New York: Academic Press, 1976).

37. J. Kamiya, "Operant Control of the EEG Alpha and Some of Its Reported Effects on Consciousness," in *Altered States of Consciousness,* ed. C. Tart (New York: John Wiley and Sons, 1969).

38. R. J. Davidson and G. E. Schwartz, "Psychobiology of Relaxation and Related States: A Multi-Process Theory," in *Behavior Control and Modification of Physiological Processes,* ed. D. Mostofsky (New York: Prentice Hall, 1976).

39. H. Benson, *The Relaxation Response* (New York: William Morrow, 1975).

40. J. Stoyva and T. Budzynski, "Cultivated Low Arousal—An Antistress Response?" in *Limbic and Automatic Nervous Systems Research,* ed. L. V. DiCara (New York: Plenum, 1974).

41. J. D. Sargent, E. E. Green, and E. D. Walters, "Preliminary Report on the Use of Autogenic Feedback Training in the Treatment of Migraine and Tension Headaches," *Psychosomatic Medicine* 35 (1973):129–35.

42. J. H. Schultz and W. Luthe, *Autogenic Therapy,* vol. 1 (New York: Grune & Stratton, 1969).

43. E. Taub, "Self-Regulation of Human Tissue Temperature," in *Biofeedback: Theory and Research,* ed. G. E. Schwartz and J. Beatty (New York: Academic Press, 1976).

44. R. S. Surwit, "Biofeedback: A Possible Treatment for Raynaud's Disease," *Seminars in Psychiatry* 5 (1973):483–90.

45. G. E. Schwartz, "Biofeedback as Therapy: Some Theoretical and Practical Issues," *American Psychologist* 29 (1973):666–73.

46. B. T. Engel and E. R. Bleecker, "Application of Operant Conditioning Techniques to the Control of the Cardiac Arrhythmias," in *Cardiovascular Psychophysiology,* ed. P. A. Obrist, A. H. Black, J. Brener and L. V. DiCara (Chicago: Aldine, 1974).

47. H. Benson, D. Shapiro, B. Tursky, and G. E. Schwartz, "Decreased Systolic Blood Pressure Through Operant Conditioning Techniques in Patients with Essential Hypertension," *Science* 173 (1971):740–42.

48. D. A. Kristt and B. T. Engel, "Learned Control of Blood Pressure in Patients with High Blood Pressure," *Circulation* 51 (1975):370–78.

49. B. T. Engel, P. Nikoomanesh, and M. M. Schuster, "Operant Conditioning of Rectosphincteric Responses in the Treatment of Fecal Incontinence," *New England Journal of Medicine* 290 (1974):646–49.

50. S. Furman, "Intestinal Biofeedback in Functional Diarrhea: A Preliminary Report," *Journal of Behavior Therapy and Experimental Psychiatry* 4 (1973):317–21.

51. R. S. Lazarus, "A Cognitively-Oriented Psychologist Looks at Biofeedback," *American Psychologist* 30 (1975):553–61.

PART FIVE

AN ECOLOGICAL
VIEW
OF HEALTH

Introduction

> Whoever wishes to pursue properly the science of medicine must proceed thus. First he ought to consider what effects each season of the year can produce ... the hot winds and the cold ... the properties of the waters ... the soil ... the mode of life of the inhabitants ...
>
> Hippocrates, *Airs Waters Places*

Throughout the two to three billion years of biological evolution, life has been shaped by the natural forces of the environment. Those characteristics of organisms that enhanced survival under existing environmental conditions were passed on to succeeding generations. The genetic inheritance and biological structure of man, therefore, reflects successive adaptations to demands of the natural environment that have prevailed through the long, slow evolution of life on earth.

About ten thousand years ago, a very brief period on the evolutionary time-scale, the environmental challenges to which early man was accustomed began to change markedly. This was occasioned by the transition from a hunter-gatherer society to a more settled mode of existence with the initiation of agriculture and the domestication of animals. This cultural transition, known as the Neolithic Revolution, and the accelerating changes through the subsequent Agricultural and Industrial revolutions, have introduced environmental challenges to which the human species has had no previous evolutionary experience. Further, these changes have occurred so rapidly, from an evolutionary perspective, that the usual mechanisms of genetic adaptation have not had time to respond to the changing environment. Therefore, we face the environmental demands of today with a genetic and biological structure essentially the same as our hunter-gatherer ancestors of ten thousand years ago. This has led some observers to comment that modern man is "biologically obsolete" and therefore must rely on social and behavioral mechanisms of adaptation.

As an example, primitive man evolved automatic physiological mechanisms mobilizing the body for physical activity in the face of environmental threats such as the charging of a wild animal. Survival very much depended on the success of this physiological preparation for combat or rapid retreat. This same fight-or-flight response continues to operate in modern man, but the environmental conditions have changed. Today this response is too often triggered by social situations in which fighting or fleeing and the preparatory physiological arousal are neither appropriate nor desirable.

Similarly, we are often estranged from the rhythms of the natural environment that conditioned our internal biological rhythms. We breathe air of a different quality and composition than that present throughout the evolution of life. We have adopted a sedentary life style after an evolutionary history demanding physical activity, and our diet is far different from that of our ancestors.

What are the consequences of facing environmental conditions different from those that have conditioned human evolution? What are the limits of human adaptation? What are the indirect and long-term costs of such adaptation? These are a few of the questions that René Dubos considers in his overview chapter "Human Ecology." His discussion takes us beyond healing and therapy per se to a broader view of the environmental and behavioral determinants of health. The perspective of health as an adaptive response to changing environments echoes the philosophy of many of the ancient systems of medicine and forms the foundation of the modern study of human ecology. Although human ecology involves both the health-promotive as well as pathogenic potentialities of human-environment interactions, recently most attention has been paid to the nefarious aspects of the environment. Epidemiologists have noted that some diseases such as heart disease, hypertension, cancer, bowel diseases, and certain nervous and mental disorders are more common in "civilized," that is, industrialized, populations than in less developed societies. Further, as societies industrialize or as people migrate to urban industrial regions, changes in life style and environment correlate with an increased incidence of these so-called diseases of civilization. It has been suggested therefore that the marked change in disease burden during the twentieth century is due to excessive adaptive demands imposed by environmental changes unprecedented in human evolution. It should not surprise us that certain physiological mechanisms selected by evolution because they were adaptive in one environment may prove to be maladaptive when the environment changes. Such maladaptive processes are now believed to figure predominantly in the diseases of industrial man and have led some to propose a shift in modern medicine from a reliance on physical and chemical interventions to a medicine based on an ecological understanding of human health and disease.

The importance of an ecological approach is becoming apparent in the new research on biological rhythms reviewed by Gay Luce. Throughout the course of evolution, the cycle of day and night, change of the seasons, and even subtle, unnoticed alterations in the earth's electromagnetic field have conditioned a myriad of circadian, lunar, and seasonal rhythms in human physiological functions. The ancients lived in close contact with these rhythms of the natural environment. The Navaho, through their basic ways of life and healing ceremonies, sought to harmonize with the rhythms of nature. Traditional Chinese physicians developed elaborate theories and techniques to correlate and coordinate the rhythms of the macrocosm with the phasic flow of energy within the human microcosm.

Much has changed, however, since our inherent biological rhythms were entrained with those of nature. Technological advances in artificial illumination, temperature control, and transportation have "liberated" modern man from the rhythms of the earth. Schedules and life styles now conform more to the societal demands for efficiency than the cues of our biological clocks. But what are the consequences of this dissociation between biological rhythms and the rhythms of nature? In reviewing the research in the emerging science of chronobiology, Gay Luce finds some support for the idea that certain states of ill health are related to a desynchronization of physiological functions. Also, individual susceptibility to disruptive environmental forces (for example, drugs, infectious agents, or surgery) appears to vary throughout the day in accordance with complex internal biochemical rhythms. Such findings suggest that a scientific understanding of our own time structure and how it is influenced by environmental factors is important to human health.

The ecological view of the human organism as an open system in constant interchange with the environment also suggests that we may be far more sensitive to subtle environmental changes than we have previously suspected. It has long been thought that the quality and nature of the air affects health. At least since Hippocratic times certain weather complexes, the so-called winds of ill repute like the foehn, Santa Ana, mistral, and khamsin, have been believed to cause a variety of complaints and symptoms. Recently, these weather complexes and the incipient symptoms have been found to be associated with minute changes in the air ion composition of the atmosphere. In "Air Ions and Health," Albert Krueger and I review the evidence suggesting that the balance and composition of these small electrically charged particles in the air are relevant, though largely unrecognized, factors in human health. Air pollution and indoor living significantly alter the ionization of the air such that the urban environment now differs markedly from the natural ion balance to which man is evolutionarily adapted. The discussion of air ionization is presented here as one example of a subtle environmental factor, suspected in ancient medicine, altered by conditions of civilization, and currently being evaluated with respect to its role in health and disease.

Of course, in recent human history not only has the physical environment been altered but so has the cultural environment and life style. In the early evolution of the human species, survival favored the physically strong, active, well-conditioned individual. Until recently a certain amount of strenuous physical activity was demanded in the course of everyday work. Today, however, there has been a rather abrupt shift towards a sedentary life style; physical activity is now an option. The emergence of a sedentary way of life is currently believed to be associated with susceptibility to certain degenerative conditions, most notably cardiovascular disease. In "Physical Activity in Health Maintenance," William Haskell, an exercise physiologist, reviews the experimental literature on exercise in sufficient detail to illustrate the problems in establishing a definitive role for exercise. The data are complex and confusing. Nevertheless, disease-related measures of mortality and morbidity as well as health-related indicators of fitness, functional capacity, and performance support the idea of measurable health benefits of physical activity. It is important to note that in many cases, even though physical activity may not prevent or alter the basic disease process, the overall functioning and well-being of the individual may be enhanced. Most of the data, however, is limited to Western forms of exercise and sport. Unfortunately there has been little scientific investigation on the health effects of the ancient Eastern physical arts such as Tai Chi Chuan, Aikido, Karate, and Yoga.

"A Renaissance of Nutritional Science," by Roger J. Williams and research associates, deals with one of the most important yet neglected aspects of our interaction with the environment— namely, nutrition. This subject has been of great concern in ancient and traditional medical systems, most of which developed elaborate theories and practices relating food intake and health. There is, however, a rather puzzling lack of real interest in the development of nutritional science within contemporary medicine, a deficiency that stands in marked contrast to the widespread, if not at times obsessive, concern with health and food in the popular culture. In an effort to dispel some of the popular as well as professional misconceptions and to rekindle interest in a scientific investigation of nutrition, Williams and his associates offer a refreshingly clear discussion of the basic principles of nutrition. For example, they contrast the myth of the "average human being with average nutritional requirements" with the fact that nutritional needs vary widely according to individual genetic predispositions. Unfortunately, nutritional science has not yet evolved to be able to deal adequately with this important aspect of human individuality. It is also commonly but incorrectly assumed that if an individual is not manifesting symptoms consistent with one of the clinically recognized nutritional deficiency diseases, then he is properly nourished. This misconception also stems from our lack of nutritional sophistication as well as the disease orientation of medical science. The concentration on identifying specific causes for diseases, for example, vitamin C deficiency in scurvy or vitamin B_1 deficiency in beriberi, has underplayed the significance of optimal nutrition in increasing the general resistance and health of the organism. According to Williams and his colleagues, suboptimal nutrition is the rule, not the exception, and a better understanding of nutritional science may permit the development of optimal nutritional environments.

Such examples of an ecological view of health suggest that the human organism is far more sensitive to the environment than has been previously understood. Further, we must consider the limitations of the human organism to adapt to environmental conditions far different from those that conditioned human evolution. This is not to suggest that we abandon civilization and "return to Nature," rather, that we adopt a more cautious and humble attitude toward our interactions with the natural environment and become more alert and vigilant to the consequences of environmental change.

By *René Dubos*

ᕞᕜ

Human Ecology

... Nowadays there is a tendency to believe that modern medicine consists exclusively of a few sensational recent discoveries—
miracle drugs, spectacular surgical techniques, sophisticated
immunization methods. This tendency is dangerous, for it deflects attention from another aspect of modern medicine which
is just as remarkable and perhaps of greater practical importance.
If the health of the public has improved in many regions during
recent decades, the improvement is due not only to certain
specialized medical procedures but also—and probably to a
greater extent—to a better understanding of the effects of man's
environment and way of life on his physiological and mental
state. Our health is better than that of our ancestors to the extent
that our lives are more in accord with what I would choose to call
biological wisdom. The scientific expression of that biological
wisdom is human ecology, i.e., knowledge of the relationships between man and the innumerable factors of his environment.

It would be easy and pleasant for me to devote this entire
[chapter] to an inventory of the progress of modern medical
science. But I feel that it will be more productive to consider in
what respects that science is inadequate, particularly when it
comes to coping with the new ecological crisis that at the present
time is threatening almost every country in the world.

The word "environment" has in our day acquired an ever

The Jacques Parisot Foundation Lecture, 1969, from WHO *Chronicle* 23,
no. 11 (November 1969):499–504. Reprinted by permission.

more tragic connotation, both in primitive agrarian societies and in industrial urban societies. It connotes, for example, malnutrition and infection in most of the poor countries, chemical pollution and mechanization of life in all the prosperous countries. The ecological crisis is everywhere so menacing and takes such varied forms that the term "human ecology" has come to be used only for certain situations that might lead to biological or mental disaster. Yet human ecology embraces far more than this tragic view of the relationships between man and his environment. Ecology teaches us that all the physical, biological, and social forces acting upon man impart a direction to his development and thus mould his nature. The body and the mind are constantly being modified, and hence shaped, by the stimuli that induce formative reactions. It is to be hoped that a time will come when human ecology will be able to pay greater attention to the positive and beneficial effects of the environment than to its pathogenic effects.

The social mechanisms whereby society tries to create a more or less artificial environment better adapted to man's needs and desires constitute an extremely important aspect of human ecology which I shall not attempt to discuss here. The other aspect of human ecology consists of the biological processes whereby the organism as a whole tries to adapt itself to environmental forces. The importance of these adaptive phenomena for health has frequently been demonstrated in the course of history. I shall mention a few examples of this.

In the narrative of his travels, Christopher Columbus speaks with admiration of the magnificent physical condition of the natives he discovered in Central America. In the eighteenth century, Cook, Bougainville, and the other navigators who ranged over the Pacific also wondered at the excellent health of the island populations of Oceania. Many other explorers were similarly impressed on their first contact with the Indians, the Africans, and, later, the Eskimos. The legend of the noble savage, healthy and happy, thus has its origin in the descriptions published by the explorers who observed certain native populations when they were still undeveloped and almost completely isolated from the rest of the world.

There was certainly a lot of false romanticism in the illusion that the noble savage was free from disease and social restrictions because he lived in a state of nature. But all the same this romantic and over-simple view of man's estate has been partly justified by the studies in physical and social anthropology conducted on what contemporary anthropologists call man the hunter. These studies were recently the subject of a symposium under that title, in the course of which descriptions were given of the characteristics of populations that live without agriculture and even without tools, except for a few primitive objects they employ to derive their sustenance from wild plants and animals. It appears that this way of life, though so close to nature and therefore lacking any medical assistance, is compatible with a good state of health. But I should like to emphasize the fact that primitive populations undergo rapid physical and mental deterioration as soon as they come into close contact with the modern world and thus lose their ancestral manners and customs. The noble savage who seemed so healthy and happy in the eighteenth century had often become a human wreck by the nineteenth.

The epidemiological facts suggest that the good health of primitive peoples, like that of wild animals, is a manifestation of a biological equilibrium between the living creature and its environment. This equilibrium persists as long as the conditions of human ecology remain stable, but is broken as soon as the conditions change. The enormous problems of malnutrition, alcoholism, and infectious disease, which caused such a rapid physical deterioration among the primitive populations in the seventeenth, eighteenth, and nineteenth centuries, recurred in all the Western countries at the outset of the Industrial Revolution, when their working classes, originating largely from agricultural regions, underwent massive and sudden exposure to conditions of life that were then new to them.

Adaptation to industrial society is now far advanced in the prosperous countries, but this is only a temporary phase. New problems are arising from the fact that the second Industrial Revolution is causing sudden and far-reaching changes in the physical environment and in everyday living, thus creating a new and as yet unstable ecological situation. The changes naturally bring their own specific dangers, which undoubtedly underlie what we nowadays call the diseases of civilization.

Indeed, we might say that in our day human ecology is undergoing an almost universal crisis because man is not yet adapted, and probably never will become adapted, either to the biological impoverishment of the very poor countries or to certain environmental influences that the second Industrial Revolution has introduced into the rich countries. It might be supposed that man, since he still has the same genetic make-up as in the past, could once again use the biological mechanisms that enabled him in the Stone Age to colonize a large part of the globe, and so could adapt himself to the conditions of physiological impoverishment or industrial intoxication of present-day life. But this is neither certain nor even probable, because the present changes are of a kind almost without precedent in human history.

Up till now, changes in the pattern of living have generally been so slow that it took several generations before they affected all classes of society. This slowness enabled the entire range of adaptive forces to be brought into play: physiological and even anatomical characteristics, as well as mental reactions and particularly social organization, little by little changed. Nowadays, on the contrary, everything changes so quickly that the processes of biological and social adaptation do not have time to come into play. Whether from the biological or the social point of view, the father's experience is now of practically no value to the son.

It is also a known fact that the human faculty of adaptation, great as it is, is not unlimited. It is quite possible that the stresses of present-day living are taking it near its extreme limits.

In the course of his evolution, man has constantly been exposed to inclement weather, fatigue, periodic famine, and infection. So as to survive these dangers, he has had to develop in his genetic code hereditary mechanisms that have facilitated certain processes of adaptation. But man now has to face dangers of another kind, without any precedent in the biological past of the human species. He probably does not possess adaptive mechanisms for all the new situations to which he is exposed. Moreover, the evolution of biological mechanisms is far too slow to keep up with the accelerated pace of technological and social change in the modern world.

It is certain, for example, that there is no possible means of adaptation to nutritional deficiences that persist for long periods. Many children in their growth phase succumb to them. If they survive, they cannot satisfactorily realize the potentialities of their genetic endowment; they are condemned for the rest of their lives to anatomical, physiological, and mental atrophy. A population continuously subjected to nutritional deficiency cannot but degenerate.

Industrial technology has introduced into modern life a range of substances and situations that man has never known in his biological past. It is probable that he will never be able to adapt himself to the toxic effects of chemical pollution and of certain synthetic products; to the physiological and mental difficulties caused by lack of physical effort; to the mechanization of life; and to the presence of a wide variety of artificial stimulants. We should probably add to this list the disturbances to natural body rhythms arising from the almost complete divorce of modern life from cosmic cycles.

There are no grounds for the fear that all deviations from the natural order that result from technological change will be dangerous to health. Far from it. It remains true, however, that the more a population is exposed to modern technology the more it appears to be subject to certain forms of chronic and degenerative disease—conditions called for precisely that reason the diseases of civilization. Premature death caused by these diseases is not due to the lack of medical care. In the U.S.A., for example, scientists and especially physicians have, paradoxically enough, a shorter life expectancy than other groups, although they belong to an economically privileged class. Certain demographic studies show that the life expectancy beyond the age of 35 may have decreased somewhat during the last few years in the big cities of the U.S.A.

Everyday life seems to give the lie to the anxieties expressed in the previous pages, since modern man appears to be just as adaptable as Stone Age man. An extraordinary number of people have survived the terrible ordeals of modern war and the concentration camps. Throughout the world it is the most crowded and polluted cities, those in which life is at its most ruthless, that attract most people, and it is their population that is increasing at the greatest rate. Men and women are working all the time in the midst of the infernal noise of machines and telephones, in an atmosphere polluted with chemical fumes and tobacco smoke.

This remarkable tolerance of man towards conditions so different from those in which he has evolved has given rise to the myth that, through technological and social progress, he can modify his way of life and his environment indefinitely and without risk. That is simply not true. As I stated earlier, modern man can only adapt himself in so far as the mechanisms of adaptation are potentially present in his genetic code. Furthermore, it is certain that in many cases the apparent ease with which man adapts himself biologically, socially, and culturally to new or unfavourable conditions constitutes, paradoxically, a threat to individual well-being and even to the future of the human race.

This paradox arises from the fact that the word "adaptation" cannot be applied unreservedly to the adjustments that enable human beings to survive and function under modern conditions. Indeed, in man sociocultural forces distort the effects of the kind of adaptive mechanisms that operate in the animal kingdom.

For the biologist, the expression "Darwinian adaptation" implies harmony between a species and a given environment, a harmony that enables it to multiply and, at the appropriate moment, to invade new territory. In the terms of this definition, man would appear to be remarkably well adapted to the conditions of life that exist both in highly industrialized societies and in developing countries, since the world's population is continuing to increase and to occupy an ever greater proportion of the land surface of the globe. However, what would constitute a biological success for another species is a serious social threat to the human species. The dangers arising from the increase in world population show clearly that the Darwinian concept of adaptation cannot be used if the well-being of humanity is taken as a criterion of its biological success.

For the physiologist, a reaction to environmental stress is adaptive when it neutralizes the disturbing effects of such stress on the body and mind. In general, physiological and psychological adaptive responses are a factor tending towards the well-being of the organism at the time when they occur. In man, however, they may in the long term have detrimental effects. Man is capable of acquiring some degree of tolerance towards environmental pollution, excessive stimuli, a harassing social life in a competitive atmosphere, a rhythm completely foreign to natural biological cycles, and all the other consequences of his living in the world of cities and technology. This tolerance enables him to resist successfully exposure to influences which, at the outset, are unpleasant or traumatic. However, in many cases such tolerance is only acquired through a set of organic and mental processes that risk giving rise to degenerative manifestations.

Man can also learn to put up with the ugliness of the environment in which he lives, with its smoky skies and polluted streams. He can live without the scent of flowers, the song of birds, the life-enhancing spectacle of nature, and the other biological stimuli of the physical world. The suppression of a number of the pleasurable aspects of life and the stimuli that have conditioned his biological and mental evolution may have no manifest deleterious effect on his physical appearance or on his efficiency as a cog in the economic or technological machine, but there is a risk that, in the long run, it may impoverish his life and lead to the gradual loss of the qualities we associate with the idea of a human being.

Air, water, soil, fire, and the natural rhythms and diversity of living species are important not only as chemical combinations, physical forces, or biological phenomena but also because it is under their influence that human life has been fashioned. They have created in man deep-rooted needs that will not change in any near future. The pathetic weekend exodus towards the countryside or the beaches, the fireplaces that are still built in overheated urban apartments, the sentimental attachments formed for animals or even plants all bear witness to the survival deep down in man of biological and emotional urges acquired in the course of his evolution, of which he cannot rid himself.

Like the giant Antaeus in the Greek legend, man loses his strength as soon as he loses contact with the earth.

Human ecology therefore requires a scientific and intellectual attitude differing from that which would be adequate in general biology and even in the other biomedical sciences, because it has to deal with the indirect and long-term effects exercised by the environment and way of life, even if those factors have no apparent immediate influence. It would be easy to illustrate the importance of those indirect and long-term effects by discussing, for example, the part played by the abundance or scarcity of food, the various forms of chemical and microbial pollution, the effects of noise or other stimuli, the density of and especially the rapid changes in the population; in brief, all the environmental forces that act on man in every social class and in every country. Here, however, I shall confine myself to pointing out that the most important effects of the environment and way of life are often difficult to recognize because they only show themselves indirectly and after a lapse of time.

The early stages of life are of exceptional importance because to a large extent they determine what the adult will become. The young organism never forgets anything. All the factors that act upon it therefore contribute to the psychosomatic formation of the individual. The younger the person, the more malleable he is and the more easily affected by environmental influences. Hence the importance of the first stages of life, including those within the womb. These long-term and indirect manifestations of the environment are still poorly understood, but it is fortunately possible and even easy to study them experimentally since in animals, as in man, perinatal conditions have a profound and often irreversible effect, bearing on the anatomical features of the adult as well as on metabolism and behaviour. Animal experiments will therefore make it possible to see what is not easily seen in man, to understand what is not obvious to our minds and, consequently, to take action with a view to alleviating certain untoward or even disastrous consequences of the influences to which man is exposed at the beginning of his life.

Of course the environment continues unceasingly to transform the organism. However, the first years of life have effects so profound and irreversible that they are the most important part of human ecology. I am emphasizing this fact because it seems to me that it should . . . encourage scientists to devote more effort to the problems of childhood. It is beyond doubt that the establishment of an atmosphere favourable to the biological and mental development of the child is the most economical way of improving world health.

A better understanding of the effect of environment at the beginning of life on growth and development gives a deeper sense to the definition of health made famous by the preamble to the World Health Organization Constitution: "Health is a state of complete physical, mental and social well-being and not merely an absence of disease or infirmity." This "positive health" advocated by WHO implies that a person should be able to express as completely as possible the potentialities of his genetic heritage. That heritage, however, can only find true expression to the extent that the environment transforms genetic potentialities into phenotypic realities. It is in this way that human ecology might finally become identified, as I expressed the hope that it could at the beginning of this [chapter], with the positive and beneficial effects of the environment.

The word "health" in the sense that I have chosen to give it describes not a state but a potentiality—the ability of an individual or a social group to modify himself or itself continually not only in order to function better in the present but also to prepare for the future. Ideal health will, however, always remain a mirage, because everything in our life will continue to change. The doctor and the public health expert are in the same position as the gardener or farmer faced with insects, moulds, and weeds. Their work is never done. Man quickly grows tired of conditions of life that had originally seemed attractive. Individually and collectively he will look for adventure, and this forces him to live under constantly new conditions, with all the unforeseen occurrences and threats to health involved in change.

There is no question, however, of turning back. A society that does not move forward quickly deteriorates. Indeed, it cannot even survive in a world where everything is in a state of flux. Civilizations can only succeed and survive by exploring the unknown and accepting the risks involved in plunging ahead into the future. Technology would soon cease to develop if a certificate of absolute safety were required for every technical innovation and every new product.

It is therefore inevitable that economic and social progress should always be accompanied by hazards to health, whatever the advances made by medicine and hygiene.

This fact gives the doctor and the hygienist a still more important social role than they have at the present moment. It consists in recognizing as swiftly as possible, and even in anticipating, the medical problems that will arise increasingly as a result of the accelerated rate of technological and economic innovation. For this purpose it is becoming urgent to set up what might be called listening posts to record the first signs of pathological disorders that might threaten to spread to society as a whole. For example, the effects of atmospheric pollution, changes in food habits, the almost universal and constant use of new drugs, and automation in industry and in every aspect of life are still unforeseeable but could doubtless be detected before health disasters become widespread. It is a matter of satisfaction that this social responsibility is already recognized in certain sectors of the public service. Thus, thorough studies of the biological effects of ionizing radiation have been undertaken with a view to developing in advance practical methods of protection against the probable consequences of the industrial use of radiation. . . . This farsighted attitude will have to be generally adopted. In the future the development of technological innovations should always include parallel scientific studies on the long-term effects of these innovations on human ecology.

As Jacques Parisot wrote, "To cure is good but to prevent is better." Humanity will only be able to avoid the hazards of the future by extending its scientific knowledge and showing greater social conscience.

By Gay G. Luce

❧ ☙

Biological Rhythms
in Health and Disease

A pilot on a long-run flight might take twice as long to react to a simulated emergency around 3 A.M. when he would ordinarily be asleep. Reports on industrial accidents of night-shift workers have shown clustering in the early hours of the morning, when bodily and mental functions are normally slowed for the sleep period. Research on rotating shifts has been inadequate to allow solid conclusions, but recent studies of task performance conducted in applied psychology laboratories in Great Britain indicated that workers do better at repeated arithmetical, attention-demanding, and decision-making tasks during the hours when body temperature is high.

Much of what man considers constant about himself and his world is actually pulsating in patterned cycles. Important cycles can be observed in plants, animals, and man's own body. Night follows day, the tides ebb and flow, the seasons change. All creatures wake and sleep, experience hunger cycles, menstrual and estrous rhythms, spring fever. Some rhythms, such as the period of the heartbeat, depend upon genetically inherited oscillators within the body. The universe is rhythmic and immersed in an endless sea of time information that influences rhythms of gravity or electromagnetic fields, barometric pressure, the electric charge

From *Britannica Yearbook of Science and the Future 1974* (Chicago: Encyclopædia Britannica, 1973), pp. 82–95. Copyright © 1973 by Encyclopædia Britannica. Reprinted by permission.

of the atmosphere, sound or cosmic radiations, and the 11-year cycles of solar flares that are reflected in the growth rings of trees.

It is surprising how little attention has been paid to these rhythms considering that our lives depend upon them. There is a tendency to read the work of biologists with detachment, ignoring the messages relevant to human welfare. Man does not migrate like birds, hibernate, or spawn, yet these researches are beginning to emphasize that he, also, has a time structure tuned to these same natural cycles. Until recent times, man lived in consonance with the tempo of nature, working by day, resting by night, and traveling only as fast as animals or sails could carry him. Modern inventions—electricity, communications, jet flight —have changed that tempo: now the mechanization of industrial society sets up schedules that are more suited to the efficiency of machines than to the adaptability of the human body. Rotation of work shifts, rapid travel across time zones, and a general disregard for regularity have brought their own problems to 20th-century man.

Studies of biological rhythms are beginning to suggest that these self-inflicted time displacements may be injurious to health in the long run. Indeed, rhythms so permeate life that they should not be overlooked when planning a trip, diagnosing an illness, conducting an experiment, or even testing the safety of a drug.

The importance of intermeshed cycles is easy to understand by the simple analogy of the body as a factory. Imagine the production schedule of the body, in which numerous enzymes, hormones, and other substances must be available in tissues that need them exactly on time, without shortage or delay. The regularity of the heartbeat requires that a complex neurochemical be ready at the nerve ends precisely at the right moment to modulate the contraction. Countless subroutines like this are intermeshed to keep the body running smoothly. Some of the production lines are so microscopic that the body seems to be unaware of them. Animal and plant researches suggest that there are many levels of rhythmicity, but the most basic cycles follow from the process of cell division. Before a cell can replicate itself the template molecule in the nucleus, DNA, must unwind itself and be synthesized anew in a series of steps that, within minutes, ends in two cells where there had been one.

Cell division in any particular tissue does not occur steadily or evenly around the clock, but in each tissue rises and falls in a daily cycle that is related to the rhythm of activity and sleep. The skin, cornea of the eye, lining of the nose and mouth, eroded by contact with the environment, must always be renewed, with the renewal cells showing greatest division during sleep. Throughout the night man and other diurnal mammals undulate on waves of changing consciousness, for sleep is profoundly rhythmic. Human beings undergo cycles of vivid dreaming and physiological changes every 90 to 110 minutes during the night. The same rhythms are evident in cats and rats, but in shorter cycles because of the faster metabolism in smaller animals.

CIRCADIAN RHYTHMS

A great deal of the research on biological rhythms has focused on circadian rhythms. The term derives from the Latin "circa diem" meaning "about a day." When left in isolation from sunlight and darkness, and all social time cues, plants, animals, and humans show cycles of activity and rest that vary within a period of 23 to 27 hours. Since we live on a planet that is strongly influenced by its sun and moon, it is not surprising to find a combination of the solar and lunar days—somewhere between 24 and 24.8 hours—imbedded in earth creatures.

Biologists have found circadian rhythms of activity and rest in organisms as primitive as paramecium and as complicated as chimpanzees. Any living thing keeps its body and activity in the proper phase with the external world, usually through some rhythmic factor such as light, which stimulates diurnal creatures like man to be wakeful and active. However, plants that were kept in deep caves and animals that were blinded or were kept in constant environments maintained a circadian cycle, although they did show evidence of drifting out of phase with the day-night rhythm of the world.

Many attempts have been made to discover man's basic cycle of waking and sleeping in the absence of all time cues. Scientists have undergone the rigors of working under primitive and difficult conditions along with the men and women volunteers who consented to live for periods of from 2 weeks to 6 months in underground caverns or in laboratory capsules. Some volunteers controlled their own illumination, while others remained either in constant bright or dim illumination. Rarely did any of these volunteers show a "short" day of less than 24 hours. Most oscillated, often between 24.8 and 26 hours, and occasionally, for a two-week period, a 48-hour day was observed. Man's basic "free-running" rhythm (so-called when there are no external time givers such as light) seemed to be longer than 24 hours, and extremely persistent.

In rodents, even more persistently, the circadian rhythm of running and rest did not disappear even when the animals were blinded, stressed with drugs, physical injury, freezing, heart stoppage, and other extreme measures. A West German botanist, Erwin Bunning, observed that the rhythm of plants raised in a constant environment was never more than about 3 hours more or less than 24 hours. Moreover, each species demonstrated a typical rhythmic period in isolation. When Bunning crossed a plant showing a 24.2-hour rhythm with one having a 25.6-hour rhythm, the hybrids had an intermediate period. This seemed to indicate that the circadian rhythm could have been inherited.

Zoologists, experimenting with unicellular organisms, insects, and mammals, found considerable evidence for circadian rhythms. Colin Pittendrigh observed, for instance, that a large batch of fruit fly larvae did not hatch randomly a few at a time, around the clock, but instead seemed to emerge from the pupae in groups at 24-hour intervals. If they were raised in continuous darkness there was no such rhythm, yet after a single flash of light into the darkness flies emerged together at 24-hour intervals. Pittendrigh concluded that the circadian rhythm must be the product of some basic molecular mechanism that has a periodicity of 23–25 hours and that, once started, would continue its oscillation in the absence of external synchronizers such as light or temperature change. This rhythm appears to be a basic adaptation to our rhythmic planet, in which the sun and moon create 24–25-hour periodic changes of light, temperature, and pressure. Indeed, rhythmicity must have been one of the first forces of natural selection some 200 million years ago when the first organisms tuned their metabolic change to the current changes of light, temperature, and humidity around them.

Many scientists believe that circadian rhythms are inherited, but a few argue that geophysical changes cause such a continuous inpouring of rhythmic information that organisms do not need inner clocks. Frank Brown, a biologist at Northwestern University and the most active proponent of a "cosmic receiving theory," pointed out that signals are beating upon us from the environment at all times.

Brown found that metabolism in crabs, and cycles of oxygen consumption in shellfish, rats, carrots, and potatoes underwent changes that correlated with unusual modifications in cosmic radiation. He showed that worms could orient themselves using the direction of a weak laboratory magnet. In 1962 Yves Rocard, a physics professor at the University of Paris, found that by holding his arm taut and balancing a stick, the nerves and muscles of the arm became sensitive to extremely small magnetic changes (gradients of 0.3–0.5 milligauss), which he measured with a magnetometer.

Isolation experiments conducted by Jürgen Aschoff and Rutger Wever in underground bunkers at the Max Planck Institute in West Germany indicated that human beings could be influenced by the earth's electromagnetic fields, although totally without conscious awareness. One experimental compartment was shielded with heavy metal plating against magnetic and electric field changes of earth, while the other compartment was not. Of the 75 volunteers who lived there none could have been aware of the difference between the compartments, yet those in the unshielded unit lived an average day of 25.25 hours while those in the shielded unit lived an average 24.8-hour day. The difference may seem negligible, yet the people experiencing the longer period had veered far enough from their usual 24-hour day to suffer notable desynchronization between the normally persistent, nearly 24-hour cycles of many body functions and their changed cycle of sleep and waking. The hours of sleep and waking tend to synchronize the phase of all the internal rhythms, and many of the volunteers noted in their diaries that they felt miserable and unhinged when their bodies were out of synchrony. When Wever turned on alternating electric fields (ten Hertz), the shielded volunteers consciously felt nothing new, yet their behavior changed so that activity and internal rhythms were more nearly synchronous. If natural electromagnetic fields help to keep us synchronized, we may ask ourselves how good it is for us to work and live in even partially shielded buildings of glass and steel.

A brief sumary of some of the circadian rhythms of man's physiology may indicate what the consonance between body state and activity can mean. It is known that body temperature rises and falls about 1½ degrees every 24 hours. Temperature rises in the morning to a daytime plateau that again may dip in midafter-

	morning adrenal gland activity kidney excretion	
	midday wakefulness heart rate respiratory rate	body temperature physical vigor
	evening blood pressure body weight blood clotting ability	
	night cell division (mitosis) and replacement)	

Circadian rhythms

During the 24-hour day certain biological processes within man, the circadian rhythms, demonstrate a regularly recurring ebb and flow. Shown above is the time of peak activity for some of these processes.

noon. In an experiment conducted by Michel Siffre of the French Institute of Speleology a volunteer who lived 4½ months in a cave involuntarily established a 48-hour day but nonetheless demonstrated a stubborn 24-hour rhythm of body temperature. When tested around the clock, it was found that man's time sense expanded during the temperature peak and that this was the best time for vigilance, quick reactions to signals, and decision-making. On the other hand, it was observed that the weakest performance came around 3 A.M., when body temperature was at its cyclic low.

ADRENAL TIDES

A normal, healthy human being who sleeps at night will secrete more than 50% of his daily quota of adrenocortical hormones into his blood in the last three hours of sleep. Some acutely depressed persons observed in round-the-clock studies did not show this rhythm until health was restored; also the rhythm was less pronounced in persons with severe cataracts until the removal of the cataracts allowed them to experience again the influence of light and darkness.

These adrenal tides are responsible for differences in responses to stress, such as a quarrel or an emergency, occurring at 3 A.M. during low tide or at 7 A.M. at high tide. Sensations of vitality or fatigue, the speed with which food is metabolized, and the sensory perceptions are all influenced by the amounts of these important hormones available to the tissues and nervous system at a given time. An inverse relationship exists between sensory keenness and the concentration of steroid hormones such as hydrocortisone. In the morning when hormone levels are high, sensitivity to subtle gradients of taste, smell, or sound is not so acute as it is by evening. Indeed, low levels of adrenocortical hormones may be part of what usually is called fatigue, for low levels occur at the end of the day, causing the body to become oversensitive to sensory inputs.

One more possible corollary to this adrenal rhythm is worth mentioning particularly in the United States where so many people worry about overweight and where the heaviest eating and drinking occurs after 6 P.M. In round-the-clock studies in which heavy protein meals were eaten at different hours, blood levels of amino acids suggested that metabolism was more efficient in the morning. Therefore, morning or midday might be a better time to eat heavily.

A DIAGNOSTIC TOOL

Circadian rhythms, of little interest to the healthy person in his daily activities, are a useful diagnostic tool to a physician. For instance, the constituents of a person's blood change significantly during the day and if an accident occurs in the mid-to-late day blood will clot faster than in the early hours of morning. Immunity to viruses and infections is not equal at all hours because the level of the blood's gamma globulin (that fraction of serum containing the most antibodies) is lower in the early hours of morning that are usually passed in sleep. Since virtually no part of the body is exempt from the tides of chemistry, it could be a matter of life or death in some cases, as when an anesthesiologist must adjust a dosage for a fragile patient without knowing how quickly the liver can detoxify the toxic substance. Animal studies have shown that the use of a muscle relaxant could be fatal at certain phases of the animals' cycles. Subsequent studies indicated that the fatalities occurred at the phase when the liver enzymes called upon for detoxification were least active.

Relevant as these rhythms may be to human medicine, they are practically uncharted for man, and most of what is known comes from studies of rodents. Such research on the phase of a particular target organ could determine whether X rays, drugs, surgery, or a trauma is helpful, harmful, or lethal. Lawrence Scheving, by giving identical doses to identical groups of rats at two-hour intervals around the clock, demonstrated that a heavy dose of amphetamines does not cause the same reaction at every hour. At 3 A.M., the peak of the nocturnal rat's activity cycle, 78% of the animals died—yet at 6 A.M. the same dose killed only 6%.

What does this imply about the testing and use of drugs? Prescriptions and instructions on over-the-counter drugs seldom mention hazards at particular times of day, and we assume that all available drugs are equally safe or effective at all hours. However, a better knowledge of circadian rhythms would allow the physician to understand possible variation. Some doctors became sensitive to the need for timing medications in the late 1920s knowing, for instance, that a large dose of insulin might be helpful to a diabetic in mid-morning but might send him into coma at midnight. In other illnesses, such as Addison's disease where the person's adrenals could not produce sufficient hormones, Alain Reinberg and his co-workers in Paris showed that replacement with synthetic hormones is most efficacious if the dosage mimics the body's normal rhythm. Thus Parisian patients began taking their hormones in the morning, instead of adhering to a former schedule of equal doses.

Treating or accurately diagnosing a patient's ailment without knowing his body time could be difficult—it might be 2 P.M. in the clinic but 9 A.M. in the night-owl patient who just awakened. In the future, doctors may require patients to precede their visits to a clinic by keeping a diary of bodily functions, energy, and moods. With the help of computers, information could be assayed to determine whether a person is showing cyclic changes, periodic symptoms, or mood cycles that he generally blames on some external cause. Such a diary, developed at the Institute of Living, a Hartford, Conn., psychiatric hospital, uncovered patterns of recovery and drug reactions which never before had been noticed in hospital patients. A detailed diary could acquaint an individual with his own rhythms and provide a way to watch changes that might predict an oncoming virus [infection].

It seems inevitable that sophisticated modern medicine soon must incorporate concepts of rhythmicity in scheduling surgery and medication. Consider a heart transplant in which it has been discovered that the donor heart is beating with a circadian rhythm in a different phase than the tissue to which it is grafted. This raises a question as to whether organ transplants need a matching of recipient and donor rhythms. In the early 1960s a British biologist, Janet Harker, did experiments with cockroaches that suggested illness might be a consequence of conflicting internal rhythms. She hypothesized that the circadian activity rhythm of the cockroach was governed by a kind of "second brain," a neurosecretory ganglion, for when this was removed the creature no longer was active in a rhythmic manner relative to light and darkness. Moreover, when this second brain was transplanted into another cockroach, the recipient adopted the activity rhythm of the donor. When the two creatures were out of phase, the recipient would develop a tumor after the transplant; but this has not been replicated.

Cancer has been called a disease of mistiming by Franz Halberg of the University of Minnesota, and others, who observed that cancer cells not only multiply more rapidly than normal cells but also do not do so in the circadian rhythm of the surrounding tissue. A number of common ailments are related to failure of timing, the most common and recognizable being cardiac arrhythmia, and menstrual irregularity. Periodic agitation among mental patients revealed underlying abnormalities in adrenal rhythms, and slight desynchronism of phase relations among body functions may be the subtle harbinger of depression.

Health care, thus, seems destined to concern itself with job schedules, travel, and the timing of meals. At present, the busy executive or vacation traveler subjects himself to stress by flying across many time zones, and then forces himself to negotiate business at once or go sight-seeing in local time even when the body feels that it is the dead of night. Many airline pilots and seasoned travelers know that they can maintain their equilibrium if they hold to a stable home-time regimen on short trips, and on longer trips allow at least a couple of days for transition. Internal disruption is particularly unpleasant and lasting because body systems seem to take different amounts of time to return to their normal relationship with the activity and sleep cycle. Persons, such as students or shift workers, may disturb phase with no immediate consequences, but long-term effects are not known.

Biologists and physiologists have conjectured that long-term disruption or free running might cause later illness or shorten the lifespan. Halberg and his co-workers subjected a group of adult rats to a single inversion of their light-dark schedule each week (equivalent to a one-way flight to Japan) and found they had shortened the animals' lifespans by an average of 6%. Pitten-drigh and Dorothea Minis of Stanford University scheduled light and darkness so that groups of fruit flies lived 27-, 21-, and 24-hour days, while another group lived in continuous light. The flies on the 24-hour schedule lived the longest.

LARKS AND OWLS

It has been postulated that pilots and crews of aircraft flying east-west routes actually shorten their lifespans. There is no way of knowing whether this is true, although some aviation studies show greater psychosomatic and mood problems in such crews than in those flying north-south runs. A voluminous literature from aviation studies, isolation chambers, and Soviet and U.S. space studies suggests that certain individuals are much more resistant to the effects of rotating shifts or east-west travel than are others. Like Bunning's plants, humans do not show exactly the same free-running circadian period when they are in isolation—some living a 24.3-hour day, others a 25.6-hour. Individual-ity of tempo is most noticeable in the way people distribute their energy across the day: some rise swiftly like larks in the early part of the day, full of vitality and cheer but then turn limp and sleepy at evening parties; others awaken slowly and reach a crescendo of activity at night, resembling the owl. Partly these patterns may be due to an inherited time structure, but they also could reflect early training or psychological factors. Yet rats in their cages show distinctive energy patterns similar to the human larks and owls. These patterns offer an individual a rough guide for timing events to his hours of strength, and avoiding strain during hours of weakness.

German studies of pilots doing simulated flight problems dur-ing transatlantic flights demonstrated that those who made the most night errors also showed the greatest physiological and sub-jective day-to-night change. Phlegmatic, stable individuals, heavy pilots who were impervious to changing mealtimes, suffered the least from irregular schedules. Ironically, the professional group that endures the most time disruption is the medical. Institutions concerned with health, the hospitals and medical schools, subject students and staff to inordinately difficult schedules, and not even the sick person is spared from a curious logistics of meals, surgery, and medication that has little regard for body time.

STRESS AND ILLNESS

A link between stress and illness always seemed plausible, but this theory went unverified until the mid-1960s when compelling statistics gathered by Thomas Holmes and Richard Rahe, of the University of Washington, Seattle, were published showing that life stresses of a certain magnitude (death, marriage, divorce, new job, buying a house) preceded illnesses of a commensurate severity. One link between stress and subsequent illness may be the disruption of internal cycles during stress, the uncoupling of rhythms from their former phase relationships in the body.

Curt P. Richter, an early worker in psychology at Johns Hopkins, suggested that the shock of a virus or trauma might cause certain cycles that were normally out of phase to become synchronized, setting up a periodic beat in the tissue. Illness such as a nine-day swelling of the joints, periodic fevers, edema, or the better known phenomenon of manic-depression, could be attributed to this disruption. Richter also observed that certain drugs (such as the female hormone estradiol, or sulfamerazine) did not affect the 4–5 day cycle of female rats until after the drug was discontinued. Then two-thirds of his animals began to show long cycles (25 days) of lethargy and weight gain, alternating with activity and weight loss. Richter and other researchers later wondered whether antibiotics, hormones, and other drugs might leave a similar cyclic aftermath in human beings, as, for example, the menstrual irregularity that sometimes follows the discontinuation of birth control pills.

The stress of psychological suffering may, itself, jostle internal rhythms so that their abnormal phase relationships place strain on organs or behavior. A series of experiments at the Institute of Living offered some insight into the way emotional and psychosomatic illnesses may develop. Charles F. Stroebel of the Institute of Living discovered that rats showed a fear response to a particular signal at a certain phase of their circadian adrenal cycle. After the fear training he noticed that a number of the animals had lost their regular 24-hour temperature peak 15 to 20 minutes later each day. After about 20 days these nocturnal animals were in a state of readiness for sleep at the hour when darkness fell in the laboratory, putting them biologically at odds with the demands of their natural environment. Moreover, monkeys that had been exposed to stresses related to loud noise or shock later showed reverberations in their bodies when left alone in their cages. Even after 28 days they re-experienced the stresses, shallow breathing and blood acidosis, at roughly the time of the original experiment. Biologists conjectured that there must be some kind of time memory in tissue, and experimented with certain organs and glands to demonsttrate this belief. An excised heart, kept in artificial nutriment, continued to accelerate and decelerate its beat, secretion, and neural responses as if it were continuing the circadian rhythm of the donor. Perhaps such memories of stress are also responsible for elusive medical symptoms, recurring at the hour when an unpleasant event had taken place.

Stroebel's experiments subsequent to the fear training in rats are worth citing in enough detail so that their possible interpretation for human illness is clear, since they demonstrate that a seemingly mild behavioral stress can cause a shift in rhythms resulting in illness. First the monkeys learned to obtain food pellets by pushing a lever to discriminate among images on a panel. Although subjected to loud noises or flashing lights, they quickly learned to turn them off by pressing another lever, clinging to the lever like a child clutching a security blanket. The annoyances then were stopped and the lever recessed in such a way that it could not be grasped. The removal of their "security level" panicked the monkeys and 14 days later they became sick.

About half of the animals resembled neurotic, psychosomatically ill humans, while the others seemed to resemble psychotics. The first sign of illness was that the reliable 24-hour brain temperature rhythm developed a longer period (24.5 hours) in the "neurotic" animals, who shifted slowly out of synchronization with their environment, doing poorly at their discrimination task. Sores on the skin and bloody stools appeared, and finally ulcers so severe that two of the monkeys later died. The other "psychotic" animals leaped from a 24-hour brain temperature rhythm to a cycle of 48 hours: they seemed out of contact with the environment, and spent their time catching imaginary insects, or masturbating, paying no attention to their tasks, to food, or to people. All of the animals suffered from insomnia, inevitable since their bodies were out of phase with light and darkness in the laboratory. When two animals from each group were given back the security lever, the neurotic animals began to recover and show their 24-hour temperature rhythm, but the psychotic animals remained out of touch, unchanged. Tranquilizers and antidepressant drugs, pulsed into the disturbed animals at 12-hour intervals, slowly began to bring them around to their 24-hour temperature rhythm. Once the temperature rhythm returned they began to act more normally.

EFFECTS OF LIGHT

Would it seem that the individual's harmony cannot be separated from the environment, particularly the alteration of night and day, the effects of light and darkness? Is it not apparent that man's own cycles are synchronized with those of earth, as are those of plants and birds through the potent effects of light? Plants count the seasons by registering the ratio of light and darkness as the days shorten into fall and lengthen into spring, a process known as photoperiodism. Some are triggered to bud by short days and long nights, some by long days and brief nights. Light inhibits or stimulates growth and budding, depending upon when it occurs in the plant's internal oscillation. Birds respond to the changing seasons by the ratio of light and darkness which penetrates the brain and affects a light-sensitive gland, the pineal. This mythical gland, sometimes known as a vestigial third eye that can be seen protruding on the skulls of lizards, responds to light by manufacturing certain neurochemicals, which in turn modify the reproductive system. Thus birds of temperate zones receive the message of increasing light, become sexually ready for mating, and migrate in a direction that is related to their hormonal state.

In the human being and other mammals, the pineal gland is buried deep within the brain, and may respond to indirect nerve messages of light. A decade of research on the pineal gland, and on the differential responses of birds to different wavelengths of light, suggests that human endocrine systems may be more influenced by seasonal light changes and by artificial light than might have been recognized. Sunlight, one of the most important cosmic forces, and artificial light, too, may guide man's physiology, for he is an open system, a being who resonates to the harmonies of earth and space whether or not his philosophy considers this possibility.

Technology is permitting man to venture into space, but he remains relatively ignorant about his own time structure and the extent to which he resonates to the clock of the earth and the solar system. What is called a physiological clock may be a collection of oscillators that tend to respond to the rhythms of earth. The time structure is only partly within the skin of the body, and the body cannot detach itself from the beat of the natural environment, even in cities of steel and glass where the time of day is a matter of choice. Internal timing may be the organization that knits together the human race, and binds it firmly to the earth and vast universe beyond.

BIBLIOGRAPHY

Colquhoun, W. P., ed. *Biological Rhythms and Human Performance.* New York: Academic Press, 1971.

Conroy, R. T. W. L., and Mills, J. N. *Human Circadian Rhythms.* Edinburgh: J. & A. Churchill, 1970.

Fraser, J. T., ed. *The Voices of Time.* New York: George Braziller, 1966.

Luce, Gay. *Body Time.* New York: Pantheon Books, 1971.

Sweeney, Beatrice M. *Rhythmic Phenomena in Plants.* New York: Academic Press, 1969.

Ward, Ritchie R. *The Living Clocks.* New York: Alfred A. Knopf, 1971.

By *Albert P. Krueger and David S. Sobel*

Air Ions and Health

In places where mountains are situated to the south, the
south winds that blow are parching and unhealthy; where
the mountains are situated to the north, there northern
winds occasion disorders and sickness . . . The winds which
must pass over mountains to reach cities do not only dry, but
also disturb the air which we breathe and the bodies of men,
so as to engender diseases.

Hippocrates, *Regimen II,* Chapters 37–38

The reactions between water, land and air during the long, slow
physical evolution of our planet have greatly affected the course
of biological evolution. To a very considerable extent this interplay is responsible for the emergence of man—a singular product
of evolution—and man, in an extremely brief span of time,
through his genius for blindly manipulating natural resources,
has attained the unique capacity to alter his total environment.
While we have begun to express serious concern for the grim consequences of our role as spoilers in disturbing ecological balances
in general, our interest is most avidly focused upon those facets of
man-engendered pollution which pose the most immediate and
direct danger to us.

We live in an ocean of air and each of us is inexorably required
to breathe in at least ten thousand liters of air every twenty-four
hours just to maintain life in our bodies. Since we are utterly dependent upon the physical and chemical properties of this air,
it isn't surprising that we now are deeply immersed in exploring

all atmospheric parameters. Characteristically, most of our efforts are devoted to the detection and control of those toxic particulates and gases contributed to the ambient air by industry and by the multitude of anthropocentric activities which require the combustion of fuels. Their threat to life is pressing and it is obvious that measures for their abatement must be developed in the immediate future. Other, more subtle atmospheric changes are in progress which, because they are less conspicuous, tend to be put aside for future consideration. Among these, one would have to list those phenomena involving small air ions.

Very shortly after the existence of atmospheric electricity was demonstrated by Franklin [1] and by d'Alibard [2] in the mid-1700s, several natural philosophers ascribed to it a variety of biological effects. For example, Father Giambattista Beccaria [3] in 1775 reported that "it appears manifest that nature makes extensive use of the atmospheric electricity for promoting vegetation." In this he was supported by Abbé Nollet [4] and Abbé Bertholon [5]. Abbé Bertholon [6] in addition concluded that the course of various diseases of man was influenced by atmospheric electricity. In 1899, Elster and Geitel [7] and J. J. Thompson [8] independently proved that atmospheric electricity depends upon the existence of gaseous ions in the air. It then became possible to develop generators for producing air ions and equipment for determining their numbers in the air. Using these technical aids, a vast amount of experimentation was undertaken to define the physical and biological properties of air ions.

There are ions in the air around us all the time, but changes in their concentration, or in the ratio of positively to negatively charged molecules, can have marked biological effects on plants and animals. Indeed, ion depletion and charge imbalance may play a significant role in a wide range of human ailments including respiratory infection in office workers and the malaise caused by weather conditions such as the khamsin winds of the Near East. Further, artificially generated air ions may prove valuable as a therapeutic modality in the treatment of burns, respiratory disorders, stomach ulcers, and nervous disorders.

Air ion formation begins when enough energy acts on a gaseous molecule to eject an electron. Most of this energy comes from radioactive substances in Earth's crust and some from the shearing forces of water droplets in waterfalls (Lenard effect) or the friction which develops when great volumes of air move rapidly over a land mass (for example, the foehn, sharav, and Santa Ana winds) or from cosmic rays. The displaced electron attaches itself to an adjacent molecule, which becomes a negative ion, the original molecule then becoming a positive ion. Molecular collisions transfer the charge, so that positive charges come to reside on molecules with the lowest ionization potential, while electrons are attracted to the species of greatest stability. Next, small numbers of molecules of water vapor, hydrogen, and oxygen cluster about the ions to form small air ions. In normal pollutant-free air over land, there are 1500 to 4000 ions/cm^3. But negative ions are more mobile and Earth's surface has a negative charge, so negative ions are repelled from the earth's surface. Thus the normal ratio of positive to negative ions is 1.2 to 1.

Certain properties of small air ions are pertinent to this discussion. They readily unite with condensation nuclei and with most classes of air pollutants to form large or Langevin ions. In both cases the biological activity of the small air ions is lost. This is true also of the combination that occurs between small air ions of opposite charge. Further, ions of like charge (unipolar ions) repel one another and tend to flow to enclosing surfaces where their ionic nature dissipates. Since they are small and carry a charge, they are deflected by electrical fields. All of these characteristics make it difficult to maintain high concentrations of small air ions and means that air ion densities are significantly altered by the indoor living and air pollution characteristic of urban life.

While the nature of air ions was under investigation by the physicists, vigorous attempts were being made by the life scientists to determine their biological effects. Although the amount of work accomplished by the biologists is a tribute to their industry, it must be admitted that many of the results reported in the literature are not convincing. Several factors in the area of experimental design served to cloak the whole field in an aura of ambiguity. Often experiments were performed with corona discharges as ion sources, neglecting the ozone and oxides of nitrogen sometimes produced along with the ions. Ion densities, temperature, and relative humidity were not monitored. Experimental subjects were not grounded; their external surfaces developed high electrostatic charges and, in consequence, repelled ions. As a rule, the air was not purified and combination of ions with air pollutants led to widely fluctuating ion densities. Clinicians assessing the value of air ions as a therapeutic modality frequently committed all or some of the errors listed above and, in addition, neglected to utilize the double-blind cross-over technique for ion administration. In view of these omissions it is not surprising that convincing proof of the role played by air ions as physiological mediators or as therapeutic agents has been slow to emerge.

In addition to these elements of uncertainty in experimental procedures, the evaluation of air ions as biologically active agents has been hampered by the widely cultivated belief that the idea is theoretically absurd. There seems to be something about the term "ion" that provokes incredulity—consider the fate of Svante Arrhenius, who first applied it in 1884 to describe atoms and molecules in aqueous solution bearing a positive or negative charge, which enabled them to migrate in an electrical field. His doctoral committee thought this idea so bizarre that they accepted his work with the greatest reluctance and granted his degree with the lowest possible grade. The major obstacle to acceptance of this magnificent concept was the requirement that fundamental differences in the properties of charged molecules (ions) and uncharged molecules be acknowledged. In the case of air ions there is no disagreement about the disparate physical nature of air ions and nonionized gaseous molecules, but there is considerable reluctance to grant that this diversity is of biological significance.

At any rate, the essence of the argument against biologically active air ions is this: The maximal ion density one can attain in a closed atmosphere is approximately 1×10^6 ions/cm^3 of air. Air contains 2.7×10^{19} nonionized molecules/cm^3, so that the ratio of small ions to nonionized molecules is 1:27 trillion. For the reasons already mentioned above, ions have a very brief life span and under the conditions ordinarily prevailing, attainable ion densities usually are considerably less than 1×10^6 ions/cm^3, making the final dilution in nonionized air greater by one or two orders of magnitude. From this unquestioned fact, the dubious conclusion has been drawn that the very sparseness of air ions places them beyond the range of biological effectiveness. The merit of this inference is more specious than real, since many biological systems respond to extremely minute chemical and physical stimuli. Two examples suffice to bear out this contention: first, the human eye can detect a flash of light when a single active quantum reaches the retina [9]; and second, the male silkworm reacts to as few as 2600 molecules of the female's sex-attractant pheromone in air containing a concentration of <200 molecules/cm^3 [10].

One further factor, that of commercial exploitation, has retarded development in the field of air ionization. During the mid-1950s air ion generators were sold directly to the public through high-powered advertising campaigns extolling their efficacy in treating a wide variety of diseases. The Federal Drug Administration brought these activities to a halt and since then has prohibited the sale of ion generators for any medical applications. This unfortunate episode has led scientists and laymen alike to conclude that the whole subject is permeated with misrepresentation or even outright fraud.

It is evident then that progress in the field of research devoted to the detection of air ion effects on living forms has been retarded by the very real difficulties attending the performance of meaningful experiments, by an unhappy example of commercial exploitation, and by the categorical rejection of the whole idea as a matter of principle on the part of many competent scientists. The technical obstacles are the major reason that we now are faced with an enormous accumulation of data of very uneven quality. The matter of rejection is not so vital, although it is disconcerting at times to find that some of our peers classify the subject with the occult arts.

THE BIOLOGICAL EFFECTS OF AIR IONS

The experimental observations taken as a whole serve to establish the fact that air ions are physiologically active and can produce functional alterations varying from barely discernible to substantial. Further, air ions are capable of evoking a wide range of response in bacteria, protozoa, higher plants, insects, animals, and man. Sometimes both positive and negative ions induce essentially the same biological reaction, in other cases they elicit opposite effects. A few selected examples will be presented to illustrate the range of biological effects of small air ions and the reader is referred to more detailed reviews of the experimental evidence [11, 12, 13].

A brief review of the effects of air ions on microorganisms reveals that both negative and positive ions (1) inhibit the growth of bacteria and fungi on solid media, (2) exert a lethal effect on vegetative forms of bacteria suspended in small droplets of water, and (3) reduce the viable count of bacterial aerosols [12].

With mammalian cells in tissue culture, Worden found that Girardi's human heart cells exposed for fourteen days to unipolar ionized atmospheres and then transplanted into nonionized atmospheres for an additional fourteen days showed adversely affected growth characteristics and rate of proliferation with positively ionized air; growth was normal with negatively ionized air. Using fibroblasts he obtained statistically significant evidence that negative ions increase and positive ions decrease the rate of proliferation. Furthermore when the fibroblasts were removed to a nonionized atmosphere, the cells previously exposed to negative ions continued to divide at an increased rate, while the cells treated with positive ions recovered slowly and eventually attained the normal rate of growth [14].

Over the past nineteen years, the Air Ion Laboratory of the University of California has conducted experiments to detect ion-induced physiological changes in plants and small animals. The subjects were maintained in a controlled microenvironment supplied with pollutant-free air, the sole variable being concentration of air ions in the ambient atmosphere. Soft β (beta) emission from tritium adsorbed on zirconium served to ionize the air without evolving toxic by-products; selection of positive or negative ions was accomplished by applying a corresponding charge to the generator electrode.

Plants appear to benefit from increases in both positive and negative ionization, and we have shown that such ionization markedly increases the rate of growth of higher plants such as barley, oats, and lettuce. With seedlings grown in chemically defined media, we found that unipolar (one charge only) ionized atmospheres containing approximately 10,000 positive or negative ions/cm³ increased the rate of growth by as much as 50 percent (as measured by integral elongation or weight), without altering the protein, sugar, or chlorophyll content of the plant. In marked contrast to growth stimulation elicited by air ions, their removal from the atmosphere resulted in a lower rate of growth, reduced turgor (pressure in plant cells), and the development of soft, fleshy leaves. Chlorophyll production was not affected [15]. Several clues to the biochemical mechanism were uncovered. Positive and negative ions expedite both the uptake of iron and its utilization in the production of ion-containing enzymes. The ions stimulate the metabolism of the high-energy compound adenosine triphosphate (ATP) in the chloroplasts and augment both nucleic acid metabolism and oxygen uptake. All of these phenomena are consistent with the observed ion-induced increase in growth rate.

Similar results were obtained when silkworm eggs and emergent larvae were exposed to ions of either charge. Hatching began earlier, larval growth accelerated, and there was increased synthesis of three enzymes (catalase, peroxidase, and cytochrome C oxidase). Spinning began earlier and cocoons were heavier [16].

Much of the work we have done with animals has been on air ion effects in the respiratory tract, and we found that air ions influence survival in respiratory diseases. High concentrations of positive ions substantially increased the death rate of mice infected with measured doses of a fungus (*Coccidoides immitis*), a bacterium (*Klebsiella pneumoniae*), or a strain of influenza virus, all administered intranasally. Ion depleted air (comparable to ion concentrations found in urban environments) also increased the death rate in mouse influenza, while a high concentration of negative ions decreased the death rate [17]. In other experiments where the influenza virus was introduced as a fine aerosol, this by-passing the protective mechanisms of the upper respiratory tract, changing ion concentrations had no influence on the death rate. This and other observations suggest that the site of action of air ions is the mucosa of the upper respiratory tract [18].

MECHANISM OF AIR ION ACTION

With regard to the mechanism underlying the response of animals to air ions, we have worked for several years on the changes in blood levels of serotonin (5-hydroxytryptamine, or 5-Ht), a powerful neurohormone capable of producing profound neurovascular, endocrine, and metabolic effects throughout the body. In the hypothalamus 5-Ht participates in various processes such as sleep, the transmission of nerve impulses, and in our evaluation of mood. We found a readily reproducible and significant change in blood 5-Ht levels in mice exposed to air ion densities of $4-5 \times 10^5$ positive or negative ions/cm^3. Positive ions raised blood levels of 5-Ht, while negative ions had the opposite effect. Additionally, we found that the brain content of free 5-Ht was responsive to the concentration of ions in the air. Because the chief metabolic route for removing serotonin (5-Ht) depends upon the enzyme monamine oxidase, we hypothesized that small negative ions stimulate, while small positive ions block the action of monamine oxidase, thus producing respectively a drop or rise in the concentration of free 5-Ht in certain tissues and eliciting a corresponding physiological response [19].

This general mechanism of air ion action has been confirmed by other investigators. Grant Gilbert at Pacific Lutheran University demonstrated that continuous treatment with negative ions produced statistically significant reductions in emotionality and brain serotonin levels in rats [20]. Jean-Michel Olivereau of the Psychophysiology Laboratory at the University of Paris conducted extensive experiments on the endocrine systems and the nervous mechanisms of rats treated for various periods of time with air ions [21, 22]. Employing elegant biochemical and histochemical techniques, he surveyed air ion action on the hypothalamus, the hypophysis, the adrenals, the thyroid, brain metabolism, behavior, eating, spontaneous activity, psychomotor performance and adaptation to stress. He concluded that air ion–induced alterations in blood levels of 5-Ht account for very significant physiological changes in the endocrine glands and central nervous systems, these, in turn, substantially alter basic physiological processes. A significant facet to Olivereau's research is his observation that negative ions exert a measurable anxiety-lessening effect on mice and rats exposed to stressful situations, a phenomenon noted by several other workers [23]. This response parallels that which follows administration to animals or man of the drug reserpine. Both reserpine and negative ions reduce the amount of serotonin in the mid-brain and this apparently accounts for the tranquilizing action.

Direct and indirect evidence supporting the theory that 5-Ht is an important mediator of air ion action on animals and humans is found in the reports of several investigators [24, 25] and is reviewed elsewhere [26, 27]. However, there is no reason to suppose that 5-Ht is the sole agent responsible for air ion–induced alteration of physiological function.

Such tentative biochemical probings are really no more than a first step in elucidating the arcane mechanisms of air ion action. We badly need to know what happens when air ions make contact with the tissues of the test organism. Our ignorance extends from the interface between the atmosphere and the cell wall to include the cellular organelles, their component enzyme systems, and almost all the tissues and organs of living forms. When we turn to the matter of air ion dosage necessary to elicit biological responses, the situation is somewhat better. Dosage constitutes a very practical element, for if extremely high ion densities are demanded, there is little likelihood of air ions playing a significant role in nature and the whole topic becomes academic or, at best, is limited to therapeutic applications. If, on the other hand, biological effects are associated with such displacements of ion densities or charge ratios as are known to occur in Earth's atmosphere, or even with relatively small shifts in ion concentrations that can be affected by ion depletion or artificial ionization in ordinary living and working quarters, the subject acquires great interest and importance.

An outstanding example of dependence of physiological response upon dosage has been reported by Bachman and his co-workers [24]. In studying the influence of air ions on the spontaneous activity of rats they noticed a curious zonal response with activity levels falling, rising, and peaking and then falling again as negative ion concentrations were increased.

Several studies, however, have demonstrated marked biological effects with lower dosage approximating natural conditions (1.5×10^3 to 4×10^3 small ions/cm³). In the experiments of Knoll and his collaborators on the effects of ions on simple visual reaction time in humans, ion concentrations of only 2×10^3 ions/cm³ produced a remarkable decrease in reaction time [28]. Deleanu and his colleagues found that relatively small ion dosages, for example, 5×10^3 to 15×10^3 ions/cm³ of air effectively influenced the development of gastric ulcers in starving rats [29]. Silverman and Kornblueh were able to detect changes in alpha frequencies of the EEG in humans exposed to only 1.8×10^3 positive or negative ions/cm³ for thirty minutes [30]. Also, a sudden increase in negative ions or a precipitate drop in positive ions within the atmospheric range of 1×10^3 to 2×10^3 ions/cm³ was reported to increase moulting in aphids [31].

In our studies mentioned above on the effect of air ions on the course of mouse influenza produced by intranasal challenge, we found that ion dosage influenced the cumulative mortality rate. Unipolar low densities of positive or negative ions (comparable to indoor and urban environments) increased the rate of death, mid-range concentrations of ions of either charge had no effect, while a reduction in mortality rates occurred when the animals were exposed to high concentrations of negative or to low concentrations of mixed ions with negative ions predominating [17].

NATURAL ION ENVIRONMENTS

We have already presented evidence that air ion concentrations comparable to those found in nature can modify physiological processes in a variety of living forms under laboratory conditions. Now it seems appropriate to ask, Do air ion–linked phenomena occur in humans outside the laboratory? This question can be answered affirmatively with some assurance in light of recent investigations of large-scale weather-related changes in air ion concentrations and charge ratios coupled with concurrent clinical studies.

To begin with, a great deal of work has been done in France,

Italy, Germany, and the U.S.S.R. on the ionic environment of spas, particularly those situated near waterfalls. The consensus seems to be that the air in many such locales, for whatever reason, contains a high concentration of small air ions with a ratio of negative to positive ions being considerably greater than normal —the Lenard effect. Bioclimatologists are inclined to attribute to this fact some of the *vis mediatrix* of these resorts. This is an attractive hypothesis, but one that is difficult to prove, since many curative modalities are brought to bear on patients simultaneously.

Turning to the adverse effects associated with certain ion environments, there have long been traditions in the folklore of nearly every country that link certain changes in weather with changes in health and behavior. One such tradition has to do with the winds of ill repute, for example, the foehn (southern Europe), sirocco (Italy), Santa Ana (United States), khamsin (Near East), and mistral (France). Wherever they prevail, their victims attribute to them the ability to induce respiratory distress of various sorts, nervousness, headache, and a multitude of other ills. So malign is their influence that when they blow, judges deal leniently with crimes of passion, surgeons postpone elective surgery, and teachers expect more than the usual fractiousness from their students.

Since the turn of the century several scientists and physicians have hypothesized that the immediate cause of such malaise is the upset in electrical balance of the atmosphere that precedes or accompanies the winds. This relationship between air ions and disease, tenuous at first, is finding support in the meteorological observations of investigators such as Robinson and Dirnfeld who studied the sharav, a weather complex afflicting the Near East and characterized by persistent wind, a rapid rise in temperature and a fall in relative humidity. Robinson and Dirnfeld measured solar radiation, temperature, relative humidity, wind velocity and direction, and the electrical state of the atmosphere before, during and after the sharav. They found that 12 to 36 hours before the characteristic changes in wind, temperature, and humidity, the total number of ions increased (from 1500 ions/cm^3 to 2600 ions/cm^3) and the ratio of positive to negative ions jumped from the normal 1.2 to 1.33. This early shift in ion density and ratio coincided with the onset of nervous and physical symptoms in weather-sensitive people and was considered the only meteorological change that could be responsible for the discomfort associated with the sharav [32].

This conclusion is supported by the extensive studies of Professor Felix Sulman and his colleagues in Jerusalem. They designate as the "serotonin hyperfunction syndrome" the cluster of signs and symptoms that afflict a considerable segment of the population a day or two before the onset of the hot, dry wind characteristic of the sharav. Individuals in this category suffer from insomnia, irritability, tension, migraine, amblyopia, edema, palpitations, precordial pain, respiratory distress, hot flashes, tremor, chills, diarrhea, polyuria, vertigo, etc. These patients display an increased output of serotonin in the urine and they experienced relief when treated with negative ions or with serotonin-blocking drugs [33, 34]. There exists, then, a scientific basis for accepting the tradition that the winds of ill repute can produce malaise in humans, that air ion imbalance is the direct meteorological incitant and that the proximate cause of the irritation syndrome is the positive air-ion-induced hypersecretion of serotonin.

Supporting laboratory evidence for the adverse effect in humans of air ion imbalances comes from a well-controlled double-blind experiment by Winsor and Beckett in which volunteer subjects developed a dry throat, husky voice, headache, itchy or obstructed nose, and a reduction in maximum breathing capacity when exposed to nasal inhalation of positive ions in concentrations of 3.2×10^4 ions/cm^3 [35].

AIR IONS AND THE
HUMAN URBAN ENVIRONMENT

In modern urban life man often faces ion conditions far different from natural ion balances, with a significant depletion of small air ions and a markedly increased ratio of positive to negative ions commonly encountered. A fourteen-day study in 1971 by B. Maczyński and others showed that in an office containing four people the small air ion concentration dropped as the day went on, falling on the average to only 34 positive ions and 20 negative ions/cm³ [36]. Central heating and air conditioning, smoking, the usual household activities of dusting and cooking all combine to lower levels of small ions in indoor environments. Further, the static electricity generated by the widespread use of synthetic fibers in clothing and room furnishing as well as stray electric fields add a different dimension to the indoor climate which is not conducive to the preservation of small air ions [37].

The effects of air pollution on air ions in the ambient atmosphere are also marked. As stated earlier, the small physiologically active air ions readily combine with gaseous and particulate pollutants to form large (Langevin) ions that are considered physiologically inert. A test in a light industrial area of San Francisco by J. C. Beckett in 1959 showed a small ion count of less than 80 ions/cm³ as compared to levels of 1500–4000 small ions/cm³ found in fresh unpolluted air [38].

The fundamental reaction is disarmingly simple: man → atmospheric pollutants; atmospheric pollutants + small air ions → air ion depletion.

That this progression has attained significant magnitude is evidenced by the fact that small air ion levels far at sea—normally very constant—are becoming appreciably lower with time, as air pollutants drift out from land. Thus while very few of our activities add small ions to the air, much of what we do culminates in ion loss. The question then amounts to this: Will the smogs, hazes, and invisible pollutants we generate with a lavish hand so reduce the small ion content of the atmosphere that plants, animals, and man must suffer harmful consequences?

Although the early results of ion depletion very likely will be unimpressive compared to the immediate and dramatic action of known toxic components of polluted air, this alone should furnish little solace. We have every reason to be aware from past experience that adverse effects may follow continued exposure to a small amount of a minor irritant (for example, organic solvents) or the long-term deprivation of an essential metabolic requirement (for example, trace elements or vitamins). People traveling to work in polluted air, spending eight hours a day in offices or factories, and living their leisure hours in urban dwellings inescapably breathe ion-depleted air for substantial portions of their lives. There is increasing evidence that this ion depletion leads to discomfort, enervation and lassitude, and loss of mental and physical efficiency. This syndrome appears to develop quite apart from the direct toxic effects of the usual atmospheric pollutants.

Physicians and environmental engineers have long suspected that the inimical effects of "dead air" in crowded rooms are due to ion depletion. In 1939, three Japanese scientists, S. Kimura, M. Ashiba, and L. Matsushima, showed that if temperature, humidity, and carbon-dioxide levels were all kept within ranges considered suitable for human comfort, but the ion level was reduced, individuals suffered from symptoms such as perspiration and depression. Further, these symptoms were promptly relieved when normal ion densities were restored by the use of ion generators [39]. Recently a team of Soviet scientists tested the effects of varying ion conditions on humans employing an impressive battery of tests to measure cardiovascular functioning, reaction time, and blood chemistry. They concluded that any enclosed compartments with "conditioned" air such as a space capsule, are likely to be depleted of ions and have a considerable excess of positive ions and that prolonged stays in such an ion environment is detrimental. The Soviet scientists recommended that ionization in such environments be increased to a more normal 2000 ions/cm^3 and that the addition of negative ions be alternated with positive or bipolar ionization [40]. The effect of various ion concentrations and charge ratios on human performance, reaction time, vigilance, and psychomotor tasks is suggestive but inconclusive and has been reviewed elsewhere [41].

ARTIFICIAL ION GENERATION:
CLINICAL APPLICATIONS

So much for the potential role of an air ion–depleted environment in man's future. There remains the more promising consideration of the environmental and medical applications of artificially generated air ions. At present there exists several means of artificially producing air ions, including corona discharge and tritium generators. These ion generators make it possible to re-establish natural and optimal microclimatic conditions in living and working quarters. Eventually air ion standards for comfort and health may be established, just as we now have set limits for temperature, relative humidity, carbon dioxide levels, etc. It may also be possible to make available highly beneficial, ion-rich microenvironments that could serve various hygienic and therapeutic functions. However, the development and use of this technology must go hand in hand with efforts to reduce air pollution from industry, automobiles, and tobacco smoke, which effectively interfere with attempts to create a balanced ionized atmosphere.

If the results of our experiments with respiratory disease in mice can be extrapolated to man, we might expect that the ion-depleted air of our offices and factories would lower resistance to influenza and perhaps other infections. Conversely, inhaling a mixture of air with, say, 4000 ions/cm^3, and with negative ions predominating, should increase resistance. A recent study in a Swiss bank indicated that this is so. In the test, 309 volunteers worked for thirty weeks in an area where the air was treated to develop a high ratio of negative to positive ions, while 362 controls worked in untreated air. During the test the ratio of days lost because of respiratory illness in the two groups was an incredible 1 to 16 [42].

Finally, one can look at some medical applications of high ion concentrations. Kornblueh and his colleagues have used negative ion therapy successfully for burn patients. Hospitalized patients were treated for 1 to 1½ hours a day, and out-patients for twenty-five to thirty minutes, to negative ion concentrations as high as 10,000 ions/cm^3. Pain, restlessness, and incidence of infection were reduced and healing promoted [43]. This application may be related to the serotonin hypothesis of air ion action. Burn patients present increased levels of serotonin (5-hydroxytryptamine) in damaged tissues and in the blood, and serotonin is known to be associated with pain under some circumstances. We have shown in laboratory animals that inhalation of negative ions increases the conversion of serotonin to 5-hydroxyindolacetic acid (a physiologically inactive metabolite), and this reaction may be involved in the relief of pain reported by burn patients treated with high concentrations of negative ions.

Another instance of laboratory observations coinciding with clinical usage is to be found in our work at the University of California and that of Palti, De Nour, and Abrahamov at Hadassah Medical School in Jerusalem. Smith and Krueger noted that the inhalation of positively ionized air by small animals contracted the smooth muscle of the tracheo-bronchial tree and decreased the operational efficiency of the mucus escalator, effects that could be duplicated by the intravenous injection of 5-HT; negative ions had the opposite effect [44]. Palti and his colleagues found that exposure to positive ions increased the respiratory rate and degree of bronchospasm in infants with asthmatic (spastic) bronchitis while treatment with negative ions produced an opposite and therapeutic effect. The negative ion therapy terminated the spastic attack after a much shorter period than that required by the conventional mode of treatment, and, in addition, no adverse side effects, common to the drug therapy, were observed with the negative ionization. Further, since the subjects in this experiment were infants under the age of one year, the possibility that the observed effects were due to psychological factors was minimized [45].

P. C. Boulatov, a Soviet investigator, has summarized his experiment work of the past thirty-five years involving the treatment of over 3,000 bronchial asthma patients with high concentrations of negative ions. He has reported that after a short period of temporary exacerbation there followed substantial improvement in the general state of the patients, a normalization of the blood picture, improved respiratory function, and a reduction in the frequency and intensity of attacks of bronchial asthma [46].

Kornblueh, the pioneer American investigator of air ion phenomena, and his coworkers obtained temporary relief of acute hay fever symptoms in patients treated with high concentrations of negative air ions. They speculated that the mode of action might be due to some physical and/or chemical effect on microscopic airborne contaminants such as dust, spores, bacteria, and pollen or to a direct physiological action on the respiratory tract [47].

More recently, Dr. A. P. Wehner reported on a closely related therapeutic modality: electroaerosols, in which minute water droplets act as a vehicle for electric charges. This therapy, used extensively in Germany and the U.S.S.R., has reportedly been applied with success in the treatment of respiratory disorders and various manifestations of autonomic dysfunction such as migraine, nervous tension, and depression [48]. Wehner also reviewed the work of K. H. Schulz, who found that negatively charged aerosols seem to stimulate the parasympathetic nervous system and therefore can help to restore autonomic balance in cases of an overstimulated activation. From these observations Schulz postulated that the effect of the ions would depend upon the state of activation of the autonomic nervous system and, further, that if the proper charge of ions is administered to a given ion "type" individual a normalization of autonomic functioning would occur [49].

In line with this theory were the findings of Monaco and Acker, who performed a large number of tests on a group of psychiatric patients and a group of nonpatients. In the psychiatric patients negative ionization decreased systolic blood pressure, increased skin resistance, and increased pulse finger volume, indicating increased parasympathetic nervous system activity. For the nonpatients only a significant decrease in pulse finger volume occurred, indicating slight increase in sympathetic nervous system activity. Thus, it appears that the negative ions had a normalizing influence, lowering activation of the psychiatric patients and increasing the activation of the nonpatients [50].

Noting the relationship between air ions and neurohormones and following the reports that negative ions produce a sedative effect, R. Ucha Udabe, R. Kertész, and L. Franceschetti at the Catholic University in Buenos Aires tried treating a large number of patients suffering from psychoneurosis and anxiety syndromes. Sessions varied from fifteen minutes to two hours and the number of treatments from ten to twenty. These authors were very impressed with the conspicuous disappearance of somatic complaints and claimed favorable results in 80 percent of their patients [51]. M. Deleanu also claims success in the treatment of gastroduodenal ulcers in animals and man using relatively low dosages of air ions (5000 to 10,000 negative ions/cm^3 and 1000–2000 positive ions/cm^3) [52].

This is only a brief review of some of the developing areas of clinical research. But based upon the evidence surveyed in this paper, it appears that air ion investigations constitute a legitimate and promising branch of biological research. As more information is acquired about the mechanisms underlying the reactions between air ions and living systems, we should be able to evaluate more clearly than at present the importance of air ions in nature and assess their potential for clinical and nonclinical applications.

REFERENCES

1. B. Franklin, *Phil. Trans.* 47 (1752):289.
2. T. F. D'Alibard, *Letter to Académie de Science* 3 (1752).
3. G. Beccaria, *Della Elettricità Terrestre Atmosferica a Cielo Sereno*, (Torino, 1775).
4. Abbé Nollet, *Mémoires d'Académie Royale de Science* (Paris, 1752).
5. Abbé P. Bertholon, *De l'électricité des végétaux* (Paris, 1783).
6. Abbé P. Bertholon, *De l'électricité du corps humain dans l'état de santé et de maladie* (Lyon, Bernuset, 1780).
7. J. Elster and H. Geitel, "Uber die Existenx Elektrischer Ionen in der Atmosphäre," *Terrestr. Magazin* 4 (1899).
8. J. J. Thompson, "On the Charge of Electricity Carried by the Ions Produced by Röntgen Rays," *Phil. Mag.* 46 (1898):528–45.
9. M. H. Pirenne, Photobiology Group Meeting at Oxford University, in *Office of Naval Research European Scientific Notes* 12 (1958): 11.
10. W. H. Bossert and E. O. Wilson, "The Analysis of Olfactory Communication among Animals," *Journal of Theoretical Biology* 5 (1963):443–69.
11. A. P. Krueger, "Preliminary Consideration of the Biological Significance of Air Ions," *Scientia* 104 (September–October 1969): 1–17.
12. A. P. Krueger, "The Biological Effects of Gaseous Ions," in *Bioclimatology, Biometeorology, and Aeroionotherapy*, R. Gualtierotti, I. H. Kornblueh, C. Sirtori, eds. (Milan: Carlo Erba Foundation, 1968).

13. G. R. Rager, *Problemes d'Ionisation et d'Aero-ionisation* (Paris: Maloine S.A. Editeur, 1975).
14. J. L. Worden, "Proliferation of Mammalian Cells in Ion-controlled Environments," *Journal of the National Cancer Institute* 26 (1961):801–11.
15. S. Kotaka and A. P. Krueger, "Studies on Air Ion-induced Growth Increase in Higher Plants, *Advancing Frontiers of Plant Sciences* 20 (1967):115–208.
16. A. P. Krueger, S. Kotaka, K. Nishizawa, Y. Kogure, M. Takenobu, and P. C. Andriese, "Air Ion Effects on the Growth of the Silk Worm (*Bombyx mori L.*)," *International Journal of Biometeorology* 10 (1966):29–38.
17. A. P. Krueger and E. J. Reed, "Effect of the Air Ion Environment on Influenza in the Mouse," *International Journal of Biometeorology* 16 (1972):209–32.
18. A. P. Krueger, E. J. Reed, M. B. Day, and K. A. Brook, "Further Observations on the Effects of Air Ions on Influenza in the Mouse," *International Journal of Biometeorology* 18 (1974):46–56.
19. A. P. Krueger, P. C. Andriese, and S. Kotaka, "Small Air Ions: Their Effect on Blood Levels of Serotonin in Terms of Modern Physical Theory," *International Journal of Biometeorology* 12, no. 3 (1968):225–39.
20. G. O. Gilbert, "Effect of Negative Air Ions upon Emotionality and Brain Serotonin Levels in Isolated Rats," *International Journal of Biometeorology* 17 (1973):267–75.
21. J. M. Olivereau, "Incidences psychophysiologiques de l'ionisation atmosphérique," Doctoral thesis, University of Paris, 1971.
22. J. M. Olivereau, "Influence des ions atmosphériques negatifs sur l'adaptation à unesituation anxiogène chez le rat," *International Journal of Biometeorology* 17 (1973):277–84.
23. J. R. Nazzaro, D. E. Jackson, and L. E. Perkins, "Effects of Ionized Air on Stress Behavior," *Medical Research Engineering* 6 (1967):25–28.
24. C. H. Bachman, R. A. McDonald, and C. J. Lorenz, "Some Effects of Air Ions on the Activity of Rats," *International Journal of Biometeorology* 10 (1966):39–46.
25. A. H. Frey, "Modification of the Conditioned Emotional Response by Treatment with Small Negative Air Ions," publication from the Institute for Research, State College, Pennsylvania, 1967.
26. A. P. Krueger, S. Kotaka, and P. C. Andriese, "Studies on the Biological Effects of Gaseous Ions: A Review." Special Monograph Series, Vol. 1, Biometeorological Research Centre, Leiden, 1966.

27. A. P. Krueger and H. B. Levine, "The Effect of Unipolar Positively Ionized Air on the Course of Coccidioidomycosis in Mice," *International Journal of Biometeorology* 10 (1967):279–88.

28. M. Knoll, J. Eichmeier, and R. W. Schon, "Properties, Measurement, and Bioclimatic Action of Small Multimolecular Atmospheric Ions," *Advanced Electronics and Electron Physics* 19 (1964): 177–254.

29. S. Cupcea, M. Deleanu, and T. Frits, "Experimentelle untersuchungen uber den einfluss der luftionisation auf pathologische veranderungen der magenschleimhaut," *Act. Biol. et Med. Germ* 3 (1959):407–16.

30. D. Silverman and I. H. Kornblueh, "The Effect of Artificial Ionization of the Air on the Electro-encephalogram," *American Journal of Physical Medicine* 36 (1957):352–58.

31. E. Haine, H. L. Konig, and H. Schmeer, "Aphid Moulting under Controlled Electrical Conditions," *International Journal of Biometeorology* 7 (1964):265–75.

32. N. Robinson and F. S. Dirnfeld, "The Ionization State of the Atmosphere as a Function of the Meteorological Elements and the Various Sources of Ions," *International Journal of Biometeorology* 6 (1963):101–10.

33. F. G. Sulman, D. Levy, A. Levy, Y. Pfeifer, E. Supersteine, and E. Tal, "Air Ionometry of Hot, Dry Desert Winds (Sharav) and Treatment with Air Ions of Weather-sensitive Subjects," *International Journal of Biometeorology* 18 (1974):313–18.

34. M. Assael, Y. Pfeifer, and F. G. Sulman, "Influence of Artificial Air Ionization on the Human Electro-encephalogram," *International Journal of Biometeorology* 18 (1974):306–12.

35. T. Winsor and J. C. Beckett, "Biological Effects of Ionized Air in Man," *American Journal of Physical Medicine* 37 (1958):83–89.

36. B. Maczyński, S. Tyczka, B. Marecki, and T. Gora, "Effect of the Presence of Man on the Air Ion Density in an Office Room," *International Journal of Biometeorology* 15 (1971):11–21.

37. I. H. Kornblueh, S. T. Swope, and F. K. Davis, "Natural Ion Levels in Enclosed Spaces," Presented at the Congress on Lacustrine Climatology, 1971, proceedings published January 1973.

38. J. C. Beckett, "Dynamics of Fresh Air," *Journal of American Society of Heating, Refrigerating and Air Conditioning* 1 (1959): 47–51.

39. S. Kimura, M. Ashiba, and I. Matsushima, "Influences of the Air Lacking in Light Ions and the Effect of Its Artificial Ionization

upon Human Beings in Occupied Rooms," *Japanese Journal of Medical Science* 7 (1939):1–12.

40. Y. G. Nefedov, B. V. Anisimov, et al., "The Aero-ionic Composition of Pressurized Cabin Air and Its Influence on the Human Body," Report Presented at Soviet Conference on Space Biology and Medicine, November 10, 1966, Proceedings pp. 32–46.

41. Bruce L. Rosenberg, "A Study of Atmospheric Ionization: Measurement of the Ion Conditions in an ATC Laboratory and a Review of the Literature of Ion Effects on Performance." Report no. NA-72-19 (Atlantic City: Federal Aviation Administration, May 1972).

42. Dr. Walter Stark, personal communication, 1974.

43. T. A. David, J. R. Minehart, and I. H. Kornblueh, "Polarized Air as an Adjunct in the Treatment of Burns," *American Journal of Physical Medicine* 31 (1960):111–13.

44. A. P. Krueger and R. F. Smith, "The Physiological Significance of Positive and Negative Ionization of the Atmosphere," *Journal of the Royal Society of Health* 79 (1959):642–48.

45. Y. Palti, E. Denour, A. Abramov, "The Effect of Atmospheric Ions on the Respiratory System of Infants," *Pediatrics* 38 (1966):404–11.

46. P. C. Boulatov, "Traitement de l'asthme bronchique par l'aéro-ionisation négative," in Gualtierotti, R., et al., see reference 12.

47. I. H. Kornblueh, G. M. Piersol, and F. P. Speicher, "Relief from Pollinosis in Negatively Ionized Rooms," *American Journal of Physical Medicine* 37 (1958):18–27.

48. Alfred P. Wehner, "Electro-Aerosols, Air Ions, and Physical Medicine," *American Journal of Physical Medicine* 48 (1969):119–49.

49. Alfred P. Wehner, "Electro-Aerosol Therapy," *American Journal of Physical Medicine*, 41 (1962):24–40, 68–86.

50. R. P. Monaco, and C. W. Acker, "Psychophysiological Effects of Ionized Air on Psychiatric Patients," *Newsletter for Research in Psychology*, 5, no. 3 (1963):23–25.

51. R. Ucha Udabe, R. Kertész, and L. Franceschetti, "Etudes sur l'utilisation des ions negatifs dans malades du système nerveux," in Gualtierotti, R., et al., see reference 12.

52. M. Deleanu, "L'Aéroionotherapie dans l'ulcère gastro-duodénal," in Gualtierotti, R., et al., see reference 12.

By *William L. Haskell*

≈§ ≥∞

Physical Activity in Health Maintenance

Generally speaking, all parts of the body which have a function, if used in moderation, and exercise in labors to which each is accustomed, become thereby healthy and well developed, and age slowly; but if unused and left idle, they become liable to disease, defective in growth and age quickly.

Hippocrates, circa 400 B.C.

Throughout history the potential health benefits of physical activity have been unjustifiably revered as well as unnecessarily maligned. Exercise enthusiasts have tended to promote vigorous physical activity as the panacea of good health while protagonists have not only ignored some obvious benefits but inappropriately stressed the potential dangers of exercise beyond that required to meet basic needs ("The most exercise I get is being a pallbearer for my more active friends"—attributed to Mark Twain). The composite results of diverse research during this century indicate that the truth, as in most health matters, lies somewhere between these two extreme views: indeed, physical activity performed on a regular basis is needed by all humans to maintain optimal health, but for certain specific disease conditions it has no benefit and for some individuals is contraindicated.

The purpose of this chapter is to summarize what is known

about the health benefits of exercise, how these benefits may be achieved and to review some of the major questions regarding physical activity and health still needing answers.

PHYSICAL ACTIVITY AND EVOLUTION

Man was designed to be physically active and throughout most of his evolution survival has favored the physically well conditioned individual. As in most animals, the requirement for effective mobility dominates our body construction. Approximately 40 percent of our body weight normally is made up of muscle with the skeleton contributing another 15 percent. Many of our important organs are of a size and design to service the muscles during exercise, such as the heart, blood vessels and lungs. The design of the nervous and endocrine systems also are the result of the body's demand for motion.

Physical stamina, strength, speed and agility were an advantage to the hunter, nomad and primitive farmer for obtaining necessary food and shelter as well as protection from his adversaries, both animal and human. Vigorous physical activity as a requirement for survival existed for thousands of years, while it has been only during the last few centuries that many men have been able to lead a sedentary life: a style indicative of success in our current culture. This abrupt change in habitual activity has not been followed by any known evolutionary adaptation in man's structure of function to compensate for the decreased demands made on the cardiovascular, respiratory, metabolic and nervous systems. Optimal function can be achieved and maintained only by regularly requiring the heart, circulation, lungs, muscles, skeleton and nervous system to respond to exercise demands.

Evidence from various sources suggests that man's evolution, favoring a physically active life style, now makes him vulnerable by accelerating the development of chronic degenerative diseases, especially those of a cardiovascular and metabolic nature. Thus, we might think of obesity, atherosclerosis (hardening of the arteries due to fatty deposits) and diabetes as, at least in part, "hypokinetic" disorders, prevention of which requires regular physical activity.

PHYSICAL ACTIVITY AND
PHYSICAL FITNESS

Whenever man shifts from a resting state to one of motion, numerous physical and chemical changes immediately take place within his body. Except for the conscious decision to move, all of these changes occur automatically and their magnitude of change is determined by the type of activity performed, the intensity of the activity relative to the individual's capacity and the duration of the activity. Also, how frequently this activity is performed will influence the degree of change it produces. How much any system or process of the body is altered by exercise will be determined by how much that system is stimulated or stressed during the actual exercise or recovery from it. Thus, when considering what the potential health benefits of physical activity might be, the type, intensity, duration and frequency of the exercise need to be specified.

Not all physical activity produces similar changes in structure and function as there is a certain amount of specificity to exercise training. To increase muscle strength and size, heavy resistance activities requiring nearly maximal strength need to be performed (weight training, isometrics, etc.). Muscle endurance is best developed by exercise of moderate intensity repeated frequently until significant fatigue occurs. To enhance cardiovascular capacity, large muscle activities requiring low resistance rhythmic movements for extended periods of time are required. Such activities are considered endurance or aerobic (with oxygen) conditioning exercises and include brisk walking, hiking, jogging, running, swimming, cycling, selected calisthenics and active sports and games. In addition to selecting the proper activity to produce desired change, the exercise needs to be performed at a sufficient intensity and duration to impose an "overload" demand on the body. If the intensity is too low or duration too short, the stress will be insufficient and no adaptation will result. It is reasonably well established that most changes occur when a biological system is stressed beyond 50 percent of its capacity.

An habitual increase in physical activity enhances an individual's capacity to perform that and similar type activities. This increase in functional capacity or physical fitness is a unique benefit of exercise in that the changes in structure and function associated with this increase in capacity cannot be achieved by other means such as diet, rest or drugs. Some of the major anatomical, physiological and biochemical alterations that contribute to an increase in functional capacity as a result of regular exercise are listed in the following table. These changes can increase muscle endurance, strength and power, capacity and efficiency of the cardiovascular system to transport blood to working muscles and more effective utilization of energy stores (substrates).

Biological Changes Contributing to an Increase in Physical Fitness Due to Physical Training

HEART AND BLOOD

Lower heart rate at rest
Lower heart rate during standardized submaximal exercise
Increased rate of heart rate recovery after standardized exercise
Larger blood volume pumped per heart beat (stroke volume)
Increased size of heart muscle (myocardial hypertrophy)
Increased strength and speed of heart muscle contraction
  (contractility)
Increased blood volume
Improved distribution of blood volume during exercise (vasomotor
  control)
Lower resting and exercise systolic and diastolic blood pressure
Increased maximal oxygen transport to muscle (aerobic capacity)

LUNGS

Increased diffusion of respiratory gases
Reduced non-functional volume of lung (residual volume)
Lower oxygen requirement of respiratory muscles during exercise

SKELETAL MUSCLES

Increased muscle glycogen content
Increased metabolic enzymatic capacity
Increased muscle mass (hypertrophy) with strength training

OTHER

Reduced sympathetic tone (catecholamines)
Reduced body fat content (adiposity)
Increased glucose tolerance
Increased anaerobic capacity (may be psychological)

A variety of other changes occurring as a result of exercise, particularly in the functioning of the nervous and hormone systems, are not well understood. It appears that in addition to improved resistance to physical stress, regular exercise also may relieve some of the detrimental physiological effects produced by psychological stresses such as anger, frustration and anxiety. It has been postulated that a variety of physical and mental disorders are caused by continued or repeated imbalance in central nervous system control. Chronic exposure to stressful situations without an acceptable outlet for a "fight or flight" response may produce an overstimulation of the sympathetic nervous system producing an excessive release of catecholamines. It is known that sympathetic stimulation and catecholamine release produces numerous changes in the cardiovascular metabolic and endocrine system requiring increased blood flow and oxygen utilization. Reduction in this sympathetic discharge, or a more acceptable utilization of catecholamines may be achieved with regular activity.

It should be emphasized that the changes summarized in the table above are associated with increased functional capacity (physical fitness) and are not necessarily synonymous with a change in health status even though certain of these alterations may be the mechanism by which some specific health benefits occur. The ability of an individual to run fast or long or to lift a heavy weight is not an absolute index of general health status.

True, he could not perform these tasks effectively if he were seriously ill, but the fact that he can perform them does not insure longevity or that he is free from a potentially serious disease.

CARDIOVASCULAR DISEASE

In North America the greatest cause of disability and death in adults is the result of a breakdown in the oxygen transport system of the body. That is, when the body is unable to move sufficient amounts of oxygen from the atmosphere to a specific organ, tissue damage occurs. The primary culprit in reducing oxygen transport capacity is the process of atherosclerosis, the laying down of fatty deposits in arteries, which impedes blood flow and the delivery of oxygen. Of particular importance is maintaining an adequate oxygen supply to both the heart muscle (myocardium) and the brain since neither of these tissues can survive without oxygen for more than four to five minutes without incurring irreversible damage. Atherosclerosis of the coronary arteries, those blood vessels which supply blood to the heart muscle (myocardium), is by far the leading cause of death in the U.S.A., resulting in nearly 1,200,000 heart attacks and 650,000 deaths annually. Another 300,000 deaths from stroke are due primarily to atherosclerosis of the cerebral arteries which supply blood to the brain.

Coronary Heart Disease

It is generally recognized in medicine that coronary heart disease (CHD) is accelerated if not caused by a variety of genetic and environmental factors working in unison to produce a reduction in myocardial oxygen supply as a result of coronary artery atherosclerosis. In addition to inactivity, elevated levels of blood fats (cholesterol and triglycerides), blood pressure, cigarette smoking, obesity, diabetes mellitus and psychological stress have been identified as CHD risk factors. The exact mechanism of how any of these habits or characteristics may produce atherosclerosis is not known.

The search for more effective approaches to prevent heart attacks has stimulated a great deal of interest in the hypothesis that an increase in habitual physical activity may reduce premature disability and death from coronary heart disease. Conclusions regarding the influence of physical activity on the pathogenesis of CHD have been based on data obtained from several types of studies: (1) a majority of the data relating inactivity to CHD risk has been derived from prospective and retrospective observational studies comparing the frequency or severity of CHD in groups of individuals classified as "least" and "more active" according to occupational or "leisure time" physical activity; (2) autopsy studies comparing the anatomic and pathologic changes of the coronary arteries and the myocardium of individuals who were reported to have participated in different levels of physical activity; (3) studies on the changes in the capacity, efficiency or reserves of the myocardium, total oxygen transport and metabolic systems due to physical conditioning; and (4) experimental studies designed to determine the influence of physical activity on biological or behavioral characteristics (CHD risk factors) possibly related to the etiology of CHD. To date, data from these studies do not provide a definitive answer to whether or not an increase in physical activity will help prevent CHD but they generally provide strong support for the idea.

OBSERVATIONAL STUDIES

A majority of the studies which have analyzed the relationship between physical inactivity and increased risk of CHD have demonstrated that both occupational and leisure time activities which involve at least moderate amounts of physical exertion on a regular basis are associated with more favorable CHD prognosis and rehabilitation [1, 2]. In general, persons reported to be more active on and off the job have fewer myocardial infarctions (heart attacks) and when they do occur they are less severe and tend to take place at an older age than their more sedentary counterparts. For example, results from the Health Insurance Plan of Greater New York suggest that both the risk of having a heart attack and dying within forty-eight hours (index of severity) are substantially greater among men classified as sedentary for on-the-job and leisure time activity than among men only slightly more active [1]. This relationship remains even when smoking habits, body weight and educational, religious and ethnic background are taken into consideration and when the comparisons are restricted to men either with no prior CHD history or no prior limitation of physical activity.

A more favorable CHD risk status was not found for more active individuals by some investigators while others have reported as much as a five-fold difference between individuals who performed one or more hours of heavy work daily as compared to those who performed none [2]. In several studies no significant difference was observed between the level of on-the-job physical activity and CHD, but individuals who developed CHD tended to be less active during non-job hours than coworkers who did not develop CHD. Also, in the follow-up study of Framingham, Massachusetts residents, when individuals were classified according to three "possible objective indicators of physical activity" (weight gain, vital capacity and resting pulse rate), those with "adverse" values for two or more of these traits had a five-fold greater mortality from CHD than those who had no "adverse" traits and were presumably the most active [3].

Except for the possibility that former athletes have a higher mortality due to accidents and other violent causes, it appears that there is little difference in the causes of death or life expectancy for former college athletes and their college classmates. It is of interest to note, however, that there appears to be a substantially lower CHD mortality rate in athletes who remained moderately or vigorously active into their later years of life than those athletes who become sedentary after college. There is no data to indicate that vigorous exercise up to and including competitive athletics by healthy individuals increases their susceptibility to CHD.

In contrast to fatal and nonfatal heart attacks, there is more of a tendency for active persons to report angina pectoris (chest pain due to inadequate oxygen supply to heart muscle) at least as frequently if not more so than their inactive counterparts. Why this difference for angina exists is not clear, but it does not appear likely that the greater exertion of the more active subjects brought out the anginal symptoms. It is very possible that the active group is living with this less threatening manifestation of the total disease process, which would have produced myocardial infarction or killed them earlier, had they not stimulated some protective adaptation by their greater activity.

Limitation of Data. The results of population studies generally confirm the hypothesis that individuals who are selected for, or who select, more active occupations and leisure time activities experience fewer and less severe CHD episodes, but they provide only indirect support for the main hypothesis in question: Does an increase in habitual physical activity by sedentary adults reduce their chance of developing clinical manifestations or prematurely dying from CHD? In these studies, individuals could have made a personal selection for, or been selected for, different activity groups as a result of factors that may also influence the frequency or severity of CHD. Such factors may include the nature of their general health in early life, body type and weight, blood pressure, responses to environmental stress and psychological make-up.

The type of activities which contribute most to the classifying of individuals as more instead of less active or sedentary in many population studies include walking on the level and upstairs, the lifting of relatively light objects, the operation of machinery or appliances, gardening or working around the house and participation in certain games or sports. The participation in "physical fitness programs" contributes very little to this classification. In most studies, only on-the-job physical activity was used for classification purposes, but it appears that both occupational and non-job physical activity need to be considered if its relationship to CHD is to be accurately determined [1].

In order for physical activity to provide some protection against CHD, it may be that the activity level does not have to be very great and that it does not have to exert a very substantial influence on physical work capacity. It seems appropriate to raise the possibility that the protective influence of physical activity might be a recurring, acute or temporary effect of reasonably low intensity activity performed on a very routine basis and not a chronic conditioning influence as is usually measured in the evaluation of physical fitness program participants. It is now necessary to answer the question: will activity of greater intensity, but performed for a shorter duration than that accounting for the differences in observational studies, provide the same or a greater degree of protection?

A definitive answer to the question of a causal relationship between increased physical activity and the prevention of CHD can be obtained only by a properly conducted longitudinal study. Individuals free from CHD clinical signs or symptoms would have to be randomly assigned to exercise and control groups and observed for an extended period of time with the number of nonfatal and/or fatal CHD events occurring in the two groups compared.

AUTOPSY STUDIES

The results of autopsy studies indicate that physical activity may reduce myocardial damage caused by ischemia but have little, if any, influence on the atherosclerosis occurring in the major coronary arteries. A collaborative study conducted by pathologists in England reported that in the hearts of 3,800 men age forty-five to seventy dying suddenly but not from CHD, there was more heart muscle damage in individuals who had engaged in "light" as compared to "active" or "heavy" job-related work [4]. Much less difference was observed in the frequency of severe coronary atherosclerosis in the large coronary vessels. Similar results have been reported by several other investigators.

STUDIES OF CARDIOVASCULAR FUNCTION

How physical activity might provide protection against CHD is not well understood, but it seems to have little influence on the atherosclerotic process occurring in the major coronary arteries. Preliminary evidence indicates that properly designed and executed exercise programs will enhance the capacity, efficiency and reserves of the heart muscle and total cardiovascular system, thus possibly increasing the heart's resistance to the detrimental influence of the atherosclerotic process and associated complications.

It is possible that physical activity can reduce the clinical manifestations of CHD without significantly altering the atherosclerotic process. If physical activity can increase the supply of oxygen to the myocardium, decrease myocardial oxygen requirement, or enhance the capacity of the heart to pump blood, an individual might be able to withstand the same or even greater disease without suffering the detrimental consequences of inadequate blood supply (ischemia), angina pectoris, myocardial infarction.

Myocardial Oxygen Supply. Physical activity might enhance myocardial oxygen supply by increasing the cross-sectional area of the coronary arteries thus diminishing the degree of obstruction caused by any given size atherosclerotic deposit (plaque). Or the reduction in coronary blood flow to a specific area of the myocardium due to atherosclerosis could be partially alleviated by stimulating the opening of new blood vessels to the compromised area (collateral circulation). Data from earlier animal studies indicated that under certain circumstances physical conditioning might produce both of these changes; however, the only systematic study reported on humans suggests no significant increase in collateral blood flow in cardiac patients who participated in an exercise program for up to one year [5]. These results do not rule out the possibility that vigorous activity performed regularly by individuals without CHD may increase the size of the major coronary vessels and reduce the detrimental impact of atherosclerosis. The answer to this possibility is critical since the atherosclerosis causing most severe heart attacks occurs in these larger vessels and any increase in their size may have a substantial preventive effect.

Myocardial Oxygen Requirement. The lower the oxygen requirement of the heart the lower the rate of coronary flow can be and still be adequate. A direct measurement of myocardial oxygen expenditure is not readily obtainable in humans, but indirect measures indicate that increased physical activity may enhance myocardial or total cardiovascular efficiency during rest and exercise. Changes produced by physical training which may result in a reduced myocardial oxygen requirement for the same level of exertion include: (1) a slower heart rate (bradycardia) during rest and submaximal exercise, (2) an increase in the amount of blood pumped with each beat (stroke volume) at rest and during exercise, (3) a decrease in systemic arterial blood pressure, (4) improved distribution of blood flow to the more active muscles, (5) an increase in systemic arteriovenous oxygen extraction and (6) a decrease in sympathetic activity as indicated by a reduction in plasma catecholamine level.

REDUCTION IN CHD RISK FACTORS

Numerous attempts have been made to determine the influence of an increase in physical activity on factors known to be related to an increased risk of acquiring or dying from CHD. To utilize data from this type of study it is necessary to make the inference that if the "risk factor" is favorably altered, the disease process is inhibited or delayed.

Blood Cholesterol and Triglycerides. The relationship between physical activity and blood fat or lipid levels, especially serum cholesterol, has not been definitively established. In most earlier studies, where exercise was reported to have a lowering effect on cholesterol, little or no information was available on the subjects' dietary habits and many had greater losses in body weight than could be accounted for by the increase in activity. Other reports include both a reduction and no change in cholesterol with an increase in physical activity when body weight is held nearly constant. The discrepancies in these results may be due to changes in dietary habits not reported by some subjects, differences in initial cholesterol levels, or variations in the characteristics of the physical conditioning programs (type, amount and intensity of activity). More research is needed where diet is stringently controlled and an adequate number of subjects are included so that the effect of conditioning programs of various intensities and durations on individuals with different initial cholesterol levels can be investigated.

It has been well demonstrated that physical activity has a substantial lowering effect on elevated triglycerides. The major change appears to occur very rapidly, within a few hours but may last only for 24 to 48 hours. Thus, in order to maintain lower triglycerides, activity must be performed at least every other day [6]. No long-term effect of exercise on triglycerides has been substantiated. It is not known whether active people maintain lower triglyceride levels than inactive people but there is some indication that this is the case.

Arterial Blood Pressure. Several investigators have reported a reduction in systolic and diastolic systemic arterial pressure in young and middle-aged men at rest and at given workloads after participation in endurance type physical conditioning programs [7]. Other investigators have not observed such changes even with training programs lasting up to seven months. Reductions appear to occur most frequently in individuals who have moderately elevated pressures to begin with and diastolic pressure seems more amenable to change than systolic. Some of the reported changes may be associated with a reduction in body weight and/or a change in diet. Additional well-controlled intervention studies are needed of the long-term effects of increased habitual physical activity on resting and more importantly the "operational" blood pressure of normal living.

Blood Coagulation and Fibrinolysis. Physical activity of light or moderate intensity (ten- to twenty-minute walk at 3 mph, or an eight-minute walk at 3.5 mph on a 5-degree grade) significantly increases, at least temporarily, the rate at which blood clots are dissolved (fibrinolytic activity). Data on more strenuous activity, especially competitive games, is less consistent, with some investigators observing increases in fibrinolytic activity or related parameters, while others have observed an opposite effect. Some of this inconsistency is probably due to differences in blood clotting evaluation techniques or the type of exercise performed. There is some suggestion that a moderate increase in habitual physical activity may have a favorable chronic effect on blood clotting mechanisms while unaccustomed strenuous exercise tends to temporarily shorten blood clotting time.

Stroke

Only two reports are available concerning the relationship between physical activity habits and the frequency or severity of strokes or cerebral vascular accidents. In both studies, individuals engaged in heavy occupational work experienced fewer strokes than their less active counterparts. Inferences from these reports are limited due to their study design. Regular exercise may reduce an individual's vulnerability to complications from a cerebral vascular lesion by (1) increasing the capability of the heart to pump more blood under a variety of stressful circumstances, (2) improving the regulation of the peripheral vascular system thus also reducing the likelihood of an inadequate oxygen supply to the brain under stress, (3) enhancing the blood clotting function, or (4) reducing arterial blood pressure. However, individuals at high risk of a stroke should be aware that the increase in systolic blood pressure produced by vigorous exercise could produce damage to blood vessels in the brain and thus care needs to be taken when they select a physical conditioning activity.

Occlusive Arterial Disease

An inadequate blood flow (and thus oxygen supply) of the lower extremities due to the arteriosclerotic process (arteriosclerosis obliterans) is a frequent cause of disability in elderly individuals of technologically advanced populations. For many persons, medications or surgical treatment is of limited value. The results of initial studies into the use of physical conditioning as a therapeutic tool for occlusive arterial disease of the lower extremities are encouraging. For example, in one study, five patients with inadequate blood flow to the lower legs and feet due to moderate arteriosclerosis obliterans were evaluated before and after a three- to eight-month physical conditioning program of intermittent walking on a treadmill [8]. This conditioning produced significant increases in the length of time a participant could walk before leg pain due to a lack of oxygen began, in maximal walking time and postexercise systolic blood pressure at the ankle. These changes were attributed to an increase in circulation of the obstructed extremity at rest and during or after exercise. Similar increases in walking ability have been reported by others.

Other Cardiovascular Diseases

Neurocirculatory asthenia (NCA) is a syndrome characterized by an abnormally low physical working capacity in spite of normal heart function. Electrocardiographic abnormalities, high heart rates, an unusually high cardiac output and a decreased extraction of oxygen by the muscles, probably due to an inadequate regulation of peripheral blood flow, are observed at rest and during exercise in individuals with NCA. Participation in an endurance type physical conditioning program substantially improves the physical working capacity of most NCA patients and normalizes their cardiovascular function. There is a need to develop methods for the early detection of the NCA syndrome since it seems readily amenable to exercise therapy.

There is no evidence that physical activity alters the damage to the heart valves caused by congenital or acquired valvular deformities. Functional damage to the valves will reduce the individual's exercise capacity and with certain valvular lesions such as aortic stenosis even moderate intensity exercise can produce a very low blood pressure resulting in dizziness, syncope or even sudden death. How much exercise an individual with valvular disease should undertake should be objectively determined by a medically monitored exercise test.

An individual with valvular disease can increase his functional capacity by improving the capacity and efficiency of the cardiovascular system without any change in valve structure or function. For example, by slowing the heart rate at rest and exercise (due to increased capacity of skeletal muscles to extract oxygen from the blood) the patient with a damaged heart valve might achieve more effective filling of the heart chambers, thus improving the amount of blood pumped with each beat.

As with valvular lesions, certain congenital or acquired defects of the heart muscle are not improved by physical training, but one's ability to function may be improved if exercise is carried out with knowledgeable medical direction. Congenital lesions that may be *worsened* by vigorous exercise or produce potentially dangerous workloads on the heart muscle include constriction of the aorta and severe restriction of the size of the heart valve. Vigorous exercise should not be performed if infection of the sac surrounding the heart (pericarditis) or of the heart muscle itself (myocarditis) is evident or even suspected. Sudden cardiac arrest has been reported in otherwise healthy people who exercised without realizing they had myocarditis. For this reason, exercise should be curtailed during any evidence of a generalized infection including that of the lungs.

CHRONIC PULMONARY DISEASE

Changes in pulmonary function take place with exercise training but regular activity does not appear to provide any protection against the development of chronic pulmonary diseases such as asthma, emphysema or bronchitis nor reverse tissue damage resulting from these diseases once it has occurred. As the result of endurance type exercise training, there is an increased efficiency in breathing during high-level exercise (amount of air breathed to obtain a given amount of oxygen is reduced). This increase in "ventilatory equivalent" is accompanied by a reduction in the volume of air needed leading to a decrease in the work of breathing, a reduced oxygen need by the respiratory muscles and a smaller blood flow to these muscles during any given amount of exercise. This improvement in breathing efficiency during exercise coupled with the improvement in cardiovascular function discussed previously results in a substantially improved working capacity for many pulmonary disease patients without directly influencing the disease process in any way.

In addition to these changes, there is some evidence that selected pulmonary patients have an increased amount of oxygen in their arterial blood at rest. This increase in arterial oxygen saturation appears to occur more frequently if patients breathe supplemental oxygen during exercise training. With asthmatic children, it has been demonstrated that respiratory exercises, gymnastics and active games or sports, will reduce the number or severity of asthma attacks, decrease the needed medication and improve functional capacity. Whether or not changes in pulmonary function occur is not clear. Some of these changes probably are psychological and occur as a result of the individual's attitude towards his disease.

DIABETES MELLITUS

Before the discovery of insulin, physical activity was the primary therapy for diabetes mellitus, but since then it has been used little or totally ignored by most physicians. The tendency has been to focus on the pharmacological and nutritional aspects with little consideration given to the possible benefit of appropriate activity. It has been well documented that a decrease in activity level increases insulin requirement and conversely, as activity increases insulin usage can be reduced. A change in insulin requirement does not necessarily mean that the severity of the disease has changed, but may only indicate some temporary alteration in carbohydrate or fat metabolism. Exercise may aid the diabetic or diabetic-prone individual by increasing glucose utilization at lower blood insulin levels. This increase in glucose uptake probably occurs in the working muscles and is related to a change in muscle metabolism resulting from physical conditioning.

Most available information demonstrates that exercise is a very useful adjunct to other forms of diabetic therapy. Unfortunately, research has concentrated on only one aspect of the total diabetic population, those patients already on insulin. Little or no research has been reported on the potential benefits of exercise on the larger number of patients who can control their diabetes with oral hypoglycemic drugs and/or proper diet. Much more information is needed on the acute and chronic influence of regular exercise on the natural history of the entire spectrum of diabetes.

OBESITY

An ideal body weight not only is aesthetically preferable in western cultures, it also has very definite health advantages. Life insurance figures, as well as numerous population studies, have convincingly demonstrated that overweight adults are much more prone to develop heart disease, stroke, high blood pressure, kidney malfunction, diabetes and numerous other life-shortening conditions than individuals of "normal or ideal" body weight. In addition to the increased workload excess fat tissue puts on the heart and circulatory system, it alters selected metabolic processes that may accelerate atherosclerosis and diabetes.

Regardless of the physiological or psychological variability of the individual, the underlying cause of all obesity is an intake of calories in excess of expenditure by the body. It is important to understand that all of the many factors (endocrine, metabolic, psychological and nutritional) which may modify the tendency to gain or lose weight operate through the common denominator of energy balance. Thus, a plethora of calories is the only explanation for obesity. The Law of the Conservation of Energy applies to the human body just as to any other machine which performs work and produces heat. When the intake of calories, whether in the form of carbohydrate, fat or protein, exceeds calorie expenditure, the excess will be stored in the body tissue as fat. A negative calorie balance (more calories used than consumed) will result in a decrease in body fat.

Until quite recently there has been a tendency to minimize the role of physical activity in weight control because of the persistence of two very common misconceptions: (1) that exercise requires relatively little calorie expenditure and therefore a change in physical activity has only a minor influence on calorie balance and, (2) an increase in physical activity always is automatically followed by an increase in appetite and food intake negating any weight-loss benefit of the exercise. Evidence exists to disprove both beliefs. Early studies on rats and more recent studies on humans have demonstrated that an increase in activity level by sedentary adults actually decreases the appetite more frequently than it increases it. Concerning the first misconception, it is essential to remember that the calories expended during exercise are cumulative from one minute to the next, hour to hour, day to day and so forth. For example, an adult weighing approximately 170 pounds will expend about 100 kilocalories while walking one mile on level terrain. This mile can be walked all at once (20 minutes at 3 mph) or may be walked some fraction at a time with the total energy expenditure remaining about the same. If such an individual would maintain the same calorie intake for one year and increase his activity level by walking one mile per day, he would lose approximately 10 pounds of fat tissue (walking 365 miles would expend 365,000 kilocalories and there are approximately 3,500 kilocalories in one pound of body fat; therefore, 365,000/3,500 = 10+ pounds). Over a three year period a reduction in body weight of 30 pounds (more than most adults are above their ideal weight) could be obtained by as little as 20 minutes of moderate exercise per day.

With increasing age there is a need for fewer calories in order to maintain body weight. Some of this reduced calorie requirement is due directly to a decrease in physical activity, but there are also several hidden effects of inactivity that further reduce caloric need. First, as the activity level is reduced there is a reduction in total muscle mass (atrophy), thus reducing the basal metabolic rate of the body. This means the body needs fewer calories to maintain itself every minute of the day. Even a very small change in this basic calorie requirement can significantly influence energy balance. A 2 to 3 percent drop in basal metabolic rate could result in a 50 kilocalorie per day change in energy balance or a change in body weight of five pounds per year. Secondly, as habitual physical activity decreases there is a decrease in functional capacity (physical fitness) and the ability to perform activities requiring higher levels of calorie expenditure. This restriction in exercise capacity tends to further reduce average calorie expenditure. The net result is a tendency to put on weight.

ORTHOPEDIC DISABILITIES

It is well established that certain minimums of physical activity are needed to support normal growth and maintain the structural and functional integrity of muscle, bone and connective tissue. This exercise stimulus is required in youth if normal growth is to occur and in adults if the strength and flexibility of these tissues are to be retained. The loss or diminution of muscle strength and joint flexibility is associated with an increased risk of various orthopedic disabilities including low back pain, muscle strains, sprains, dislocations and fractures.

Inactivity alters both skeletal muscle size and composition. As the muscle atrophies from disuse, it loses some of its strength and speed of contraction. Since muscles help support the body against gravity and help stabilize joints like the knee and shoulder during trauma, adequate muscle tone or strength helps protect against injury. With advancing age, good muscle strength can help protect against accidents by enabling the individual to better support or catch himself in situations which otherwise could have resulted in a fall. Also, by maintaining good joint (muscle and connective tissue) flexibility through stretching exercises, the likelihood of a muscle tear or joint injury (sprain) is decreased.

Studies on the effect of weightlessness have confirmed earlier findings that periods of inactivity result in a loss of calcium from bones. Such a loss decreases the strength of bone and increases the chances of fracture during an accident. Since part of the changing structure of bones with increasing age is due to a loss of calcium, periods of inactivity by the elderly accelerate the aging process.

PSYCHOLOGICAL BENEFITS

One of the most often cited benefits of a regular program of physical activity by enthusiastic participants is that they feel better. They report having more energy after exercise, they feel more relaxed and most mention an increased ability to cope with the problems of living. Objective measurements of such psychological changes are difficult to obtain; however, there is no doubt that many participants do temporarily enhance their psychological status by engaging in one of a variety of conditioning or vigorous leisure time activities. For many individuals, young and old alike, improvements in physical fitness and appearance by regular exercise yield improvements in self-esteem and self-confidence.

Even though few mental health experts disagree with the importance of physiologic well-being in the maintenance of emotional health, there is no evidence that the biologic changes produced by physical training specifically protect against or reverse basic mental or neurological dysfunction. Selected physical activities can provide a socially acceptable outlet for aggression or tension for mental patients that might otherwise be vented in a self-destructive manner. Patients who are depressed or who demonstrate high levels of anxiety due to chronic disease such as coronary heart disease do improve psychologically with exercise training. The fact that with exercise training they have demonstrated to themselves that they are not invalids probably is responsible for most of this improvement.

Regular physical activity may improve an employee's adjustment to his job. Many of the federal government employees who participated regularly in a noon-time exercise program reported an improved attitude towards their work, improved their productivity as evaluated by peers and supervisors and had an improved self-image [9]. These changes could not be accounted for by improvements in physical working capacity and must be due to changes in mental attitude.

SUMMARY

The implications of this brief review should be quite clear: not enough is known about the relationship between physical activity and health status throughout life. There is a great need for improved communications among individuals investigating the many parameters of health maintenance. Such cooperation among physicians, physiologists, psychologists, physical educators and public health personnel could provide answers to many unanswered questions in this complex area of investigation. Simple summary statements regarding this intricate inter-relationship between physical activity and health status should be interpreted with caution; otherwise the perpetuation of misunderstanding and folklore will occur. In summary:

1. With the advent of modern technology there has been a general decrease in physical activity by adults and an increase in disability and death due to chronic disease. That these two events have occurred during the same time does not denote a cause-and-effect relationship between them.

2. There is reasonably consistent evidence from a variety of studies that moderate-intensity endurance type activity may be of value in coronary heart disease prevention and rehabilitation. Similar but more limited evidence exists for stroke and occlusive arterial disease.

3. Regular exercise may improve the functional capacity of

patients with chronic lung disease but it does not alter the pathological process of tissue destruction.

4. Physical activity can be a useful adjunct to the more traditional treatment of diabetes mellitus by medication and diet.

5. Calorie expenditure by means of increased exercise is an important component of a successful long-term weight control program for many people. Successful control of obesity may affect disability and death resulting from coronary heart disease, stroke, diabetes and hypertension.

6. Proper exercise may reduce disability associated with orthopedic problems, especially during old age. Of particular importance is the potential prevention or relief of low back pain by maintaining abdominal strength and low back flexibility.

7. No evidence exists as to any benefit provided in the prevention or treatment of infectious diseases. In most instances, vigorous exercise should be avoided during bouts of infection (especially if the suspected cause is a virus).

8. Exercise may not directly influence certain chronic disease processes but may improve the adaptation of the organism to the limitations resulting from them.

REFERENCES

1. S. Shapiro, E. Weinblatt, C. W. Frank, R. V. Sager, "Incidence of Coronary Heart Disease in a Population Insured for Medical Care (HIP): Myocardial Infarction, Angina Pectoris, and Possible Myocardial Infarction." *American Journal of Public Health* 59 (supplement) (1969):1–101.

2. W. J. Zukel, R. H. Lewis, P. E. Enterline, R. C. Painter, L. S. Ralston, R. M. Fawcett, A. P. Meredith, and B. Peterson, "A Short-term Community Study of the Epidemiology of Coronary Heart Disease: A Preliminary Report on the North Dakota Study," *American Journal of Public Health* 49 (1969):1630–39.

3. W. B. Kannel, "Habitual Level of Physical Activity and Risk of Coronary Heart Disease," Proceedings of the International Symposium on Physical Activity and Cardiovascular Health, *Canadian Medical Association Journal* 96 (1976):811.

4. J. N. Morris and M. D. Crawford, "Coronary Heart Disease and Physical Activity of Work: Evidence of a National Necropsy Survey," *British Medical Journal* 2 (1958):1485–96.

5. R. J. Ferguson, et al., "Effect of Physical Training on Treadmill Capacity, Collateral Circulation and Progression of Coronary Disease," *American Journal of Cardiology* 34 (1974):764.

6. L. B. Oscai, et al., "Normalization of Serum Triglycerides and Lipoprotein Electrophoretic Patterns by Exercise," *American Journal of Cardiology* 30 (1972):775.

7. J. L. Boyer and F. W. Kasch, "Exercise Therapy in Hypertensive Men." *Journal of the American Medical Association* 211 (1970): 1668.

8. J. S. Skinner and D. E. Strandness, "Exercise and Intermittent Claudication," *Circulation* 36 (1967):23.

9. D. C. Durbeck et al., "The National Aeronautics and Space Administration vs. Public Health Service Health Evaluation and Enchancement Program," *American Journal of Cardiology* 30 (1970):784.

By Roger J. Williams, James D. Heffley,
Man-Li Yew, and Charles W. Bode

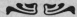

A Renaissance
of Nutritional Science

INTRODUCTION

There is a wide spectrum of uninformed inexpert opinion regarding the practical importance of quality nutrition in our daily lives. At one extreme are the food enthusiasts, including faddists; at the other is the majority of practicing physicians who through the fault of their medical school training tend to ignore all, but the most elementary aspects of nutrition, and to avoid becoming involved in a field so characterized by intricacies, uncertainties, and ignorance.

Those who have medical training are in a unique position; they alone have the background necessary to grasp fully the deep-seated significance of nutrition in relation to health and disease. Unfortunately, however, medical science has not developed and nurtured nutritional science [1], and the public has all too often discovered that those who should know the most about nutrition know very little.

There have been, of course, far-sighted physicians who have been interested in nutrition and have contributed a substantial part of what is presently known. They have often chided their

From *Perspectives in Biology and Medicine* 17 (1973):1–15. Copyright © 1973 by The University of Chicago Press. Reprinted by permission.

colleagues—generally, but not always, with soft voices—largely to no avail. These physicians who are really interested in nutrition often lack prestige and tend to operate outside the mainstream of medicine. In addition, an increasing number of those who are medically trained carry out investigations which impinge strangely on nutrition, yet because of their training they are not nutritionally oriented.

As a result of decades of neglect of nutritional science by medical science, what we would regard as sophisticated well-rounded nutritional science does not exist. Senator Schweiker, a layman, has recognized this severe deficiency and has introduced a bill authorizing the appropriation of $5 million annually to provide nutritional education in medical schools.

Expert sophisticated nutritional science necessarily involves a basic understanding of biochemistry, physiology, and pathology and an ability to deal in depth with the functioning and interrelationships of all the nutrients—minerals, trace minerals, amino acids, vitamins, etc. Not only this, but it must also encompass the biological nature of the human beings who are to be nourished, including the inheritance factors which affect their nutrition. As with other branches of science, its development must depend on interdisciplinary interest and intercommunicating specialized experts. Many tools, including those of mathematics, are now available with which to study human beings and their biological uniqueness. What is needed is the incentive, interest, and support of such investigations.

Sophisticated nutritional science, when developed, will recognize four basic facts which have not entered the mainstream of medical thinking. These four facts will be presented briefly, not with the claim that they are completely new or previously unheard of, but rather that they are crucial to the development of nutritional science and are commonly neglected.

I. Food Is a Part of Our Environment

Once stated, the above proposition becomes so obvious as not to require defense. We get oxygen from the air we breathe, water from the fluid we drink, and an assortment of about 40 or more essential nutrients from the food we consume. Those all become a part of our internal environment, the *milieu intérieur* that Claude Bernard talked about in the last century.

The mere recognition of this fact raises serious questions. What happens to cells and tissues if this nutritional environment is not well adjusted? May not the quality of the nutritional environment have a profound effect on health [2]? Can we afford to monitor carefully and scientifically other aspects of our environment like air and water, at the same time giving inexpert stepmotherly attention to the most complex part? From a practical standpoint, in what ways is this complex nutritional environment most subject to damaging deterioration?

II. Suboptimal Nutrition Prevails in Nature

Because nutritional science has been neglected, another crucial consideration has not been grasped. It is the fact that it is very common indeed for organisms in nature to live continuously under suboptimal nutritional conditions. This may happen during embryonic stages of development, but is most certainly the rule during postembryonic stages of life.

Among higher organisms, those receiving the best nutrition are the very young, the sprout nurtured by the seed, the embryos of mammals and fowls, and the suckling young. Nature has ordained it so that good nutrition is often furnished; otherwise the young would not survive. When, however, organisms pass from these early stages to become corn growing in a field, partially grown fowls or mammals, children of school age or younger, there is no automatic way in which they get what they need, and suboptimal nutrition prevails.

That suboptimal nutrition is common throughout the biological kingdom can be made clear by a few examples. A half-ounce cake of compressed yeast, if given good nutrition continuously, will yield in 1 week over a billion tons of yeast. This kind of nutrition is not supplied to yeast cells in nature. Corn growing in a field may produce all the way from less than 1 bushel up to 150 or more bushels per acre, depending on the quality of the environment furnished. Practically speaking, this environment is always suboptimal. Young weanling rats fed grain diets which were thought "normal" 50 years ago develop slowly, gaining weight at the rate of 1–2 grams per day. Now, when we know more about rat nutrition, they may be expected to develop rapidly and gain, if well fed, 5–7 grams per day. Some organisms commonly get in nature better nutrition than others, but in general adult organisms do not get nutrition of such high quality that it could not be improved.

No doubt the same principles apply to human beings. Large segments of the world population subsist on nutrition which is very far from optimal. The cells and tissues of our bodies (like those of other species, including all plants and animals) commonly compete for food essentials, and it certainly cannot be assumed that even in more advanced countries these cells and tissues automatically get precisely the right assortment of individual nutrients. This is a particularly dangerous assumption when applied to a highly industrialized culture in which processed and preserved foods are consumed and scientific nutrition is neglected.

We often get passable nutrition for the cells and tissues of our bodies because we are surrounded by plants and animals which furnish us food. These plants and animals have in their metabolic machinery the very same building blocks—minerals, amino acids, and vitamins—that we have in our cellular machinery. The removal of some of these building blocks during processing and preservation can only cause damage, and this damage cannot be repaired by partial replacement.

The acceptance of the idea that suboptimal nutrition is universal is enough by itself to change one's entire outlook. Nutrition now becomes something that is always subject to improvement. "Normal nutrition" becomes a relatively meaningless expression; if it means anything, it is some level of suboptimal nutrition. If nutrition were optimal, it certainly would not be "normal."

III. Individuality Is a Crucial Factor in Nutrition

A third vital consideration neglected by a backward nutritional science, in spite of its tremendous practical importance, is individuality in nutrition. Lucretius wrote about 2,000 years ago: "What is one man's meat is another's poison," but medical science in its general neglect of realistic nutrition has not sought to explore the roots and determine the full significance of this ancient saying.

The bearing of individuality on the practical application of nutrition can be indicated by this illustration. The following five statements are probably true. (1) The majority of adults require 750 mg or less of calcium per day. (2) The majority of adults require 10 mg or less of iron per day. (3) The majority of adults require 800 mg or less of lysine per day. (4) The majority of adults require 1 mg or less of thiamine per day. (5) The majority of adults require 1.5 mg or less of riboflavin per day.

If we attempt to collect and tabulate these five bits of information, we may arrive at the following table. This, however, is completely spurious.

Daily Needs of the "Majority of Adults" (Spurious)

Calcium	750 mg or less
Iron	10 mg or less
Lysine	800 mg or less
Thiamine	1 mg or less
Riboflavin	1.5 mg or less

To explain how this collective tabulation is invalid and that the collective data do not necessarily apply to not more than about 3 percent of the supposed population, we may start with an imagined population of 1,000 adults. If the first statement regarding calcium needs is strictly and literally true, 499 out of the 1,000 adults may have calcium needs higher than 750 mg and, hence, strictly speaking must be excluded from the tabulation. If the second statement is likewise strictly true, 250 more may have iron needs above 10 mg and, hence, cannot with strictness be included. If the third, fourth, and fifth statements are likewise true, 125, 62, and 31 additional individuals may be successively eliminated from the collective estimates, leaving a residue of only 33 out of 1,000 to whom all five estimates must apply.

If our illustration had included a large number of nutrient items, the percentage for whom the collective estimates certainly apply would decrease to the vanishing point, regardless of the exact method of calculation. If 30 nutrients were involved, for example, calculating on the same basis as above shows that all but about five members of the entire estimated world population would be excluded from the collective estimates. If the five original estimates were correct for "80 percent of adults" instead of the "majority of adults," the collected estimates would apply not to "80 percent of adults" but to about 33 percent. If in this case there were 30 nutrient items involved, the collected estimates would apply to only one adult in 806 instead of "80 percent of adults."

Those who neglect this principle may concern themselves unwittingly with the nutrition of a minuscule part of the whole population—those whose needs are above average in each of dozens of respects.

This discussion would be merely academic if individual needs were clustered around narrow limits, but this is very far from the case. When the Food and Nutrition Board considered several years ago the desirability of publishing the ranges of human needs, they were confronted by the fact that these ranges were not known. The studies essential to such determinations had not, in many cases, been made.

The situation is about the same at the present time. We have found definitive, though not necessarily ample, evidence with respect to range of needs of 10 nutritional items as presented in the following table.

For 10 other items—magnesium, iron, copper, iodide, vitamin A, vitamin D, vitamin E, ascorbic acid, pyridoxine, cobalamine—there is some indirect evidence about differences in requirements but little about ranges. In the cases of vitamin A [14, pp. 143–146; 15; 16], vitamin D [17, 18, 19], ascorbic acid [20, 21, 22], and pyridoxine [23, 24, 25], the evidence is that the ranges are probably very wide if the entire population is included. For 16 other nutrients, about which there can be no serious question, we find no information whatever regarding ranges of human needs. The presumption, on the basis of the definitive information available, is that the needs for all nutrients vary on the average over a fourfold range.

Ranges of Daily Human Needs for Certain Nutrients

NUTRIENT	RANGE	NO. SUBJECTS	REFERENCE
Tryptophan	82–250 mg (3-fold)	50	3, 4
Valine	375–800 mg (2.1-fold)	48	3, 5
Phenylalanine	420–1,100 mg (2.6-fold)	38	3, 6
Leucine	170–1,100 mg (6.4-fold)	31	3, 7
Lysine	400–2,800 mg (7-fold)	55	3, 8, 9
Isoleucine	250–700 mg (2.8-fold)	24	3, 10
Methionine	800–3,000 mg (3.7-fold)	29	3, 9
Threonine	103–500 mg (4.8-fold)	50	3, 11
Calcium	222–1,018 mg (4.6-fold)	19	12
Thiamine	0.4–1.59 mg (3.9-fold)	15	13

These data cannot be neglected in any intelligent realistic approach to human nutrition. To do so can result only from living in a dream world where the "hypothetical average man" is of most vital concern and real individuals are banished.

An inspired writer in the *Heinz Handbook of Nutrition* wrote 13 years ago as follows:

Individual organisms differ in their genetic makeup and differ also in morphologic and physiologic aspects, including their endocrine activity, metabolic efficiency, and nutritional requirements. . . . It is often taken for granted that the human population is made up of individuals who exhibit average physiologic requirements and that a minor proportion of this population is composed of those whose requirements may be considered to deviate excessively. Actually there is little justification in nutritional thinking for the concept that a representative prototype of *Homo sapiens* is one who has average requirements with respect to all essential nutrients and thus exhibits no unusually high or low needs. In the light of contemporary genetic and physiologic knowledge and the statistical interpretations thereof, the typical individual is more likely to be one who has average needs with respect to many essential nutrients *but who also exhibits some nutritional requirements for a few essential nutrients which are far from average* [26] [italics supplied].

This statement, however, has barely rippled the waters of the dyed-in-the-wool nutritionists. The time has come, we believe, when far more serious attempts will be made not only to know more about the ranges of human needs, but also to determine for individuals what needs they may have which are "far from average." In the case of some nutrients, this can be done now, but to make substantial progress in this area will require a major effort. Medical science must come to the rescue, applying to the job a substantial proportion of the resources it has been furnished. Automated equipment and computerized techniques will be widely used in this effort.

Acceptance of the facts of individuality greatly magnifies the possibilities of improving the suboptimal nutrition which is so widespread. People who are regarded as in relative good health may be living with suboptimal nutrition in a generalized sense; more pointedly, however, they are very likely to be functioning at a low level of efficiency because their nutrition is suboptimal in specific ways which can be not only determined but also corrected.

These considerations lay the groundwork for a grand eye-opening with respect to the importance of expertly monitored nutrition for people in general as well as the tremendous role it can play in medical practice. Instead of assuming, as physicians are prone to do, that patients automatically are well nourished, it will become accepted as common knowledge that generally speaking they are not, even if they do escape beriberi, pellagra, scurvy, and kwashiorkor. It will be realized that with human beings as with experimental animals [27], there is an enormous variability on the part of individuals to subsist on diets of mediocre or poor quality.

The genetotrophic concept, now 23 years old, is of vital concern in this discussion [28]. The basic idea may be simply expressed as follows: Diseases which have hereditary roots (this may be a widely inclusive category) may exist because the individuals concerned have unusual nutritional needs that are not easily met. If this is so, then meeting these needs should abolish the diseases in question.

It is well recognized in biological science that specific organisms require suitable environments if they are to thrive. The genetotrophic concept is an application of this principle. Certain individuals, it proposes, must have special nutritional environments if they are to thrive.

In spite of the fact that genetotrophic diseases may well include most noninfectious diseases, the validity or nonvalidity of this postulate has received practically no attention. The word genetotrophic is in medical dictionaries, but that is about as far as the matter has progressed. This could not possibly have happened if medical science were alert to the principles of nutrition. The soundness of the genetotrophic idea has never been questioned; it simply has not been tested for its applicability to any common disease.

It has been found inadvertently to be valid in some cases. In phenylketonuria, for example, fully adequate diets low in phenylalanine are not found naturally, but when these are compounded and furnished children suffering from phenylketonuria, the difficulty is controlled.

Certain rats with a hereditary need for high levels of manganese develop on ordinary diets severe inner ear difficulties. When these animals are artificially furnished high manganese diets, the inner ear difficulties do not appear [29–31]. There are probably a number of other isolated examples that could be cited, but what medical science needs to ascertain, by using expertise that is not generally cultivated, is whether individuals who are peculiarly susceptible to heart disease, obesity, arthritis, dental disease, mental disease, alcoholism, muscular dystrophy, multiple sclerosis, and even cancer, can be benefited by nutritional adjustments. How can we possibly know if medical science, taking the vital facts of individuality into account, does not try seriously to find the answer?

IV. In Nutrition, Teamwork Is Essential

The fourth basic fact in nutrition which has been sadly neglected by medical science is that of the essential "teamwork" among nutrients. Because this principle has been neglected, a wholly unscientific concept has been widely accepted with respect to what a nutrient may be expected to do.

The basic error, tacitly accepted, may be expressed as follows. Nutrients—amino acids, minerals, and particularly vitamins—are potential "medicines," and should be tested accordingly, using statistical methods and suitable placebo controls to determine their efficacy in combating diseases. If they prove to be "specifics" for particular diseases, well and good; if not, they must be regarded as medically worthless. In defense of this way of thinking is the historical fact that individual nutrients have in some cases acted like medicines—thiamine for beriberi, ascorbic acid for scurvy, niacinamide for pellagra. However, the parallel between these vitamins and "medicines" is more apparent than real, as careful consideration will show.

Following this erroneous reasoning, it is concluded that since specific individual nutrients are ineffective when tested in this way against specific common ailments, these nutrients are worthless for combating disease. It is easy to conclude also that there should be no substantial concern regarding the intake of these nutrients on the part of patients.

The joker in the argument is that while no nutrient by itself is an effective remedy for any common disease, the nutrients acting as a team are probably effective in the prevention of a host of diseases. Against infective diseases, the teamwork may serve to increase resistance. The reasonableness of this broad claim becomes apparent if we accept the postulate that when the environment of our body cells and tissues is adequate and perfectly adjusted, the cells and tissues will perform all their functions well, and a disease-free condition will be promoted.

It must be emphasized that adequate nutrition must involve the complete chain of nutrients. If a diet is missing one link in the nutritional chain, it may be as worthless for supporting life as if it were missing 10 links. One nutrient—mineral, amino acid, or vitamin—added as a supplement to a food can bring no favorable effect unless the food contains some of all the other nutrients or unless they are available from the reserves of the person being nourished.

It is now well recognized, for example, that while thiamine does act as a remedy for beriberi, it does so because in the diet of polished rice the weakest link in the chain is its thiamine content; thiamine alone will do no good if the other members of the nutrition chain are absent. It is a well-authenticated fact that to bring back health to a victim of beriberi, pellagra, or scurvy, complete nutrition—the complete chain or team—is essential. Manifestly, the nutritional chain is as strong as its weakest link. Every nutrient in the list acts like a gear in a complicated machine. There are no nutrients (or gears) which are dispensable.

To seek to educate the public as the Wheat Flour Institute has done [32, p. 14] by teaching that vitamin A, thiamine, niacin, riboflavin, vitamin C, vitamin D, protein, calcium, and iron are the "key nutrients" is to miseducate. Is there any evidence to suggest that phosphate, magnesium, zinc, vitamin B_6, vitamin B_{12}, and pantothenic acid are not key nutrients? Actually, the list of key nutrients is a long one. Every essential nutrient is a separate key which operates only when the other keys are also available.

The development of nutritional science will reveal, we believe, a clear-cut distinction between medicines and nutrients. The physiological effects of medicines can be ascribed to their ability to enter into metabolic machinery and interfere with enzyme systems. This can happen to the detriment of parasites, and presumably in a beneficial way when the host tissues are concerned. Nutrients, on the one hand, act constructively as building blocks for enzyme systems. If a medicine were to act constructively, it would cease to be medicine. It would be a nutrient.

Those who would lightly dismiss the teamwork principle as exemplifying the "shotgun approach" fail to appreciate that biologically every kind of organism in existence derives from its environment all of its nutritional essentials as a team. An organism typically derives whatever nutrients it needs simultaneously, not *ad seriatim*. If the teamwork principle exemplifies the "shotgun approach," it can hardly be condemned on this basis. This approach has a very long and honorable history. It has been used consistently and universally ever since life on earth began.

It is no coincidence that those nutrients so often stressed in elementary "nutritional education" of the past include conspicuously those which have historically acted like "medicines." These are undeniably important, but to think of them as *"the* key nutrients" is to deny the teamwork principle.

Nutrients as physiological agents must be judged on the basis of how they participate in teamwork. A substance suspected of being an indispensable nutrient cannot be excluded on the basis of its ineffectiveness when tested as a "medicine." Nutrients can be extremely valuable, particularly in preventive medicine, but not unless they are used with intelligent appreciation of how they work as members of a team.

Those who recognize fully the validity of the teamwork principle cannot be complacent about the possible existence of nutritional "unknowns." If there are still unrecognized cogs, they must be identified before the operation of the whole machinery can be adequately controlled and studied. Unless there are important alternative ways in which organisms bring about metabolism, the furnishing of each of the nutrients we know about depends upon all the other nutrients being available. Laboratories that are pharmaceutically oriented tend to be interested in any new "medicine," but the search for unknowns in human nutrition is relatively quiescent. That these may exist is suggested by our inability to grow cells at will in chemically defined media in tissue culture. If medical science were fully alert, it would be very much concerned with the problem.

A reflection of the lack of appreciation of the teamwork principle is the reliance placed upon food composition tables. These tables as ordinarily presented in government publications and elsewhere give no hint of the existence of a large indispensable team of coordinated nutrients. They give only fragmentary information which is easily misleading. Judgments as to the nutritional value of a food based on such tables are subject to serious error, especially when processed foods are involved and when nutrient items listed include prominently those which have commonly been added as fortification—thiamin, riboflavin, niacin, and iron.

"Nutrition surveys" [33] reflect the same neglect of the teamwork principle. The nutritional adequacy of the food consumed in different localities cannot be judged adequately on the basis of its content of thiamin, riboflavin, niacin, and iron, particularly when these are the nutritional elements used to "enrich" bread and cereals.

In our laboratories we have recently studied an alternative criterion for judging food values [34]. This is by measuring what we call the "trophic" or beyond-calorie value. Experimentally we ascertain how much new tissue the food in question can produce, beyond that produced in control animals where carbohydrate is supplied in place of the tested food. This method, which inevitably involves biological testing, measures the effective presence of the entire team necessary for tissue building and repair, including the unknowns if they exist.

BROAD SIGNIFICANCE OF THESE FOUR CRUCIAL FACTS

The four facts we have outlined—food is a part of our environment; suboptimal nutrition is ubiquitous; individuality is crucial in nutrition; and teamwork is essential in nutrition—cannot be seriously disputed, and they are far from trivial. When they are accepted, as they must be, there will be a revolution not only in nutritional science, but also in all of medicine, particularly when it is concerned with prevention.

When these four facts are duly considered and nutritional science developed, many currently accepted ideas will be weighed in the balance and found wanting, as either meaningless or misleading and essentially false. Such statements as the following are often made or tacitly accepted. "People in America get good nutrition." "Food contains an abundance of all the minerals, vitamins, etc. that are needed." "Food composition tables adequately reveal food values." "Nutrition surveys will tell us wherever there is malnutrition." "The recommended daily allowances of the Food and Nutrition Board are a safe guide to all nutrient needs." "If you want nutritional advice, ask your physician."

In the light of the four facts we have emphasized, these statements are puerile and are accepted only in ignorance. The fact, which must be faced, is that nutrition is an involved and intricate matter, and at present no one knows just what optimal nutrition is or how precisely to find out. Abundant incentives exist for attempting to reach this goal [35]. Such an objecive must await the further development of nutritional science.

The general acceptance of the four facts we have outlined will result in far more intelligent regulations on the part of the Food and Drug Administration. This body is naturally influenced greatly by current medical opinion, and it will change its attitudes as medical thinking changes. At present the Food and Drug Administration credits physicians with an expertise they should possess but do not. Their regulations too often reflect the backwardness of nutritional science.

The four facts we have discussed are simple ones. They can be and need to be understood even by adolescents. The menace of faddism and charlatanism can only be overcome by education, but it has to be education at a much higher level than has been customary. When the public is reasonably well informed, and medical science has adopted nutritional science as its own, faddism will tend to disappear, and people can get dependable nutritional advice from their physicians.

The prevention of disease, an objective which is inherent in better nutrition and the development of nutritional science, is as old as Hippocrates, who advocated nutrition first, then drugs, then surgery.

Prevention of disease—by every means at our disposal—is the wave of the future in medicine. The expertness medical science has developed in preventing infectious disease will spread to the prevention of noninfective disease. The economies resulting from prevention in terms of health and wealth will be enormous [36]. Prevention of a disease in an individual, when the means are known, may cost only a few cents or a few dollars, while if the disease is allowed to strike, the cost in money alone may easily run into the thousands of dollars. A gram of prevention is worth a kilogram of cure. The development of nutritional science is the principal highway that will lead to the prevention of noninfective disease.

Scientifically, nutritional science is a mere shadow of what it will be when medical science throws its weight behind its development by promoting a health-oriented instead of a disease-oriented discipline.

One relatively open area for scientific investigation is that of intercellular symbiosis [37]. There are probably many substances, of which glutamine, other "nonessential" amino acids, inositol, lipoic acid, and coenzyme Q are examples, which are considered nonessential for the "normal human being" who produces them endogenously. In the light of our discussion of individuality and the genetotrophic concept, however, these nutrients may be crucially needed by certain individuals whose endogenous processes may be somewhat impaired. It appears, for example, that victims of heart disease often are unable to produce enough coenzyme Q to keep their heart muscle unimpaired [38].

All the nutrients we have mentioned above, as well as others, are potential additions to the armamentarium of future physicians who wish to prevent and treat disease by sophisticated nutritional means.

A well-developed nutritional science which recognizes the hard facts of individuality will also delve into many other problems such as the matter of imbalances, the role of intestinal microorganisms in the nutrition of individuals, the question of the incidence and importance of defective enzymatic systems in the digestive tract [2, pp. 189–190], the large problem of malabsorption as it relates to the nutrition of individuals, and the broad question of the overall effects of slow or rapid development during youth on future health and well-being during adulthood.

Another area of great concern to those who would embrace sophisticated nutritional science is that of the basic functioning of some of the well-established nutrients like vitamin A, vitamin A acid, vitamin E, and vitamin C. Because enzymology is a relatively active field, the functioning of many of the B vitamins is relatively well understood, but the physiological function of the vitamins which were originally designated by the first, third, and fifth letters of the alphabet, still presents serious enigmas.

Another area of great scientific interest is the relationship of nutrition to hormone production. It is well known, for example, that thyroid hormone production may be limited by the availability of dietary iodine. Is insulin production, for example, ever limited by dietary lack of sulfur-containing amino acids, or are there other hormones the building of which may be impaired because of nutritional lacks? Development of sophisticated nutritional science will inevitably help solve the major problem of the biochemical functioning of hormones and the general problems of endocrinology.

Of great practical interest is the question of how expert nutritional adjustments can come into play in protecting against pollution. The well-recognized fact that ascorbic acid protects animals against lead poisoning and the recent finding that vitamin E protects animals against atmospheric pollutants [39, 40] call attention to this important potentiality. The broad problem of pollution includes iatrogenic pollution of the internal microenvironments and that produced by self-medication and self-indulgence in tobacco, marijuana, caffeine, and alcohol. All of the foreign elements which enter into the *milieu intérieur* are capable of affecting the nutritional status of the individual concerned.

Still another area of great practical interest and one that cannot be explored without regard for the facts of individuality and the other facts we have discussed is that of the self-selection of food.

Some nutritionists have stated dogmatically that there is no instinct which guides one in his choice of food. This extreme position in our opinion is just as untenable as the opposite one, namely, "instinct always guides us to select the right food." Somewhere between these two extremes lies the truth, and it needs to be ascertained. It is known that in healthy animals total food consumption (also water consumption) is often well controlled by internal forces. It is also known that impairment of the adrenals greatly affects salt consumption and the ability to taste salt [41, 42]. Some recent studies show that rats have a mechanism in which the brain is involved for selecting essential amino acids [43, 44]. Their food consumption is also affected by the amino acid levels in the blood [45]. It is known that in humans excessive sugar or fat or salt consumption may lead to nausea and rejection.

Experiments have shown that healthy young children given a wide selection of wholesome foods will provide themselves with reasonably good nutrition. Such experiments beg the question of how well the selection will work if some of the foods are not so wholesome! It is a common observation that if children are given a choice of beverage—milk, sweetened chocolate milk, or a cola drink—a large percentage will choose most unwisely. It seems probable this unwise selection is based, in part at least, upon previous poor nutrition of that portion of the brain which plays a role in food selection. Body wisdom is probably not fostered by the consumption of deficient foods. The whole problem of whether and to what extent human beings have internal mechanisms which help them select food wisely needs exploration, along with the question of whether nutritional adjustments can improve faulty choice mechanisms.

The problem of prenatal nutrition requires, in our opinion, special attention, taking into account all of the four facts we have stressed. Nutrition during the reproductive period is more exacting than at other times. It has been found consistently that diets which will successfully maintain adult animals may not be adequate for reproduction. This has been demonstrated in rats, mice, dogs, cats, foxes, monkeys, chickens, turkeys, and fish. For this reason one might suspect that in a world where suboptimal nutrition generally prevails, pregnant women are often inadequately nourished. Nature tries to provide growing fetuses with good environments, but it is powerless to do so if the necessary raw materials are absent from the food consumed. Prenatal nutrition merits extensive and careful study because for reasons we cannot detail here it is probable that infertility, miscarriages, "spontaneous" abortions, premature births, birth deformations, minor birth defects, and mental retardation often have their roots in the suboptimal environment pregnant women furnish the embryos when they eat carelessly or follow inexpert advice [2, chap. 4]. Even if the hereditary cards are stacked somewhat against one, this does not mean in the light of the genetotrophic concept that expert nutritional help could not obviate the potential difficulty.

REFERENCES

1. R. J. Williams, *Perspectives in Biology and Medicine* 14 (1971):608.
2. R. J. Williams, *Nutrition Against Disease* (New York: Pitman, 1971).

3. W. C. Rose, *Nutritional Abstracts Review* 27 (1957):631.

4. R. M. Leverton, N. Johnson, J. Pazur, and J. Ellison, *Journal of Nutrition* 58 (1956):219.

5. R. M. Leverton, M. R. Gram, E. Brodovsky, M. Chaloupka, A. Mitchell, and N. Johnson, *Journal of Nutrition* 58 (1956):83.

6. R. M. Leverton, N. Johnson, J. Ellison, D. Geschwender, and F. Schmidt, *Journal of Nutrition* 58 (1956):341.

7. R. M. Leverton, J. Ellison, N. Johnson, J. Pazur, F. Schmidt, and D. Geschwender, *Journal of Nutrition* 58 (1956):355.

8. E. M. Jones, C. A. Baumann, and M. S. Reynolds, *Journal of Nutrition* 60 (1956):549.

9. S. G. Tuttle, S. H. Bassett, W. H. Griffith, D. B. Mulcare, and M. E. Swendseid, *American Journal of Clinical Nutrition* 16 (1965):229.

10. M. S. Swendseid, I. Williams, and M. S. Dunn, *Journal of Nutrition* 58 (1956):495.

11. R. M. Leverton, M. R. Gram, M. Chaloupka, E. Brodovsky, and A. Mitchell, *Journal of Nutrition* 58 (1956):59.

12. F. R. Steggerda and H. M. Mitchell, *Journal of Nutrition* 31 (1946):407.

13. L. B. Pett, *Journal of Public Health* 36 (1945):69.

14. R. J. Williams, *Biochemical Individuality* (New York: John Wiley, 1956).

15. R. J. Williams and R. B. Pelton, *Proceedings of the National Academy of Sciences* 55 (1966):125.

16. M. Z. Rodriguez and M. I. Irwin, *Journal of Nutrition* 102 (1972): 909.

17. T. D. Spies and H. R. Butt, in *Diseases of Metabolism,* ed. G. D. Garfield (Philadelphia: W. B. Saunders, 1953), p. 473.

18. F. Albright, et al., *American Journal of Diseases of Childhood* 54 (1937):529.

19. C. I. Reed, et al., *Vitamin D* (Chicago: University of Chicago Press, 1939).

20. A. B. Kline, *Journal of Nutrition* 28 (1944):413.

21. R. J. Williams and G. Deason, *Proceedings of the National Academy of Sciences* 57 (1967):1638.

22. Man-Li Yew, *Proceedings of the National Academy of Sciences* 70 (1973):969.

23. C. J. Malory and A. H. Parmelee, *Journal of the American Medical Association* 154 (1954):405.

24. A. D. Hunt, et al., *Pediatrics* 13 (1969):140.

25. L. E. Rosenberg, *New England Journal of Medicine* 281 (1969): 145.
26. B. T. Burton, ed., *The Heinz Handbook of Nutrition* (New York: McGraw-Hill, 1959).
27. R. J. Williams and R. B. Pelton, *Proceedings of the National Academy of Sciences* 55 (1966): 126.
28. R. J. Williams, E. Beerstecher, Jr., and L. J. Berry, *Lancet* 1 (1950): 287.
29. R. M. Hill, et al., *Journal of Nutrition* 41 (1950): 359.
30. C. W. Ashling, et al., *Anatomical Records* 136 (1960): 157.
31. L. S. Hurley and G. J. Everson, *Proceedings of the Society of Experimental Biology and Medicine* 102 (1959): 360.
32. *Eat to Live* (Chicago: Wheat Flour Institute, 1970).
33. Interdepartmental Committee on Nutrition for National Defense, *Manual for Nutritional Surveys*, 2 ed. (Bethesda, Md.: National Institute of Health, 1963).
34. R. J. Williams, J. D. Heffley, M.-L. Yew, and C. W. Bode, *Proceedings of the National Academy of Sciences* 70 (1973): 710.
35. R. J. Williams, paper presented to the National Academy of Sciences, October 1971.
36. C. E. Weir, "An Evaluation of Research in the United States on Human Nutrition," *Benefits from Nutrition Research* (Washington, D.C.: U.S. Department of Agriculture, 1971).
37. R. J. Williams, *Texas Report of Biology and Medicine* 19 (1961): 245.
38. K. Folkers, et al., *International Journal of Vitamin Research* 40 (1970): 380.
39. B. D. Goldstein, R. D. Buckley, R. Cardenas, and O. J. Balchum, *Science* 169 (1970): 605.
40. J. N. Roehm, J. G. Hadley, and D. B. Menzel, *Archives of Internal Medicine* 128 (1971): 88.
41. C. P. Richter, *American Journal of Psychiatry* 97 (1941): 878.
42. G. C. Supplee, R. C. Bender, and O. J. Kahlenberg, *Endocrinology* 30 (1942): 355.
43. Q. R. Rogers and A. E. Harper, *Journal of Comparative Physiology and Psychology* 72 (1970): 66.
44. P. M. B. Leung and Q. R. Rogers, *Live Sciences* 8 (1969): 1.
45. Y. Peng and A. E. Harper, *Journal of Nutrition* 100 (1970): 429.

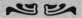

Supplemental Bibliography

It is a great source of frustration to an editor not to be able to include in an already lengthy book some additional articles and points of view. Therefore, partly as a service to readers and partly as a way to put my mind at ease, I have appended this bibliography. The listings are grouped to correspond to the five parts of the book. The articles and books included are, with a few exceptions for special emphasis, ones not already listed as references in the preceding essays.

HOLISTIC APPROACHES TO HEALTH

Antonovsky, Aaron. "Breakdown: A Needed Fourth Step in the Conceptual Armamentarium of Modern Medicine." *Social Science & Medicine* 6 (1972):537–44.

Audy, J. Ralph. "Man-Made Maladies and Medicine." *California Medicine* 113 (November 1970):48–53.

———. "Measurement and Diagnosis of Health." In *Environ/Mental: Essays on the Planet as Home,* edited by Paul Shephard and Daniel McKinley, pp. 140–61. Boston: Houghton Mifflin, 1971.

Beeson, Paul B. "McKeown's *The Role of Medicine:* A Clinician's Reaction." *Milbank Memorial Fund Quarterly* 55 (Summer 1977):365–71.

Belloc, Nedra B. "Relationship of Health Practices and Mortality." *Preventive Medicine* 2 (1973):67–81.

Belloc, Nedra B., and Breslow, Lester. "Relationship of Physical Health Status and Health Practices." *Preventive Medicine* 1 (1972):409–21.

Bennet, Glin: "Scientific Medicine?" *Lancet,* August 24, 1974, 453–56.

Berliner, Howard S. "Emerging Ideologies in Medicine." *Review of Radical Political Economics* 9 (Spring 1977):116–24.

Black, Peter McL. "Must Physicians Treat the 'Whole Man' for Proper Medical Care?" *The Pharos* 39 (January 1976):8–11.

Bluestone, Naomi. "Don't Be a Litter-bug: Dispose of Health Appropriately." *New England Journal of Medicine* 293 (July 17, 1975):148–50.

Blum, Henrik L. *Expanding Health Care Horizons*. Oakland, Calif.: Third Party Associates, 1976.

Boyce, Tom, and Michael, Max: "Nine Assumptions of Western Medicine." *Man and Medicine* 1 (Summer 1976):311–35.

Breslow, Lester. "A Quantitative Approach to the World Health Organization Definition of Health: Physical, Mental and Social Well-being." *International Journal of Epidemiology* 1 (1972):347–55.

———. "Research in a Strategy for Health Improvement." *International Journal of Health Services* 3 (1973):7–16.

Burnum, John F. "Outlook for Treating Patients with Self-Destructive Habits." *Annals of Internal Medicine* 81 (1974):387–93.

Cardus, David. "Towards a Medicine Based on the Concept of Health." *Preventive Medicine* 2 (1973):309–12.

Carlson, Rick J. *The End of Medicine*. New York: John Wiley & Sons, 1975.

Cassel, John: "The Contribution of the Social Environment to Host Resistance." *American Journal of Epidemiology* 104 (August 1976): 107–23.

Cassell, Eric J. "Preliminary Explorations of Thinking in Medicine." *Ethics in Science & Medicine* 2 (1975):1–12.

———. *The Healer's Art: A New Approach to the Doctor-Patient Relationship*. Philadelphia: J. B. Lippincott, 1976.

Chapman, John S. "Health and Medicine." *Archives of Environmental Health* 28 (June 1974):356–57.

Cheraskin, E., and Ringsdorf, W. M. *Predictive Medicine: A Study in Strategy*. Mountain View, Calif.: Pacific Press, 1973.

Cochrane, A. L. *Effectiveness and Efficiency: Random Reflections on Health Service*. The Nuffield Provincial Hospitals Trust. London: Oxford University Press, 1972.

"The Concept of Health." *The Hastings Center Studies* 1, no. 3 (1973).

"Concepts of Health and Disease." *The Journal of Medicine and Philosophy* 1, no. 3 (September 1973).

Dubos, René. "Bolstering the Body Against Disease." *Human Nature* 1 (August 1978):68–72.

———. "Health and Creative Adaptation." *Human Nature* 1 (January 1978): 74–82.

————. *Mirage of Health.* New York: Anchor Press, 1959.

Engel, George L. "The Best and the Brightest: The Missing Dimension in Medical Education." *The Pharos* 36 (October 1973):129–33.

————. "The Nature of Disease and the Care of the Patient: The Challenge of Humanism and Science in Medicine." *The Rhode Island Medical Journal* 45 (May 1962):245–51.

————. "The Need for a New Medical Model: A Challenge for Biomedicine." *Science* 196 (April 8, 1977):129–36.

————. "Too Little Science: The Paradox of Modern Medicine's Crisis." *The Pharos* 39 (October 1976):127–31.

————. "A Unified Concept of Health and Disease." *Perspectives in Biology and Medicine* 3 (1960):459–85.

Feinstein, Alvan R. *Clinical Judgment.* Huntington, N.Y.: Robert E. Krieger, 1967.

Fielding, Jonathan E. "Health Promotion—Some Notions in Search of a Constituency." *American Journal of Public Health* 67 (November 1977):1082–85.

Fink, Donald L. "Holistic Health: Implications for Health Planning." *American Journal of Health Planning* 1 (July 1976):23–30.

Freymann, John Gordon. "Medicine's Great Schism: Prevention vs Cure: An Historical Interpretation." *Medical Care* 13 (July 1975): 525–36.

Fuchs, Victor R. *Who Shall Live?: Health, Economics, and Social Choice.* New York: Basic Books, 1974.

Glazier, William H. "The Task of Medicine." *Scientific American* 228 (April 1973):13–17.

Hamburger, Jean. *The Power and the Frailty: The Future of Medicine and the Future of Man.* New York: Macmillan, 1973.

Handler, Seymour. "Bring Back the Mustard Plaster." *Minnesota Medicine* 54 (December 1971):973–79.

Hayes-Bautista, David, and Harveston, Dominic S. "Holistic Health Care." *Social Policy* 7 (March/April 1977):7–13.

Hinkle, Lawrence E. "Studies of Human Ecology in Relation to Health and Behavior." *Bioscience* 15 (August 1965):517–20.

Hoke, Bob. "Promotive Medicine and the Phenomenon of Health." *Archives of Environmental Health* 16 (February 1968):269–78.

Horrobin, David. *Medical Hubris: A Reply to Ivan Illich.* Montreal: Eden Press, 1977.

Howard, Jan, and Strauss, Anselm, eds. *Humanizing Health Care.* New York: John Wiley & Sons, 1975.

Illich, Ivan. *Medical Nemesis: The Expropriation of Health.* New York: Pantheon Books, 1976.

Ingelfinger, Franz J. "The Physician's Contribution to the Health System." *New England Journal of Medicine* 295 (September 2, 1976): 565–66.

Kaslof, Leslie. *Wholistic Dimensions in Healing: A Resource Guide.* New York: Doubleday, 1978.

Kass, Leon R. "Regarding the End of Medicine and the Pursuit of Health." *The Public Interest* 40 (Summer 1975): 11–42.

Knowles, John, ed. *Doing Better and Feeling Worse: Health in the United States.* New York: Norton, 1977.

Kuhn, Thomas S. *The Structure of Scientific Revolutions.* 2nd ed., enlarged. International Encyclopedia of Unified Science, vol. 2, no. 2. Chicago: University of Chicago Press, 1970.

Laframboise, H. L. "Health Policy: Breaking the Problem Down into More Manageable Segments." *Canadian Medical Association Journal* 108 (February 3, 1973): 388–93.

Lalonde, Marc. *A New Perspective on the Health of Canadians.* Ottawa: Government of Canada, 1974.

Ledermann, E. K. *Philosophy and Medicine.* Philadelphia: J. B. Lippincott, 1970.

Levin, Lowell S.; Katz, Alfred H.; and Holst, Erik. *Self-Care: Lay Initiatives in Health.* New York: Prodist, 1976.

Levine, Myra E. "Holistic Nursing." *Nursing Clinics of North America* 6 (June 1971): 253–64.

McDermott, Walsh. "Medicine: The Public Good and One's Own." *Perspectives in Biology and Medicine* 21 (Winter 1978): 167–86.

McKeown, Thomas. "Determinants of Health." *Human Nature* 1 (April 1978): 60–67.

———. *The Modern Rise of Population.* New York: Academic Press, 1976.

———. *The Role of Medicine: Dream, Mirage or Nemesis?* London: Nuffield Provincial Hospitals Trust, 1976.

McKinlay, John B. "A Case for Refocussing Upstream—The Political Economy of Illness." *Applying Behavioral Science to Cardiovascular Disease,* proceedings of a conference, June 17–19, 1974. Seattle, Wash.: American Heart Association, 1974, pp. 7–17.

McKinlay, John B., and McKinlay, Sonja M. "The Questionable Contribution of Medical Measures to the Decline of Mortality in the United States in the Twentieth Century." *Milbank Memorial Fund Quarterly* 55 (Summer 1977): 405–28.

Menninger, Roy W. "Psychiatry 1976. Time for a Holistic Medicine." *Annals of Internal Medicine* 84 (May 1976):603–04.

Miller, James. G. *Living Systems.* New York: McGraw-Hill, 1978.

Neale, Ann. "An Analysis of Health." *The Kennedy Institute Quarterly Report* 1 (Autumn 1975):1–9.

Pellegrino, Edmund D. "Philosophy of Medicine: Problematic and Potential." *The Journal of Medicine and Philosophy* 1 (1976):5–31.

Powles, John. "The Effects of Health Services on Adult Male Mortality in Relation to the Effects of Social and Economic Factors." *Ethics in Science & Medicine* 5 (1978):1–13.

Preventive Medicine USA: Health Promotion and Consumer Health Education. A Task Force Report sponsored by the John E. Fogarty International Center and The American College of Preventive Medicine. New York: Prodist, 1976.

Rasmussen, Howard. "Medical Education: [Revolution or Reaction." *The Pharos* 38 (April 1975):53–59.

Rushmer, Robert F. *Humanizing Health Care: Alternative Futures for Medicine.* Cambridge, Mass.: MIT Press, 1975.

Sheldon, Alan. "Toward a General Theory of Disease and Medical Care." In *Systems and Medical Care,* edited by Alan Sheldon, Frank Baker, and Curtis P. McLaughlin. Cambridge, Mass.: MIT Press, 1970.

Sobel, David S., and Hornbacher, Faith L. *An Everyday Guide to Your Health.* New York: Grossman, 1973.

Sokolowska, Magdalena. "Two Basic Types of Medical Orientation." *Social Science & Medicine* 7 (1973):807–15.

Suchman, Edward A. "Health Attitudes and Behavior." *Archives of Environmental Health* 20 (1970):105–10.

Thomas, Lewis. *The Lives of a Cell: Notes of a Biology Watcher.* New York: Viking, 1974.

Twaddle, Andrew C. "The Concept of Health Status." *Social Science & Medicine* 8 (1974):29–38.

Waitzkin, Howard. "A Marxist View of Medical Care." *Annals of Internal Medicine* 89 (1978):264–78.

White, Kerr L., ed. *Life and Death and Medicine.* San Francisco: W. H. Freeman, 1973.

Wilson, Michael. *Health Is for People.* London: Darton, Longman & Todd, 1975.

Zola, Irving K. "Healthism and Disabling Medicalization." In *Disabling Professions,* edited by Ivan Illich. London: Marion Boyars, 1977.

ANCIENT SYSTEMS OF MEDICINE

Ackerknecht, Erwin H. *Medicine and Ethnology.* Bern: Verlag Huber, 1971.

————. "Natural Diseases and Rational Treatment in Primitive Medicine." *Bulletin of the History of Medicine* 19 (May 1946):467–97.

Agren, Hans. "A New Approach to Chinese Traditional Medicine." *American Journal of Chinese Medicine* 3 (1975):207–12.

Alland, Alexander, Jr. *Adaptation in Cultural Evolution: An Approach to Medical Anthropology.* New York: Columbia University Press, 1970.

Burang, Theodore. *The Tibetan Art of Healing.* London: Watkins, 1973.

Castiglioni, Arturo. "Neo-Hippocratic Tendency of Contemporary Medical Thought." *Medical Life* 41 (March 1934):115–46.

Chen, Paul C. Y. "Medical Systems in Malaysia: Cultural Bases and Differential Use." *Social Science & Medicine* 9 (1975):171–80.

Coulehan, John L. "Navajo Indian Medicine: A Dimension in Healing." *The Pharos* 39 (July 1976):93–96.

Davis, Devra Lee. "The History and Sociology of the Scientific Study of Acupuncture." *American Journal of Chinese Medicine* 3 (1975): 5–26.

Eisenberg, Leon. "Disease and Illness: Distinctions Between Professional and Popular Ideas of Sickness." *Culture, Medicine and Psychiatry* 1 (1977):9–23.

Fabrega, Horacio, Jr. *Disease and Social Behavior: An Interdisciplinary Perspective.* Cambridge, Mass.: MIT Press, 1974.

Galdston, Iago. "The Decline and Resurgence of Hippocratic Medicine." *Bulletin of the New York Academy of Medicine* 44 (October 1968):1237–56.

Gruner, O. Cameron. "The Interpretation of Avicenna." *Annals of Medical History* 3 (1921):354–58.

————. *A Treatise on the Canon of Medicines of Avicenna.* New York: Augustus M. Kelley, 1970.

Hameed, Abdul, ed. *Theories and Philosophies of Medicine,* 2nd ed. New Delhi: Institute of History of Medicine and Medical Research, 1973.

Horton, Robin. "African Traditional Thought and Western Science." *Africa* 37 (1967):50–71, 155–87.

Jaeger, Werner. *Paideia: The Ideals of Greek Culture,* vol. 3. New York: Oxford University Press, 1944.

Supplemental Bibliography

Jilek, W. G.: "From Crazy Witch Doctor to Auxiliary Psychotherapist—The Changing Image of the Medicine Man." *Psychiatric Clinics* 4 (1971):200–20.

Kiev, Ari, ed. *Magic, Faith, and Healing: Studies in Primitive Psychiatry Today.* New York: Free Press, 1969.

Kiev, Ari. "Primitive Holistic Medicine." *International Journal of Social Psychology* 7 (1962):58–61.

————. *Transcultural Psychiatry.* New York: Free Press, 1972.

Kleinman, Arthur M. "Some Issues for a Comparative Study of Medical Healing." *International Journal of Social Psychiatry* 19, nos. 3–4 (1973):159–65.

————. "Toward a Comparative Study of Medical Systems: An Integrated Approach to the Study of the Relationship of Medicine and Culture." *Science, Medicine, and Man* 1 (1973):55–65.

————. "The Symbolic Context of Chinese Medicine: A Comparative Approach to the Study of Traditional Medical and Psychiatric Forms of Care in Chinese Culture." *American Journal of Chinese Medicine* 3 (1975):103–24.

Kleinman, Arthur; Eisenberg, Leon; and Good, Byron. "Culture, Illness and Care: Clinical Lessons from Anthropological and Cross-Cultural Research." *Annals of Internal Medicine* 88 (1978):251–58.

Kleinman, Arthur; Kunstader, Peter; Russel, Alexander E.; and Gale, James L. *Medicine in Chinese Cultures.* Washington, D.C.: Fogarty International Center, 1975.

Kluckhohn, Clyde, and Leighton, Dorothea. *The Navaho.* Cambridge, Mass.: Harvard University Press, 1947.

Lambo, Thomas Adeoye. "Psychotherapy in Africa." *Human Nature* 1 (March 1978):32–39.

————. "Psychotherapy in Africa." *Psychotherapy and Psychosomatics* 24 (1974):311–26.

————. "Traditional African Cultures and Western Medicine." In *Medicine and Culture,* edited by F. N. L. Poynter. London: Wellcome Institute of the History of Medicine, 1969.

Landy, David, ed. *Culture, Disease and Healing.* New York: Macmillan, 1977.

Leighton, Alexander, and Leighton, Dorothea. "Elements of Psychotherapy in Navaho Religion." *Psychiatry* 4 (1941):515–23.

————. *The Navaho Door,* Cambridge, Mass.: Harvard University Press, 1945.

Leighton, Alexander; Prince, Raymond D.; and May, Rollo. "The Therapeutic Process in Cross-Cultural Perspective—A Symposium." *American Journal of Psychiatry* 124 (March 1968):57–69.

Leslie, Charles, ed. *Asian Medical Systems.* Berkeley: University of California Press, 1976.

Leslie, Charles. "Modern India's Ancient Medicine." *Trans-Action* (June 1969):46–55.

———. "The Professionalization of Ayurvedic and Unani Medicine." *Transactions, New York Academy of Science,* Series II, 30 (1968): 559–72.

Leslie, Charles, ed. "Theoretical Foundations for the Comparative Study of Medical Systems: A Conference." *Social Science & Medicine* 12 (April 1978):67–138.

Li, C. P. "A New Medical Trend in China." *American Journal of Chinese Medicine* 3, no. 3 (1975):213–21.

Luckert, Karl W. "Traditional Navaho Theories of Disease and Healing." *Arizona Medicine* 29 (July 1972):570–73.

Majno, Guido. *The Healing Hand: Man and Wound in the Ancient World.* Cambridge, Mass.: Harvard University Press, 1975.

McLachlan, Gordon, and McKeown, Thomas, eds. *Medical History and Medical Care: A Symposium of Perspectives.* London: Oxford University Press, 1971.

Medical Anthropology Newsletter, published by the Society for Medical Anthropology, 1703 New Hampshire Avenue, N.W., Washington, D.C.

Needham, Joseph. *Science and Civilization in China,* vol. 6. Cambridge: Cambridge University Press, in press.

Needham, Joseph, and Gwei-Djen, Lu. "Chinese Medicine." In *Medicine and Culture,* edited by F. N. L. Poynter. London: Wellcome Institute of the History of Medicine, 1969.

———. "Problems of Translation and Modernisation of Ancient Chinese Technical Terms." *Annals of Science* 32 (1975):491–502.

Neuburger, Max. "Vis Medicatrix Naturae." *Medical Life* (1932):657–92.

Palos, Stephan. *The Chinese Art of Healing.* New York: Herder and Herder, 1971.

Porkert, Manfred. *The Theoretical Foundations of Chinese Medicine,* Cambridge, Mass.: MIT Press, 1974.

Poynter, F. N. L., ed. *Medicine and Culture.* London: Wellcome Institute of the History of Medicine, 1969.

Risse, Guenter B. "Shamanism: The Dawn of a Healing Profession." *Wisconsin Medical Journal* 71 (December 1972):18–23.

Sandner, Donald F. "Navaho Medicine." *Human Nature* 1 (July 1978):54–62.

Smith, Adolph E., and Kenyon, Dean H. "Acupuncture and A.T.P.: How They May Be Related." *American Journal of Chinese Medicine* 1, no. 1 (1973):91–97.

Snow, Loudell F. "Sorcerers, Saints and Charlatans: Black Folk Healers in Urban America." *Culture, Medicine and Psychiatry* 2 (1978): 69–106.

Temkin, Owsei. "The Scientific Approach to Disease: Specific Entity and Individual Sickness." In *Scientific Change,* edited by A. C. Crombie. New York: Basic Books, 1963.

Torrey, E. Fuller. *The Mind Game: Witchdoctors and Psychiatrists.* New York: Bantam, 1973.

Unschuld, Paul Ulrich. "Medico-Cultural Conflicts in Asian Settings: An Explanatory Theory." *Social Science & Medicine* 9 (1975):303–12.

————. "Western Medicine and Traditional Healing Systems: Competition, Cooperation or Integration?" *Ethics in Science and Medicine* 3 (1976):1–20.

Young, Allan A., ed. "Rethinking the Western Health Enterprise: A Conference." *Medical Anthropology* 2 (Spring 1978):1–124.

Zimmer, Henry R. *Hindu Medicine.* Baltimore: Johns Hopkins University Press, 1948.

UNORTHODOX MEDICINE

Barlow, Wilfred. *The Alexander Technique.* New York: Alfred A. Knopf, 1973.

Boyd, Linn J. *A Study of the Simile in Medicine.* Philadelphia: Boericke and Tafel, 1936.

Collipp, Platon J. "The Efficacy of Prayer: A Triple-Blind Study." *Medical Times* 97 (May 1969):201–04.

Coulter, Harris L. *Divided Legacy: A History of the Schism in Medical Thought,* vols. 1–3. Washington, D.C.: Wehawken, 1974–1977.

Dean, Stanley R., ed. *Psychiatry & Mysticism.* Chicago: Nelson-Hall, 1975.

Edmunds, H. Tudar, ed. *Some Unrecognized Factors in Medicine,* 2nd ed. Wheaton, Ill.: Theosophical Publishing House, 1976.

Feldenkrais, Moshe. *Awareness Through Movement: Health Exercises for Personal Growth.* New York: Harper & Row, 1972.

Firman, Gregory J., and Goldstein, Michael S. "The Future of Chiropractic: A Psychosocial View." *New England Journal of Medicine* 293 (September 1975):639–42.

Frank, Jerome D. "The Medical Power of Faith." *Human Nature* 1 (August 1978):40–47.

———. *Persuasion and Healing*, rev. ed. Baltimore: Johns Hopkins University Press, 1973.

———."Psychotherapy of Bodily Disease." *Psychotherapy and Psychosomatics* 26 (1975):192–202.

Garfield, Charles A., ed. *Rediscovery of the Body*. New York: Dell, 1977.

Goldstein, Murray, ed. *The Research Status of Spinal Manipulative Therapy*. Bethesda, Md.: Dept. of Health, Education, and Welfare, 1975.

Hayes-Bautista, David E. "Marginal Patients, Marginal Delivery Systems, and Health Systems Plans." *American Journal of Health Planning* 1 (January 1977):36–44.

Inglis, Brian. *The Case for Unorthodox Medicine*. New York: G. P. Putnam's, 1969.

Joyce, C. R. B., et al. "The Objective Efficacy of Prayer: A Double-Blind Clinical Trial." *Journal of Chronic Disease* 18 (1965):367–77.

Kane, R. L.; Leymaster, C.; Olsen, D.; et al. "Manipulating the Patient: A Comparison of the Effectiveness of Physician and Chiropractor Care." *Lancet* 1 (1974):1333–36.

Kaufman, Martin. *Homeopathy in America*. Baltimore: Johns Hopkins University Press, 1971.

Korr, Irvin M. "Osteopathy and Medical Evolution." *The Journal of the American Osteopathic Association* 61 (March 1962):515–26.

Krieger, Dolores. "Therapeutic Touch: The Imprimatur of Nursing." *The American Journal of Nursing* 75 (May 1975):784–87.

Krippner, Stanley, and Villoldo, Alberto. *The Realms of Healing*. Millbrae, Calif.: Celestial Arts, 1976.

Kruger, Helen. *Other Healers, Other Cures: A Guide to Alternative Medicine,* Indianapolis: Bobbs-Merrill, 1974.

Luce, John M. "Chiropractic: Its History and Challenge to Medicine." *The Pharos* 41 (April 1978):12–17.

Mason, R. C.; Clark, G.; Reeves, R. B.; and Wagner, B. "Acceptance and Healing." *Journal of Religion and Health* 8 (1969):123.

McCorkle, T. "Chiropractic: A Deviant Theory of Disease in Contemporary Western Culture." In *Medical Care,* edited by W. R. Scott and E. H. Volkart. New York: John Wiley & Sons, 1966.

Meek, George W., ed. *Healers and the Healing Process*. Wheaton, Ill.: The Theosophical Publishing House, 1977.

Reed, Louis S. *The Healing Cults*. Chicago: University of Chicago Press, 1932.

Roland, Charles G. "Does Prayer Preserve?" *Archives of Internal Medicine* 125 (April 1970):580–87.

Rolf, Ida P. *Rolfing: The Integration of Human Structures.* Santa Monica, Calif.: Dennis-Landman Publishers, 1977.

Rose, Louis. *Faith Healing.* Baltimore: Penguin Books, 1971.

Roth, Julius A. *Health Purifiers and Their Enemies.* New York: Prodist, 1977.

Shealy, C. Norman. *Occult Medicine Can Save Your Life.* New York: Dial Press, 1975.

Simonton, O. Carl; Matthews-Simonton, Stephanie; and Creighton, James. *Getting Well Again.* Los Angeles: J. P. Tarcher, 1978.

Simonton, O. Carl, and Simonton, Stephanie S. "Belief Systems and Management of the Emotional Aspects of Malignancy." *Journal of Transpersonal Psychology* 7 (1975):29–47.

Sobel, David S. "Gravity and Structural Integration." In *The Nature of Human Consciousness,* edited by Robert Ornstein. San Francisco: W. H. Freeman, 1973.

Theosophical Research Centre. *The Mystery of Healing.* Wheaton, Ill.: Theosophical Publishing House, 1958.

Tinbergen, Nikolaas. "Ethology and Stress Diseases." *Science* 185 (July 5, 1974):20–27.

Wallis, Roy, and Morley, Peter, eds. *Marginal Medicine.* New York: Free Press, 1976.

Wardwell, Walter I. "Limited, Marginal, and Quasi-Practitioners." In *Handbook of Medical Sociology,* edited by H. Freeman, S. Levine, and L. G. Reeder. Englewood Cliffs, N.J.: Prentice-Hall, 1972.

Weatherhead, Leslie D. *Psychology, Religion and Healing.* New York: Abingdon Press, 1972.

TECHNIQUES OF SELF-REGULATION

Adler, Herbert M., and Hammett, V. "The Doctor-Patient Relationship Revisited: An Analysis of the Placebo Effect." *Annals of Internal Medicine* 78 (1973):595–98.

Barber, Theodore X., ed. *Advances in Altered States of Consciousness and Human Potentialities,* vol. I. New York: Psychological Dimensions, 1976.

Benson, Herbert. *The Relaxation Response.* New York: William Morrow, 1975.

Biofeedback and Self-Control 1970–1978. Aldine Annuals on the Regulation of Bodily Processes and Consciousness. Chicago: Aldine-Atherton, 1970–1978.

Birk, Lee, ed. *Biofeedback: Behavioral Medicine.* New York: Grune & Stratton, 1973.

Brena, Stephen. *Yoga & Medicine,* Baltimore: Penguin Books, 1972.

Byerly, Henry. "Explaining and Exploiting Placebo Effects." *Perspectives in Biology and Medicine* 19 (Spring 1976):423–36.

Davidson, Richard J., and Schwartz, Gary E. "The Psychobiology of Relaxation and Related States: A Multi-Process Theory." In *Behavior Control and Modification of Physiological Activity,* edited by David Mostofsky. Englewood Cliffs, N.J.: Prentice-Hall, 1976.

Gellhorn, Ernst, and Kiely, William F. "Mystical States of Consciousness: Neurophysiological and Clinical Aspects." *The Journal of Nervous and Mental Disease* 154 (1972):399–405.

Glueck, Bernard C., and Stroebel, Charles F. "Biofeedback and Meditation in the Treatment of Psychiatric Illnesses." *Comprehensive Psychiatry* 16, no. 4 (1975):303–21.

Hirai, Tomio. *Psychophysiology of Zen.* Tokyo: Igaku Shoin, 1974.

Kuvalayananda, Swami, and Vinekar, S. L. *Yogic Therapy: Its Basic Principles and Methods.* New Delhi: Government of India, Ministry of Health, 1971.

Mahoney, J. J., and Thoresen, C. E. *Self-Control: Power to the Person.* Monterey, Calif.: Brooks/Cole, 1974.

Ornstein, Robert E. *The Psychology of Consciousness.* San Francisco: W. H. Freeman, 1973.

Ornstein, Robert E., ed. *The Nature of Human Consciousness.* San Francisco: W. H. Freeman, 1973.

Pelletier, Kenneth. *Mind as Healer, Mind as Slayer.* New York: Dell, 1977.

Pomerleau, O.; Bass, F.; and Crown, V. "The Role of Behavior Modification in Preventive Medicine." *New England Journal of Medicine* 292 (June 12, 1975):1277–81.

Schwartz, Gary E., and Beatty, Jackson, eds. *Biofeedback: Theory and Research.* New York: Academic Press, 1977.

Seyle, Hans. *The Stress of Life,* rev. ed. New York: McGraw-Hill, 1976.

Shapiro, Arthur K. "Factors Contributing to the Placebo Effect: Their Implications for Psychotherapy." *American Journal of Psychotherapy* 73 (Supplement) (1964):73–88.

Simeons, A. T. W. *Man's Presumptuous Brain.* New York: E. P. Dutton, 1960.

Stoyva, Johann. "Self-Regulation and the Stress-Related Disorders: A Perspective on Biofeedback." In *Behavior Control and Modification of Physiological Activity,* edited by David Mostofsky. Englewood Cliffs, N.J.: Prentice-Hall, 1976.

Stroebel, Charles F., and Glueck, Bernard C. "Biofeedback Treatment in Medicine and Psychiatry: An Ultimate Placebo?" *Seminars in Psychiatry* 5 (November 1973):379–93.

Tart, Charles T., ed. *Altered States of Consciousness.* New York: John Wiley & Sons, 1969.

AN ECOLOGICAL VIEW OF HEALTH

Boyden, S. V., ed. *The Impact of Civilization on the Biology of Man.* Toronto: University of Toronto Press, 1970.

Burkitt, D. P. "Some Diseases Characteristic of Modern Western Civilization." *British Medical Journal* 1 (1973):274–78.

Burkitt, D. P., and Trowell, H. C., eds. *Refined Carbohydrate Foods and Disease.* New York: Academic Press, 1975.

Dubos, René. "The Disease of Civilization: Achievements and Illusions." In *Mainstreams of Medicine: Essays on the Social and Intellectual Context of Medical Practice,* edited by Lester King. Austin: University of Texas Press, 1973.

————. "Health and Environment." *American Review of Respiratory Disease* 108 (1973):761–66.

————. *Man Adapting.* New Haven: Yale University Press, 1972.

————. *Man, Medicine, and Environment.* New York: New American Library, 1968.

Eckholm, Erik P. *The Picture of Health: Environmental Sources of Disease.* New York: Norton, 1977.

Halberg, F.; Halberg, J.; and Halberg, E. "Reading, 'Riting, 'Rithmetic and Rhythms: A New Relevant R in the Educative Process." *Perspectives in Biology and Medicine* 17 (1973):128–41.

Hall, Ross H. *Food for Nought: The Decline in Nutrition.* New York: Harper & Row, 1974.

Krueger, Albert P., and Sigel, Sheelah. "Ions in the Air." *Human Nature* 1 (July 1978):46–52.

Luce, Gay Gaer. *Body Time, Physiological Rhythms and Social Stress.* New York: Bantam, 1973.

Ott, John N. *Health and Light: The Effects of Natural and Artificial Light on Man and Other Living Things.* Old Greenwich, Conn.: Devin-Adair, 1973.

Soyka, Fred. *The Ion Effect.* New York: E. P. Dutton, 1977.

Sulman, Felix G. *Health, Weather and Climate.* New York: S. Karger, 1976.

Tromp, Solco W. *Medical Biometeorology.* New York, Elsevier, 1963.

Williams, Roger J. *Nutrition Against Disease.* New York: Bantam, 1973.

————. "Nutritional Individuality." *Human Nature* 1 (June 1978):46–53.

————. *Physician's Handbook of Nutritional Science,* Springfield, Ill.: Charles C. Thomas, 1975.

Wurtman, Richard J. "The Effects of Light on the Human Body." *Scientific American* 233 (July 1975):68–77.

Acknowledgments

This book is in part a record of my own education. There are many people who have generously contributed both to my education and to the book, and I would like to thank some of them. First, there are the contributors themselves who put up with what must at times seemed like interminable editing. Then there are my colleagues at The Institute for the Study of Human Knowledge and, in particular, Robert Ornstein, whose critical open-mindedness was a welcome example. I would also like to thank my associates at the Health Policy Program of the University of California, San Francisco, including George Brown, Rick Carlson, Pat Franks, Howard Brody, and especially Philip Lee, whose interest in these subjects grew along with mine. And special thanks to Richard Grossman for his early encouragement as a publisher and later as a colleague.

Contributors

HERBERT BENSON, M.D. is Associate Professor of Medicine at Harvard Medical School and a Fellow of the American College of Cardiology. He is Program Director of the Clinical Research Center and head of the Hypertension Section at Beth Israel Hospital in Boston. Dr. Benson has done extensive research in cardiology, operant conditioning of blood pressure, and the physiology of the relaxation response. He is also the author of the book *The Relaxation Response*.

HOWARD BRODY, M.D., Ph.D. is a resident in family practice at the University of Virginia. He received a fellowship from the Institute on Human Values in Medicine and the National Endowment for the Humanities. His doctorate in the philosophy of medicine dealt with the placebo effect and mind-body relationships. He is author of *Ethical Dimensions in Medicine*.

HARRIS L. COULTER, Ph.D. is a private historian, translator, interpreter, and author of the three-volume *Divided Legacy: A History of the Schism in Medical Thought*. He is currently living in Washington, D.C., and working on a book on the development of twentieth-century medicine.

RENÉ DUBOS, Ph.D. is Professor Emeritus of Environmental Biomedicine at the Rockefeller University. His early research involved the development of antimicrobial drugs and more recently he has been investigating the effects that environmental forces—physiochemical, biological, and social—exert on human life. Dr. Dubos is author of over twenty books including *The Mirage of Health, Man Adapting, So Human an Animal,* and *Beast or Angel: Choices That Make Us Human.* He also serves as an advisory editor to the magazine *Human Nature*.

JEROME D. FRANK, M.D., Ph.D. is Professor Emeritus of Psychiatry, Department of Psychiatry and Behavioral Sciences at The Johns Hop-

Contributors

kins University School of Medicine. One of his major research interests has been the elucidation of the healing components shared by methods of psychotherapy, about which he has written a book, *Persuasion and Healing.*

BERNARD GRAD, Ph.D. is a research biologist and Associate Professor, Department of Psychiatry, at McGill University. In addition to his experimental studies on the biological effects of the laying on of hands, his research activities have been in the areas of endocrinology, oncology, and gerontology.

ROBERT J. HAGGERTY, M.D. is Roger I. Lee Professor of Public Health (Health Services and Pediatrics) at Harvard University. His interests lie in social medicine, medical education, health education, and family stress and health. He is coauthor of *Child Health and the Community.*

WILLIAM L. HASKELL, Ph.D. is Clinical Assistant Professor of Medicine, Stanford Heart Disease Prevention Program at Stanford University School of Medicine. His research interests include the early identification of cardiovascular disease with exercise stress testing and the role of exercise in the prevention and rehabilitation of coronary heart disease.

W. H. S. JONES, Litt. D. was Bursar and Steward of St. Catharine's College, Cambridge, and Corresponding Member of The Historical Section of the Royal Society of Medicine.

ALBERT P. KRUEGER, M.D. is Emeritus Professor of Bacteriology and Emeritus Lecturer in Medicine, at the University of California, Berkeley. For over 20 years he has directed the Air Ion Research Laboratory and investigated the biological effects of air ions.

SWAMI KUVALAYANANDA was Director of Research, Kaivalyadhama S.M.Y.M. Samiti, Lonavla, India.

GAY LUCE, Ph.D. has served as an editor and writer for the President's Scientific Advisory Committee and N.I.M.H. Her books include *Biological Rhythms in Psychiatry and Medicine, Body Time,* and *Current Research in Sleep and Dreams.* She is at present codirector of S.A.G.E., a holistic program for people over age 65 located in Berkeley, California.

MANFRED PORKERT, Ph.D. is Associate Professor and a Director for the Institut für Ostasienkunde at München Universität in Germany. His research has included extensive investigations of Chinese philosophy and science, the technical literature of Taoism and, above all, the traditional Chinese healing system, as presented in his book *The Theoretical Foundations of Chinese Medicine: Systems of Correspondence.*

Contributors

JOHN W. POWLES, M.B.B.S. is a member of the Faculty of Community Medicine of the Royal College of Physicians (U.K.) and a faculty member of the Departments of Social and Preventive Medicine and Social Work at Monash University, Melbourne, Australia. His research interests include exploring the connection between the modern way of life and mortality trends.

DONALD F. SANDER, M.D. is a training analyst at the C. G. Jung Institute of San Francisco and has a private practice in psychiatry. Over the past eight summers he has done field studies with Navaho medicine men and has just completed the book *Navaho Symbols of Healing*.

GARY E. SCHWARTZ, Ph.D. is Associate Professor, Department of Psychology, Yale University, and Department of Psychiatry, Yale University School of Medicine. His current research interests are biofeedback and self-regulation, with applications to the study and treatment of psychosomatic and affective disorders. He is an editor of *Consciousness and Self-Regulation: Advances in Research*, and *Biofeedback: Theory and Research*.

DAVID S. SOBEL, M.D., M.P.H. is a Fellow in the Health Policy Program at the University of California School of Medicine, San Francisco. He also serves as medical director of The Institute for the Study of Human Knowledge.

ILZA VEITH, Ph.D. is Professor and Vice-Chairman of the Department of the History of Health Sciences and Professor of the History of Psychiatry, Department of Psychiatry, at the University of California, San Francisco. In addition to her numerous articles on the history of medicine and psychiatry, Dr. Veith has written about the history and philosophy of Far Eastern medicine including *Medizin in Tibet, Acupuncture Therapy: Current Chinese Practice,* and a commentary and translation of the ancient Chinese medical text *The Yellow Emperor's Classic Internal Medicine.*

S. L. VINEKAR, B.A. (Hons.) M.B.B.S. was Joint Director of Research, Kaivalyadhama S.M.Y.M. Samiti, Lonavla, India.

ROGER J. WILLIAMS, Ph.D., D.Sc. is Emeritus Professor of Chemistry at the University of Texas at Austin and former Director and Research Scientist at the Clayton Foundation Biochemical Institute, where his coworkers include Drs. James D. Heffley, Man-Li Yew, and Charles W. Bode. He was the first to identify, isolate, and synthesize pantothenic acid, one of the B vitamins, and he also did pioneer work on folic acid. He is author of several books, including *Biochemical Individuality, Nutrition Against Disease,* and *Physician's Handbook of Nutritional Science.*